2005–6

Pocket Book of Infectious Disease Therapy

2005–6

Pocket Book of Infectious Disease Therapy

John G. Bartlett, M.D.

Professor of Medicine
Chief, Division of Infectious Diseases
Johns Hopkins University School of Medicine
Baltimore, Maryland

 LIPPINCOTT WILLIAMS & WILKINS
A **Wolters Kluwer** Company
Philadelphia · Baltimore · New York · London
Buenos Aires · Hong Kong · Sydney · Tokyo

Acquisitions Editor: Jim Merritt
Developmental Editor: Raymond E. Reter
Purchasing Manager, Clinical and Healthcare: Jennifer Jett
Typesetter: Maryland Composition Company, Inc.
Printer: Victor Graphics

© 2004 by LIPPINCOTT WILLIAMS & WILKINS
530 Walnut Street
Philadelphia, PA 19106-3780 USA
LWW.com

Printed in Canada

ISBN: 0-7817-7406-3

First Edition, 1990	Sixth Edition, 1995	Tenth Edition, 2000
Second Edition, 1991	Seventh Edition, 1996	Eleventh Edition, 2001–2002
Third Edition, 1992	Eighth Edition, 1997	Twelfth Edition, 2004
Fourth Edition, 1993	Ninth Edition, 1998	Thirteenth Edition, 2005–2006
Fifth Edition, 1994		

00 01 02 03
2 3 4 5 6 7 8 9 10

PREFACE

The *2005–06 Pocket Book of Infectious Disease Therapy* is intended for physicians and other care providers who manage adult patients with infectious diseases. These include internists, generalists, surgeons, obstetricians, gynecologists, medical subspecialists, and surgical subspecialists.

This book has the same lofty goals as the first eleven editions: to provide standards of care for the management of infectious disease with particular emphasis on antimicrobial agents, their selection, dosing regimens, costs, and side effects. As with prior editions, there is extensive use of recommendations from various authoritative sources such as the Centers for Disease Control and Prevention (CDC) and the *Medical Letter on Drugs and Therapeutics* and from official statements of learned societies such as the American College of Physicians/American Society of Internal Medicine (ACP/ASIM), the American Heart Association (AHA), the American Thoracic Society (ATS), the Infectious Diseases Society of America (IDSA), and the Surgical Infection Society (SIS).

The 2005–06 edition has extensive additions, deletions, and revisions. Tabular material has been updated to account for recently approved antibiotics and new recommendations for management. This edition includes topical issues such as MRSA (USA 300 strain), Avian influenza, Acinetobacter Hepatitis B virus (HBV), hepatitis C virus (HCV), and bioterrorism. It also contains the new guidelines for pyogenic meningitis, diabetic foot infections, healthcare-associated pneumonia, surgical prophylaxis, fungal infections, bacteruria and management of infections associated with international travel. Antimicrobials introduced since the eleventh edition that are now included are entecavir (Baraclude), rifamaxin, (Xifaxan), tinidazole (Tindamax), tigecycline (Tygacil) and micafugin (Mycamine).

The HIV/AIDS section has been deleted because of space constraints and the availability of an alternative resource: *Medical Management of HIV Infection* by this author.

The reader is encouraged to notify the author (1830 Monument Street, Room 437, Baltimore, MD 21205, 410-955-7634) if there are errors, differences of opinion, or suggested additions.

CONTENTS

ANTIMICROBIAL AGENTS

PREVENTIVE TREATMENT

NONBACTERIAL INFECTIONS

SPECIFIC INFECTIONS

ANTIMICROBIAL AGENTS

PREPARATIONS AND RECOMMENDED DOSING REGIMENS FOR ANTIMICROBIAL AGENTS

(Adapted from Drug Information 03, American Hospital Formulary Service, 2003; Physicians' Desk Reference, 57th Edition, 2003; and Drug Information for the Health Care Professional, USP DI, 23rd Edition, 2003)

Agent (generic) Pregnancy category*	Trade names	Dosage form	Usual adult regimen and AWP**
Acyclovir Category C***	Zovirax	5% ointment; 2 & 15 g tubes	Topical q3h • 2 g @ $37.00
		200 mg cap	200 mg po; × 3–5/d • 200 mg @ $1.00
		400 & 800 mg tabs	400 mg po bid 800 mg po × 5/d • 800 mg @ $4.00
		200 mg/5 mL susp 500 & 1000 mg vials (IV)	200–800 mg po × 3–5/d 15–30 mg/kg/d IV over 1 hr q8h • 500 mg @ $74
Adofovir Category C	Hepsera	10 mg tab	10 mg po qd × 48–92 wks • 10 mg @ $18.00
Albendazole Category C	Albenza	200 mg tabs	400 mg po bid • 200 mg @ $1.49
Amantadine Category C	Symmetrel Symadine	100 mg cap 50 mg/5 mL soln	200 mg qd or 100 mg bid (treatment or prophylaxis); 100 mg/d age >65 yr • 100 mg @ $1.40
Amikacin Category D	Amikin	0.1, 0.5 & 1 g vials	15 mg/kg/d IV × 1/d or q8–12h • 500 mg @ $6–18
Aminosalicylic acid* Category C	Paser granules	4 g packet	150 mg/kg/d po q6–12h • 4 gm packet @ $4.00
Amoxicillin Category B	Amoxil, Trimox, Wymox	250 & 500 mg caps 125 & 250 mg/5 mL susp	250–500 mg po tid • 500 mg @ $0.60 • 875 mg @ $1.00
Amoxicillin + clavulanate Category B	Augmentin	125/31 & 250/62 mg/5 mL susp 125/31 & 250/62 mg chewable tab 250/125 & 500/125 mg tab 1000/62.5 mg tab 875/125 mg tab	250–500 mg po tid (amoxicillin) • 875/125 mg @ $6.00 • 500/125 mg @ $5.00 • 1000/62.5 @ $3.01 875/125 mg po bid
Amphotericin B Category B	Fungizone	50 mg vial	0.3–1 mg/kg/d IV over 4–6 hr • 50 mg @ $20.00

Continued

1

Agent (generic) Pregnancy category*	Trade names	Dosage form	Usual adult regimen and AWP**
Amphotericin B lipid complex Category B	Abelcet (ABLC)	100 mg vials	5 mg/kg/d IV • 100 mg @ $240.00
	Amphotec (ABCD)	50 & 100 mg vials	3–4 mg/kg/d IV • 100 mg @ $160
Amphotericin B liposomal Category B	AmBisome	50 mg vials	3–5 mg/kg/d IV Usually 5 mg/kg/d • 50 mg @ $196
Ampicillin Category B	Omnipen Totacillin	250 & 500 mg caps 125, 250 & 500 mg/5 mL susp	250–500 mg po qid • 250 mg @ $0.23 • 500 mg @ $0.40
Ampicillin sodium Category B	Omnipen-N Polycillin-N Totacillin-N	0.125, 0.25, 0.5, 1, 2 & 10 g vials	1–2 g IV q4–6h (up to 8 g/d) • 2 g @ $ 6–13
Ampicillin + sulbactam Category B	Unasyn	1:0.5 & 2:1.0 g vials (amp:sulbactam)	1–2 g IV q6h (ampicillin) • 2:1 g @ $31–62
Atovaquone Category C	Mepron	750 mg/5 mL susp	750 mg po bid w/food • 210 mL (21 day supply) @ $18/5 mL
Atovaquone + proguanil Category C	Malarone	250 mg atovaquone + 100 mg proguanil tabs	Malaria treatment—4 tabs/d × 3 days (single daily dose) • 250/100 mg @ $5.00
		62.5 mg atovaquone + 25 mg proguanil tabs (pediatrics)	Malaria prevention—1 tab/ day Take with food
Azithromycin Category B	Zithromax	250 & 600 mg tab Z Pak with 6 250 mg tabs Tri Pak with 3 500 mg tabs Z max 2000 mg slurry 500 mg vial	500 mg po first day, then 250 mg q24h × 4 or 500 mg po qd • 250 mg @ $8.00 • 500 mg @ $16 • 600 mg @ $19.00 • Tri Pak @ $47 • Z Pak @ $47 Z max 2000 mg slurry Z max @ $47 500 mg IV qd • 500 mg @ $28.00
Aztreonam Category B	Azactam	0.5, 1 & 2 g vials	0.5–2.0 g q q 6–8 h • 1 g @ $22
Bacitracin*	Baci-IM Baciguent	50,000 unit vial 500 units/g ointment 15, 30, 120 & 454 g	10,000–25,000 units IM q6h; 25,000 units po q6h (C. difficile colitis) • 50,000 units @ $18
Butoconazole	Femstat	2% vaginal cream, 3 single doses	1 dose hs × 3 • 5 g @ $34.62
Capreomycin Category D	Capastat	1 g vial	1 g/day IM or IV • 1 g @ $26.60

Continued

2

Agent (generic) Pregnancy category*	Trade names	Dosage form	Usual adult regimen and AWP**
Carbenicillin indanyl sodium Category B	Geocillin	382 mg tab (with 118 mg indanyl sodium)	382–764 mg po q6h • 382 mg @ $2.50
Caspofungin Category C	Cancidas	50 & 70 mg vials	70 mg IV (initial dose), then 50 mg/d IV (daily dose) • 50 mg @ $388
Cefaclor Category B	Ceclor Roniclor	250 & 500 mg parvules 125, 187, 250 & 375 mg/5 mL susp 125, 187, 250 & 375 mg chewable tabs	250–500 mg po tid • 500 mg @ $4
	Ceclor ER	375 & 500 mg extended-release tabs	375 or 500 mg po q12h • 500 mg ER @ $4
Cefadroxil Category B	Duricef Ultracep	500 mg cap 1 g tab 125, 250 & 500 mg/ 5 mL susp	0.5–1 g po qd or bid • 500 mg @ $7 • 1000 mg @ $13
Cefamandole Category B	Mandol	1, 2 & 10 g vials	0.5–3 g IM or IV q4–6h (up to 12 g/d) • 2 gm @ $2
Cefazolin Category B	Ancef, Kefzol Zolicef	0.25, 0.5, 1, 5, 10 & 20 g vials	0.5–2 g IV q6–8h • 1 g @ $5.60
Cefdinir Category B	Omnicef	300 mg caps 125 mg/5 mL susp	300 mg bid or 600 mg qd (bid usually preferred) • 300 mg @ $4.50
Cefditoren Category B	Spectracef	200 mg tabs	200–400 mg bid po pc • 200 mg @ $2
Cefepime Category B	Maxipime	0.5, 1 & 2 g vials	0.5–2 g IV q12h • 1 g @ $18 • 2 g @ $36
Cefixime Category B	Suprax	100 mg/5 mL susp	400 mg po qd or bid • 5 mL @ $4.60
Cefotaxime Category B	Claforan	0.5, 1, 2 & 10 g vials	2–12 g/d IV or IM q6–8h • 2 g @ $20
Cefotetan Category B	Cefotan	1, 2 & 10 g vials	1–2 g IM or IV q12h • 1 g @ $15
Cefoxitin Category B	Mefoxin	1, 2 & 10 g vials	0.5–2 g IM or IV q4–6h • 1 g @ $15
Cefpodoxime proxetil Category B	Vantin	100 & 200 mg tabs 50 & 100mg/5 mL susp	100–400 mg po bid • 200 mg @ $6
Cefprozil Category B	Cefzil	250 & 500 mg tabs 125 & 250 mg/5 mL susp	0.25–1 g po qd or bid, usually 500 mg qd or bid • 500 mg @ $9

Continued

Agent (generic) Pregnancy category*	Trade names	Dosage form	Usual adult regimen and AWP**
Ceftazidime Category B	Fortaz, Tazidime Ceptaz, Tazicef	0.5, 1, 2 & 6 g vials	1–3 g IM or IV q8–12h, up to 8 g/d • 1 g @ $15 • 2 g @ $28
Ceftibutin Category B	Cedax	400 mg tabs 90 & 180 mg/5 mL susp	400 mg/d • 400 mg @ $9
Ceftizoxime Category B	Cefizox	1 & 2 g vials	1–4 g IM or IV q8–12h, up to 12 g/d • 2 g @ $24
Ceftriaxone Category B	Rocephin	0.25, 0.5, 1, 2 & 10 g vials	1–2 g/d up to 4 g/d IV or IM q24h • 1 g @ $51
Cefuroxime Category B	Zinacef, Kefurox	0.75 & 1.5 g vials	0.75–1.5 g IM or IV q6–8h up to 4.5 g/d • 1.5 g @ $10.00
Cefuroxime axetil Category B	Ceftin	0.125, 0.25 & 0.5 g tabs, 125 & 250 mg/5 mL susp	250–500 mg po bid • 250 mg @ $5.00 • 500 mg @ $10
Cephalexin Category B	Keflex, Keftab, Cefanex	0.25 & 0.5 g caps 0.25 & 0.5 g tabs 125 & 250 mg/5 mL suspension	250–500 mg po qid • 250 mg @ $0.70 • 500 mg @ $1.50
Cephradine Category B	Velosef	250 & 500 mg caps	0.5–1 g po qid–bid • 500 mg @ $2
Chloramphenicol	Chloromycetin	0.5% soln	Topical
Chloramphenicol sodium succinate	Chloromycetin sodium succinate	1 g vial	0.5–2 gm IV q6h usually 1 g q6h • 1 g @ $7.60
Chloroquine HCl Category C	Aralen HCl	250 mg amp (200 mg base)	160–200 mg base IM q6h
Chloroquine PO_4 Category C***	Aralen PO_4	500 mg tab (300 mg base) 250 mg tab (150 mg base)	300–600 mg (base) qd–q wk • 250 mg @ $2.50 • 500 mg @ $4.00
Cidofovir Category C carcinogenic and teratogenic in animals	Vistide	375 mg/5 mL vial	5 mg/kg IV q2 wk • 375 mg @ $888
Cinoxacin Category B	Cinobac	250 & 500 mg caps	250–500 mg po bid or qid usually 1 g/d • 500 mg @ $3

Continued

Agent (generic) Pregnancy category*	Trade names	Dosage form	Usual adult regimen and AWP**
Ciprofloxacin Category C***	Cipro	250, 500 & 750 mg tabs 500 mg XR tabs 50 & 100 mg/mL susp. 0.3% ophth ointment 3.5 g 0.1–1% otic drops 10 mL 0.3% ophth soln 2.5, 5 & 10 mL	500–750 mg po bid • 500 mg @ $6 • 750 mg @ $6 • 500 mg XR @ $7 • 1000 mg XR @ $10
	Cipro IV	200 & 400 mg vials	200–400 mg IV q12h • 200 mg @ $16
Clarithromycin Category C	Biaxin Biaxin XL	250 & 500 mg tabs, 125 & 250 mg/5mL, susp. 500 mg tab	250–500 mg po bid • 250 mg @ $4.50 • 500 mg @ $4.50 1 g po qd • 500 mg XL @ $5.00
Clindamycin Category B	Cleocin	75, 150 & 300 mg caps	150–300 mg po qid • 300 mg @ $6
Clindamycin PO$_4$ Category B	Cleocin PO$_4$	150, 300, 600 & 900 mg vials	600 mg IV q8h up to 2.7 g/d • 600 mg @ $11 • 900 mg @ $14
Clindamycin topical gel/soln	Cleocin T	1% gel, 25 & 50 g tube 1% soln 30, 60 mL	Topical 1–2 ×/d • 25 g @ $62.38
Clindamycin vaginal cream Category B	Cleocin VC	2% cream 40 g tube 100 mg vaginal tabs	Topical: 1/day × 7 days Tab qd × 3 • 40 gm tube @ $55 • 100 mg @ $16.00
Clofazimine	Lamprene	50 & 100 mg caps	100–300 mg po qd usually 300 mg/d (leprosy) • 50 mg @ $0.20
Clotrimazole Category C	Mycelex, Lotrimin, Gyne- Lotrimin	1% cream; 15, 30 & 45 g; 1% lotion 10 mg troches 200 mg vaginal tabs	Topical 1–5 ×/d 200 mg vaginal tab 1 qd × 3 • 1% cream 30 g @ $7.00 • 200 mg tab @ $3.00 • 10 mg troche @ $0.50
Colistimethate Category B	Coly-Mycin S Coly-Mycin M	Otic drops—5, 10 mL 150 mg vial (IV)	Topical 3–4×/d 2.5–5.0 mg/kg/d IV q6–12h • 150 mg @ $64
Co-trimoxazole	(see trimethoprim- sulfamethoxazole)		
Crotamiton	Eurax	Cream: 60 g Lotion: 2 & 16 oz	Topical × 1 or 2 • 60 g @ $13.36
Cycloserine Category C	Seromycin	250 mg caps	250–500 mg po bid • 250 mg @ $4
Dapsone Category C		25 & 100 mg tabs	25–100 mg po qd • 100 mg @ $0.25

Continued

5

Agent (generic) Pregnancy category*	Trade names	Dosage form	Usual adult regimen and AWP**
Daptomycin Category B	Cubicin	500 mg vial	4 mg/kg/d • 500 mg @ $168
Dicloxacillin Category B	Dycill, Dynapen Pathocil	250 & 500 mg caps 62.5 mg/5 mL susp	0.25–0.5 g po qid usually 500 mg qid • 500 mg @ $1.20
Diethyl-carbamazine	Hetrazan (only available from Lederle Labs)	50 mg tab	6–13 mg/kg/d, 1–3 doses
Diloxanide	Furamide (only available from CDC)		500 mg po q8h
Dirithromycin	Dynabac	250 mg tabs	500 mg po qd • 250 mg @ $4
Docosanol Category C	Abreva	2 g tube	Apply 5×/d • 2 g @ $13
Doxycycline Category D	Vibramycin, Doxy Vibra-tabs Doxy tabs Doxy 100, 200 Adoxo	50 & 100 mg cap 50, 75, 100 mg tab 50 mg/5 mL susp 100 & 200 mg vial	100 mg po qd or bid, usually bid • 100 mg @ $5 100 mg IV q12h • 100 mg @ $14.80
Drotrecogin Category C	Xigris	5 & 20 mg vials	24 mcg/kg/h × 96 hrs • 20 mg @ $1082 (about $8000/course)
Eflornithine	Ornidyl	200 mg/mL vial (100 mL)	400 mg/kg/d IV q6h 100 mg/kg po q8h
Emetine HCl	available from CDC	65 mg/mL (1 mL vial)	1–1.5 mg/kg/d up to 90 mg/d; IM or deep SC injection
Entecavir Category C	Baraclude	0.5–1.0 gm tabs	0.5 –1.0 mg po qid empty stomach • 5 mg @ $23.70
Ertapenem Category B	Invanz	1 g vial	1 g IV q24h • 1 g @ $60
Erythromycin Category B Erythromycin base	E-mycin, ERYC, Ery-Tab, Erythro, EES, Erythrocot MyE Wintrocin, Robimycin A/T/S, Emgel, Erycette, Erygel, etc	250 mg cap 250, 333 & 500 mg tabs 250, 333, 500 mg EC 2% and 3–5% topical gel 30 & 60 g soln 60 mL	250–500 mg po tid–qid • 500 mg @ $0.27 • 500 mg EC @ $2.50 Topical for acne • 2% gel 30 g @ $32.02
Erythromycin estolate Avoid in pregnancy	Ilosone	250 mg cap 500 mg tab 125 & 250 mg/5 mL susp	250–500 mg po qid
Erythromycin ethylsuccinate	EES	200 & 400 mg tabs 200 & 400 mg/5 mL susp	400–800 mg po qid • 400 mg @ $0.23

Continued

Agent (generic) Pregnancy category*	Trade names	Dosage form	Usual adult regimen and AWP**
Erythromycin gluceptate	Ilotycin gluceptate	1 g vial	250 mg–1 g IV q6h • 1 g @ $7.70
Erythromcin lactobionate	Erythrocin lactobionate	0.5 & 1 g vials	250–500 mg IV q6h • 1 g @ $8
Erythromycin stearate	Erythrocin stearate, Wyamycin S	250 & 500 mg tabs	250–500 mg po qid • 500 mg @ $0.26
Ethambutol Category B	Myambutol	100 & 400 mg tabs	15–25 mg/kg po qd • 400 mg @ $2.25
Ethionamide Category C	Trecator-SC	250 mg tab	0.5–1 g/d po in 1–3 daily doses • 250 mg @ $3
Famciclovir Category B	Famvir	125, 250 & 500 mg tabs	125 mg q12h, 500 mg q8h • 500 mg @ $8
Fluconazole Category C	Diflucan	50, 100, 150 & 200 mg tabs 10 mg/mL susp 200 & 400 mg vials	100–200 mg po qd or bid • 100 mg @ $9 • 200 mg @ $15 200–400 mg IV qd • 200 mg @ $107.00
Flucytosine	Ancobon	250 & 500 mg caps	25–33 mg/kg po qid • 500 mg @ $8.60
Foscarnet Category C	Foscavir	24 mg/mL 250, 500 mL	40–60 mg/kg IV q8h (induction) 90–120 mg/kg IV qd (maintenance) • 6 g @ $83
Fosfomycin Category B	Monurol	3 g sachet	3 g × 1 • 3 g @ $38.00
Furazolidone		100 mg tabs	100 mg po q6h
Ganciclovir Category C	Cytovene Cytovene	0.5 g vial 250 & 500 mg cap	5 mg/kg IV bid (induction) or qd (maintenance) • 500 mg @ $38 1000 mg po tid • 500 mg @ $10
Gatifloxacin Category C***	Tequin	200 & 400 mg tabs 200 & 400 mg vials	400 mg po qd • 400 mg @ $10 400 mg IV qd • 400 mg @ $38
Gemifloxacin Category C***	Factive	320 mg tab	320 mg po qd × 5d (AECB) or 7 days (pneumonia) • 320 mg @ $19

Continued

Agent (generic) Pregnancy category*	Trade names	Dosage form	Usual adult regimen and AWP**
Gentamicin Category C	Garamycin G-Mycin Jenamicin	20, 60, 80 & 120 mg vials	1.5–2.0 mg/kg IV or IM q8h or 5 mg/kg qd • 80 mg @ $5
Griseofulvin Category C	Gris-PEG Fulvicin Grisfulvin V Grisfulvin Griseof	Microsize: 250 & 500 mg tabs, 125 mg/5 mL susp Ultramicrosize: 125, 250 mg tabs	500 mg–1 g/d po • 500 mg @ $1 330–750 mg/d po • 250 mg @ $1.40
Hydroxy- chloroquine Category C	Plaquenil	200 mg tab (155 mg hydroxychloroquine)	400 mg weekly (malaria prophylaxis) 200–600 mg/d • 200 mg @ $1.09
Idoxuridine	Herplex Liquifilm	0.1% ophth drops in 15 mL	1 qtt q1h (day) & q2h (night) • 15 mL @ $21.00
Imipenem/cilastatin Category C	Primaxin	0.25, 0.5 & 0.75 g vials (imipenem: cilastatin is 1:1)	0.25–1 g IV q6h • 500 mg @ $31.40
Immunoglobulin			
IVIG	Gamimune-N 10% (Bayer) Gammagard SD (Baxter) Sandoglobin (Novartis)	1, 5, 10 & 20 mg/kg vials 10 gm vial 1 & 12 g vials	Parvovirus: 0.4 g/kg IV qd × 5 ITP 0.4–1 g/kg days 1, 2, 14 then q 2–3 wks AWP: 1 g @ • $95 (Novartis) • $101.00 (Bayer) • $50 (Baxter)
Hyperimmune globulins			
Hepatitis B	Bay Hep B (Bayer) Nabi-HB (Nabi)	0.5 mL syringe 5 mL vial 1 & 5 mL vials	0.06 mL/kg IM • 0.5 mL syringe @ $78.00
Rabies	Bay Rab (Bayer) Imogam Rab (Aventis)	2 & 10 mL vials 2 & 10 mL vials	20 IU/kg IM 150 units/mL half in wound site and half IM gluteal • 150 units @ $175.00
Vaccinia	VIG Obtain via CDC	Vials 404-639-3356	0.6 mL/kg IM, average 40 mL IM over 24–36 hr
Tetanus	BayTet (Bayer)	250 mL syringe	Prophylaxis: 250 units IM Contaminated wound of > 24 hrs: 500 units IM Tetanus: 3,000–10,000 units IM • 250 unit syringe @ $131.00
Varicella	VZIG	25 & 625 unit vials 800-843-7477	> 40 kg: 625 units IM 30–40 kg 500 units IM • 625 unit vial @ $726.00

Continued

Agent (generic) Pregnancy category*	Trade names	Dosage form	Usual adult regimen and AWP**
<u>Interferon</u> Category C Alfa-2a	Roferon-A (Roche)	3, 9, 18 & 36 mil unit vials	3 mil units 3×/wk (HCV) 30–35 mil units/wk (HBV) • 3 mil units @ $38.18 1 mil units intralesion (condylomata) 3×/wk
Alfa-2b	Intron A (Schering)	3, 5, 10, 18, 25 & 50 mil unit vials	As above • 3 mil units @ $48.83
Peginterferon alfa-2b	PegIntron (Schering)	1 mL vial with 100, 160, 240 & 300 μg/mL	1.5 μg/kg SC q wk + ribavirin (Schering) • 177 μg @ $273.00
Peginterferon alfa 2a	Pegasys (Roche)	1 mL vial with 180 μg/mL	180 mcg SC q wk + ribivirin (Roche) • 180 mcg @ $364.00
Iodoquinol	Yodoxin	210 & 650 mg tabs	650 mg po tid • 650 mg @ $0.89
Isoniazid Category C***	Tubizid	100 & 300 mg tabs 50 mg/5 mL (oral soln)	300 mg po qd • 300 mg @ $0.16
	Nydrazid	1 g vial (IM)	300 mg IM qd • 1 gm vial @ $20
Isoniazid + rifampin	Rifamate	INH 150 Rif 300 mg cap	2 tabs po qd • 1 tab @ $2.60
Isoniazid + rifampin + pyrazinamide	Rifater	INH 50 mg + Rif 120 mg + PZA 300 mg tabs	6 tabs/d (>120 lb) • 1 tab @ $2
Itraconazole Category C	Sporanox	100 mg cap	100–200 mg po qd or bid usually 200–400 mg/d with food • 100 mg @ $9.30
		10 mg/mL oral soln 150 mL	100 mg po qd or bid on empty stomach • 100 mg @ $9.30
		250 mg vials	200 mg IV bid × 4 doses, then 200 mg IV qd • 250 mg @ $168
Ivermectin Teratogenic in animals	Stromectol	3 mg tab	4–5 tabs po × 1 • 3 mg @ $5.40
Ketoconazole Category C	Nizoral	200 mg tab	200–400 mg/d po q12–24h up to 1.6 g/d • 200 mg @ $3.03
		2% cream; 15, 30 & 60 g 2% shampoo, 120 mL	Topical qd–bid • 30 g @ $28.32
Lamivudine Category C	Epivir HBV	100 mg tab 5 & 25 mL soln	100 mg po qd (HBV) • 100 mg @ $6

Continued

Agent (generic) Pregnancy category*	Trade names	Dosage form	Usual adult regimen and AWP**
Levofloxacin Category C***	Levoquin	250, 500 & 750 mg tabs	500 mg po qd • 750 mg @ $17 • 500 mg @ $11
		500 & 750 mg vials	500 mg IV qd • 750 mg @ $60 • 500 mg @ $40
Lincomycin Category B	Lincocin	300 mg vial	0.6–2.4 g IV q8h • 300 mg @ $10
Lindane	Kwell	1% Lotion, 16 oz 1% Shampoo, 60 and 480 mL	Apply and wash after 4 min (lice) or 8–14 hr (scabies) • 16 oz @ $90
Linezolid Category C	Zyvox	600 mg tabs 100 mg/5 mL oral susp 600 mg vials	600 mg po or IV q12h • 600 mg tab @ $63 • 600 mg IV @ $85
Lomefloxacin Category C***	Maxaquin	400 mg tab	400 mg po qd • 400 mg @ $7
Loracarbef Category C	Lorabid	200 & 400 mg pulvules 100 & 200 mg/5 mL susp	200–400 mg po bid • 400 mg @ $6
Mafenide	Sulfamylon	8.5% cream 2, 4 & 14.5 oz cans	Topical qd or bid • 4 oz @ $45.35
Mebendazole Category C	Vermox	100 mg tab	100 mg po × 1–2 up to 2 g/d • 100 mg @ $6
Mefloquine Category C*** Avoid in first trimester	Lariam	250 mg tab	1250 mg po × 1 (treatment) 250 mg po q wk (prophylaxis) • 250 mg @ $11
Meropenem Category B	Merrem	500 mg and 1 g vials	1 g IV q8h • 1 g @ $60
Methenamine hippurate Category C	Hiprex Urex	1 g tab	1 g po bid • 1 g @ $1.50
Methenamine mandelate Category C	Mandelamine	0.35, 0.5 & 1 g tabs	1 g po qid • 1 g @ $0.50
Metronidazole Category B Contraindicated in first trimester	Flagyl, Protostat Metronid	250, 375, 500 & 750 mg tabs	250–500 mg po tid or 0.5–1.0 g po bid • 250 mg @ $2.50 • 500 mg @ $4.00
	Metro IV, Flagyl IV	500 mg vial	0.5–1 g IV q12h • 500 mg @ $15.42
	Metrogel-vaginal	0.75% gel, 70 g	Topical—bid • 70 g @ $54.44

Continued

Agent (generic) Pregnancy category*	Trade names	Dosage form	Usual adult regimen and AWP**
Micafungin	Mycamine	50 mg vial	150 mg IV • 50 mg @ $112
Miconazole	Monistat, Buza cream, Cruex, Desenex, Micatin	2% cream, 15, 30, 35 & 85 mg spray vaginal cream 100 & 200 mg as vaginal supply	0.2–1.2 g IV q8h Vaginal-hs × 3–7 days • 2% cream 35 gm @ $13 • 2% spray 3.5 oz @ $5.00 • Vaginal supply 100 mg $12/7 days
Minocycline Category D	Minocin Dynacin	50, 75 & 100 mg caps 75 & 100 mg tabs 50 mg/5 mL syrup 100 mg vial	100 mg po bid • 100 mg @ $1.70 100 mg IV q12h • 100 mg @ $46.38
Moxifloxacin Category C***	Avelox	400 mg tabs 400 mg vials	400 mg po qd • 400 mg @ $10 400 mg IV qd • 400 mg @ $44
Mupirocin	Bactroban	2% ointment—1 g tubes (single use)	Topical bid, 1/2 contents in each nostril • 15 g @ $36
Nafcillin Category B	Nafcil, Nallpen	0.5, 1, 2 & 10 g vials	0.5–3 g IV q4–6h up to 12 g/d • 2 g @ $15
Nalidixic acid Category C***	NegGram	0.25 & 0.5 g tabs 250 mg/5 mL susp	1 g po qid • 500 mg @ $2
Neomycin Category C	Neo-Tabs Neo-Fradin	500 mg tab 125 mg/5 mL soln 1% ointment	1–4 g po tid • 500 mg @ $1.24
Nitazoxamide	Alinia	Susp 100 mg/5 mL 500 mg tab	Adult—500 mg po q6–12h or 1 gm bid × 3 days • 500 mg @ $13.50
Nitrofurantoin Category B	Macrodantin, Faran Furadantin Macrobid	Macrocrystals: 25, 50 & 100 mg caps Microcrystals: 50 & 100 mg caps; 50 & 100 mg tabs 25 mg/5 mL susp	50–100 mg po q6h Suppressive treatment: 50–100 mg qd • 50 mg @ $1.20 • 100 mg @ $2.00
Nitrofurazone	Furacin	0.2% gauze strips	Topical (burns) • 28 g @ $15
Norfloxacin Category C***	Noroxin	400 mg tab	400 mg po bid • 400 mg @ $4.00
Novobiocin	Albamycin	250 mg cap	250 mg–1 g po bid–qid, up to 2 g/d

Continued

Agent (generic) Pregnancy category*	Trade names	Dosage form	Usual adult regimen and AWP**
Nystatin Category B	Mycostatin	100,000 units/mL susp 60 & 480 mL	5 mL swish, swallow 5–10 mL po 3–5 × daily
	Mycostatin	500,000 units tab	• 500,000 unit tab @ $0.70
	Nystatin	100,000 unit/g cream 15 & 30 g	Topical
	Bio-statin	50,000, & 100,000 U caps	• 30 gm @ $29
	Nystatin	500,000 U tab	
	Mycostatin	100,000 U vaginal tab	
Ofloxacin Category C***	Floxin	200, 300 & 400 mg tabs	200–400 mg po bid • 400 mg @ $7
Oseltamivir Category C	Tamiflu	75 mg caps	75 mg bid (treatment) 75 mg qd (prophylaxis) • 75 mg @ $8
Oxacillin Category B	Bactocill, Oxacill Prostaphlin	250 & 500 mg caps 250 mg/5 mL soln 0.25, 0.5, 1, 2, 4 & 10 g vials	2–4 g/d po qid • 1 g @ $9 0.5–4 g IM or IV q4–6h, up to 12 g/d
Paromomycin Category C	Humatin	250 mg cap	2–4 g/d po q6–12h • 250 g @ $3.20
Peginterferon alfa 2b	Peg-Intron	50, 80, 120, 150 mcg vials	1.0 mg/kg/wk SC monotherapy 1.5 mg/kg/wk SC with ribavirin • 150 mg vial @ $407
alfa 2a	Pegasys	180 mcg/ml	180 mcg/wk SC • 180 mcg @ $364
Penciclovir	Denavir	1.5 g tube	Apply q2h during day • 1.5 g @ $26
<u>Penicillin G and V</u> Category B		(1 unit = 0.6 µg)	
Crystalline G potassium	Penicillin G for injection Pfizerpen	1, 2, 3, 5, 10 & 20 mil unit vials	0.5–5 mil units IV q4–6h
Crystalline G sodium	Penicillin G sodium for injection	5 mil unit vial	0.5–5 mil units IV q4–6h
Benzathine	Bicillin (in U.K.) Bicillin L-A Permapen	3 mil unit vial 600,000 units/mL vial (1, 2 & 4 mL vials)	1.2–2.4 mil units IM • 1.2 mil units @ $42
Benzathine + procaine	Bicillin C-R	Benzathine: procaine/mL 150,000:150,000 units/mL (10 mL) 300,000:300,000 units/mL (1, 2 & 4 mL) 450,000:150,000 units/mL (2 mL)	1.2–2.4 mil units IM • 0.3 mil units @ $16

Continued

Agent (generic) Pregnancy category*	Trade names	Dosage form	Usual adult regimen and AWP**
Procaine	Crysticillin Pfizerpen Wycillin	3 mil units (10 mL) 6 mil units (12 mL) 600,000 units/mL (1, 2 & 4 mL syringe)	0.3–2.4 mil units IM q6–12h • 1.2 mil units @ $17
Phenoxymethyl penicillin (V)	Pencil V Pen V	125, 250 & 500 mg tabs 125 & 250 mL/5 mL susp	250–500 mg po qid • 250 mg @ $2 • 500 mg @ $4
Pentamidine Category C	Pentam 300 Nebupent	300 mg vial 300 mg aerosol	4 mg/kg/d IV qd (treatment) • 300 mg @ $98 300 mg/d/mo (prophylaxis) • 300 mg @ $98
Permethrin Category B	Elimite, Nix, Permethrin, RID spray Lice-ENZ	1%, 5% cream 1% liquid 0.5% resp spray	Apply and wash after 10 min (lice) or 8–14 hr (scabies) • 60 g @ $30 • 5 oz spray @ $5
Piperacillin Category B	Pipracil	2, 3, 4 & 40 g vials	1–6 g IV q4–6h, up to 24 g/d • 4 g @ $17
Piperacillin + tazobactam Category B	Zosyn	2:0.25 g; 3:0.375 g, 4:0.5 g vials (piperacillin:tazobactam)	3 g (pip) IV q6h • 3 g @ $17
Polymyxin B Category B	Aerosporin Poly Rx	(1 mg = 10,000 units) 500,000 unit vial 200,000 units + 40 mg neomycin	0.75–1.25 mg/kg IM or IV q12h • 500,000 units @ $14
Praziquantel Category B	Biltricide	600 mg tab	20–75 mg/kg/d po in 3 doses • 600 mg @ $12
Primaquine Category C		15 mg (base) tab	15 mg po qd • 26 mg @ $2
Primaquine + chloroquine Category C	Aralen with primaquine	45 mg (primaquine)+ 300 mg (chloroquine) tab	45/300 mg tab weekly
Pyrantel Category C	Pin-X	144 mg/mL; 30 & 60 mL	11 mg/kg × 1 • 30 mL @ $8
Pyrazinamide Category C***	Generic	500 mg tab	15–30 mg/kg/d po in 2–4 doses, usually 500 mg tid • 500 mg @ $1.20
Pyrimethamine Category C	Daraprim	25 mg tab	25 mg po q wk or daily up to 200 mg/d • 25 mg @ $0.58
Pyrimethamine + sulfadoxine Category C	Fansidar	Sulfa 500 mg + pyrimeth 25 mg	1 tab/wk 3 tabs (1 dose) • tab @ $4.20

Continued

Agent (generic) Pregnancy category*	Trade names	Dosage form	Usual adult regimen and AWP**
Quinine dihydrochloride Category X	(available from CDC 404-639-3670)	IV	600 mg IV q8h
Quinine sulfate Category X	Quinamm, Quiphile, Quindan, Quin-amino	200, 300 & 325 mg caps 162.5, 260 & 325 mg tabs	325 mg po bid • 325 mg @ $1 650 mg po q8h
Quinupristin/ dalfopristin (No data)	Synercid	10 mL vials: 150 mg quinupristin + 350 mg dalfopristin & 180/420	7.5 mg/kg IV q8–12h; mix in 250 mL D5W, infuse over 1 hr via central catheter • 500 mg @ $127
Ribavirin Category X	Copegus (Roche) (+ INF 2a)	200 mg caps	< 75 kg: 400 mg po AM and 600 mg PM > 75 kg: 400 mg bid • 200 mg @ $8
	Rebetol (Schering)	200 mg caps	• 200 mg @ $12
	Rebetron (Schering) (+ INF 2b)	200 mg caps	Genotype 1 < 75 kg: 400 mg po AM and 600 mg po PM > 75 kg: 600 mg po bid Genotype 2 & 3: 400 mg po bid 200 mg ribavirin + interferon alfa 2b @ $804.00 (1 wk)
Rifabutin Category B	Mycobutin	150 mg caps	300 mg/d po • 150 mg @ $6.50
Rifamaxin	Xifaxan	200 mg tab	300 mg po tid × 3d • 200 mg @ $4
Rifampin Category C	Rifadin, Rimactane	150 & 300 mg caps	600 mg po qd (TB) • 300 mg @ $2.20
	Rifamate	300 mg caps with 150 mg INH	600 mg po qd or bid (other indications) • 300/150 mg @ $2.60
	Rifater	120 mg tabs with 50 mg INH and 300 mg pyrazinamide	6 tabs/d • 1 tab @ $2
	Rifadin-IV	600 mg vial	600 mg/d IV • 600 mg @ $90
Rifapentine Category C	Priftin	150 mg tabs	600 mg po q wk • 150 mg @ $3
Rimantadine Category C	Flumadine Rimantid	100 mg tab 50 mg/5 mL syrup	100 mg po bid (treatment or prophylaxis) 100–200 mg/d age >65 yrs • 100 mg @ $2.20
Spectinomycin	Trobicin	2 & 4 g vials	2 g IM × 1
Streptomycin Category D		1 g vials	1–2 g/d IM • 1 g @ $10

Continued

Agent (generic) Pregnancy category*	Trade names	Dosage form	Usual adult regimen and AWP**
Sulfonamides			
Category C—caution in last trimester, contraindicated at term			
Trisulfa-pyrimidines	Sulfadiazine	500 mg tab	0.5–1 g po qid • 500 mg @ $1.40
Silver sulfa-diazine	Silvadene	1% cream, 20, 50, 85 & 1000 g	Apply qd or bid • 50 g @ $8.22
Sulfadiazine		0.5 g tab	0.5–1 g po qid • 500 mg @ $1.44
Sulfamethox-azole	Gantanol Urobak	0.5 g tab	0.5–1 g po bid or tid
Sulfamethoxazole phenazopyridine	Azo-Gantanol	0.5 g sulfa + 0.1 g phenazopyridine	0.5–2 g po bid or tid
Sulfapyridine		0.5 g tab 0.25 g/5 mL susp	0.5–1 g po bid–qid
Sulfasalazine	Azulfidine, Azulfidine EN tabs	0.5 g tab	0.5–1 g po bid–qid • 500 mg @ $0.50
Sulfisoxazole	Gantrisin, Soxa Gulfasin	0.5 g tab	1–2 g po qid • 500 mg @ $0.50
Sulfisoxazole-phenazopyridine	Azo-Gantrisin	0.5 g sulfa + 0.05 g (50 mg) phenazopyridine	1 g po qid
Telithromycin	Ketek	400 mg tab 300 mg tab	• 800 mg qd @ $9.20 • 400 mg @ $4.60 • 300 mg @ $4.60
Terbinafine Category B	Lamisil Desenex	1% cream; 12, 24, 30 & 60 g 250 mg tab	Topical bid • 24 g @ $10 1 tab qd • 250 mg @ $10
Tetracyclines Category D			
Sumycin	Tetracycline	250 & 500 mg cap	250–500 mg po qid • 500 mg @ $0.20
Doxycycline Category D	Vibramycin, Monodix	100 mg tab 50 & 100 mg caps	100–200 mg po qd or bid • 100 mg @ $3.00
	Adoxa	100 & 200 mg vials	100 mg IV q12h • 100 mg @ $14.60
Minocycline	Minocin	50 & 100 mg caps	100 mg po bid • 100 mg @ $1.70
	Dynacin	100 mg vial	100 mg IV q12–24h
Oxytetracycline	Terramycin	50 & 125 mg/mL with lidocaine (IM)	0.5–1 g/d IM q12h
Tinidazole	Tindamax	250 & 500 mg tabs	2 gm with food • 500 mg @ 4.60
Thiabendazole Category C	Mintezol	500 mg tab	1–3 g/d po • 500 mg @ $1.25
Ticarcillin Category B	Ticar	1, 3, 6, 20 & 30 g vials	1–6 g IV q4–6h up to 24 gm/d • 3 g @ $14

Continued

15

Agent (generic) Pregnancy category*	Trade names	Dosage form	Usual adult regimen and AWP**
Ticarcillin + clavulanic acid Category B	Timentin	3 g ticarcillin + 0.1 g CA vials	3–6 g (ticarcillin) IV q4–6h, up to 24 g/d • 3.1 g @ $16
Tigecycline	Tygacil	50 mg vial	100 mg IV × 1, then 50 mg IV q12h
Tobramycin Category C	Nebcin Tobrex	20, 60, 80 & 120 mg vials	1.5–2.0 mg/kg IM or IV q8h or 5 mg/kg qd • 80 mg @ $24
Tolnaftate	Aftate, Tinactin Absorbine Jr	1% gel 15 g 1% cream 15 g 1% powder 45, 150 g 1% liquid 10, 45, 120 mL	Topical bid • 4 oz spray @ $3.11 • 30 g cream @ $8.68
Trifluridine	Viroptic	1% ophthalmic soln; 7.5 mL	1 drop q2h • 7.5 mL @ $89.11
Trimethoprim Category C	Proloprim, Primsol	100 mg tabs 50 mg/5 ml po soln	200 mg/d po in 1–2 doses • 100 mg @ $1
Trimethoprim-sulfamethoxazole Category C	Bactrim, Septra Cotrim, Cofatrim Sulfatrim, Triazole, Uroplus, Trisulfam, Sulfamar, Sulfamethoprim	Trimethoprim: sulfa 40:200 mg/5 mL susp 80:400 mg tabs 160:800 mg DS tabs 16 mg:80 mg/mL (IV) (5, 10, 20 mL vials)	2–20 mg/kg/d (trimethoprim) po or IV in 3–4 daily doses • SS @ $1 • DS @ $2 • 80:16 mg @ $21
Trimetrexate	Neutrexin	200 mg vial	45 mg/m^2 IV q24h • 200 mg @ $1,320
Valacyclovir Category C***	Valtrex	500 & 1000 mg caplets	1000 mg po tid (zoster) 500 mg po bid (recurrent HSV) • 500 mg @ $4.45 • 1000 mg @ $8
Valganciclovir Category C	Valcyte	450 mg tab	900 mg po bid + food × 3 wks, then 900 mg • 450 mg @ $30
Vancomycin Category C	Vancocin	125 & 250 mg caps 250 mg/5 mL; 20 mL 500 mg/6 mL; 120 mL	125 mg po qid (C. difficile colitis) • 125 mg @ $9
	Vancocin HCl IV	0.5 g vial (IV) 1 g liquid (po)	0.5–1 g IV q12h usually 2 g/d • 1 g @ $35
Voriconazole Category D	Vfend	50 & 200 mg tabs 200 mg IV vials	200 mg po q12h • 200 mg @ $32 6 mg/kg IV q12h × 2 then 4 mg/kg q12h infused over 1–2 h • 200 mg @ $109

Continued

16

Agent (generic) Pregnancy category*	Trade names	Dosage form	Usual adult regimen and AWP**
Zanamivir Category C	Relenza	"Rotadisk" inhalation devise with 5 mg doses × 4	2 inhalations of 5 mg bid (4 doses/d) × 5 days (treatment) • 5 × 4 disk @ $56.73

*Classification for use in pregnancy based on FDA categories: Ratings range from "A" for drugs that have been tested for teratogenicity under controlled conditions without showing evidence of damage to the fetus, to "D" and "X" for drugs that are definitely teratogenic. The "D" rating is generally reserved for drugs with no safer alternatives. The "X" rating means there is absolutely no reason to risk using the drug in pregnancy.

Category	Interpretation
A	Controlled studies show no risk. Adequate, well-controlled studies in pregnant women have failed to demonstrate risk to the fetus.
B	No evidence of risk in humans. Either animal findings show risk, but human findings do not, or, if no adequate human studies have been done, animal findings are negative.
C	Risk cannot be ruled out. Human studies are lacking, and animal studies are either positive for fetal risk, or lacking as well. However, potential benefits may justify the potential risk.
D	Positive evidence of risk. Investigational or postmarketing data show risk to the fetus. Nevertheless, potential benefits may outweigh the potential risk.
X	Contraindicated in pregnancy. Studies in animals or humans, or investigational or postmarketing reports, have shown fetal risk which clearly outweighs any possible benefit to the patient.

**Average wholesale price (AWP) as of July 2005 usually rounded to nearest dollar

***Acyclovir—Recommended only for life threatening disease, but record through pregnancy registry suggests safety

Chloroquine—Preferred for malaria prophylaxis

Fluoroquinolones—All fluoroquinolones are contraindicated in pregnancy

Isoniazid—Delay prophylaxis until postpartum unless high risk (HIV, recent contact or radiograph with old lesions). Give with pyridoxine

Mefloquine—Appears to be safe in second and third trimester

Pyrazinamide—Safety in pregnancy not established INH, RIF, and EBM regimen preferred unless resistance suspected

Valacyclovir—Same as acyclovir

PREFERRED ANTIMICROBIAL AGENTS FOR SPECIFIC PATHOGENS

(Adapted from: Medical Letter Treatment Guidelines 2004; 2:13)

Organism	Usual disease	Preferred agent(s)	Alternatives (in random order)
Acinetobacter baumanii (CID 2003;37:214; AAC 2003;47:1681 CID 2003; 36:1268)	Sepsis (esp line sepsis) Pneumonia-ventilator Burn wound sepsis	Imipenem/meropenem; amikacin; ampicillin-sulbactam; ceftazidime	Ciprofloxacin, tetracycline (4); antipseudomonad penicillin (2); aztreonam; colistin/polymyxin; tigecycline; sulfa-trimethoprim Note: Some sensitive only to polymyxin or colistin
Actinobacillus actinomycetemcomitans	Actinomycosis	Penicillin; amoxicillin	Clindamycin; tetracycline (4); erythromycin; cephalosporins (5);
	Endocarditis	Penicillin + aminoglycoside (1)	Cephalosporin (5) + aminoglycoside (1)
Actinomyces israelii (also *A. naeslundii*, *A. odontolyticus*, and *Arachnia proprionica*)	Actinomycosis	Penicillin G; amoxicillin	Clindamycin; tetracycline (4); macrolide (8)
Aeromonas hydrophila (CID 2001;32:331)	Diarrhea (see p 268)	Fluoroquinolone (6); sulfa-trimethoprim × 3d	Tetracycline (4); gentamicin
	Bacteremia	Imipenem/meropenem Fluoroquinolone (6) Sulfa-trimethoprim	Cephalosporin (3rd generation) (5); tigecycline
	Cellulitis/myositis/ osteomyelitis	Fluoroquinolone (6) Sulfa-trimethoprim	
Afipia felix (see *Bartonella henselae*)			
Alcaligenes xylosoxidans (AAC 1996;40:772)	Meningitis, septicemia	Imipenem/meropenem Antipseudomonad penicillin (2)	Ceftazidime; sulfa-trimethoprim; doxycycline; ticarcillin-clavulanic acid

Continued

Organism	Usual disease	Preferred agent(s)	Alternatives (in random order)
Anaplasma phagocytophilum—(see Ehrlichia phagocytopila)			
Areanobacterium haemolyticum (Clin Micro Rev 1997;10:125)	Pharyngitis, chronic ulcers	Penicillin; macrolides (2)	Clindamycin; doxycycline
Babesia microti (NEJM 2000;343: 1454; AAC 2002;46:1163)	Babesiosis	Atovaquone (750 mg po q12h) + azithromycin (500 mg × 1, then 250 mg/d × 7) Quinine (650 mg po tid × 7 d) plus clindamycin (600 mg po qid × 7 d)	
Bacillus anthracis (JAMA 2002; 287:2236)	Inhalation anthrax	Ciprofloxacin IV, Levofloxacin IV or doxycycline IV plus 1–2 other agents: vancomycin, clindamycin, rifampin, penicillin, imipenem/ meropenem, ertapenem, clarithromycin, chloramphenicol; then oral ciprofloxacin (500 mg bid) levofloxacin (500 mg qd) or oral doxycycline (100 mg bid) to complete 60 days	In vitro sensitivity of strain for bio-terrorism will dictate recommendations Other fluoroquinolones are probably comparable to ciprofloxacin; cipro, levo, pen and doxy are FDA-approved for anthrax Steroids: Role is unclear; some treat 100 days Duration based on presumed inhalation exposure
	Cutaneous anthrax	Ciprofloxacin 500 mg bid or levofloxacin 500 mg qd or doxycycline 100 mg bid × 60 days	
	Prophylaxis	Ciprofloxacin 500 mg bid or levofloxacin 500 mg qd or doxycycline 100 mg bid × 60 days	

Continued

Organism	Usual disease	Preferred agent(s)	Alternatives (in random order)
Bacillus cereus	Food poisoning	Not treated	
	Endophthalmitis	Intravitreal clindamycin 450 μg and/or gentamicin 200–400 μg	Imipenem; fluoroquinolones (6)
Bacillus species (Medicine 1987;66:218)	Septicemia (comp host) Endocarditis	Vancomycin	Imipenem/meropenem; clindamycin
Bacteroides bivius (*Prevotella bivia*)	Female genital tract infections	Metronidazole; clindamycin; cefoxitin; cefotetan; beta-lactam-BLI (7)	Chloramphenicol; antipseudomonad penicillin (2); imipenem/meropenem
"*B. fragilis* group" (*B. distasonis, B. fragilis, B. ovatus, B. thetaiotamicron, B. vulgatus*) (CID 2002;35:S126)	Abscesses Bacteremia Intra-abdominal sepsis	Metronidazole; beta-lactam-BLI (7); imipenem/meropenem/ ertapenem	Clindamycin; antipseudomonad penicillin (2); cefoxitin; tigecycline
"*B. melaninogenicus* group" (*Prevotella melaninogenicus, P. intermedius*)	Oral-dental, pulmonary, female genital tract infections	Metronidazole; clindamycin; beta-lactam-BLI (7)	Imipenem/meropenem cefoxitin; tigecycline
Bartonella bacilliformis	Bartonellosis (Oroya fever)	Chloramphenicol 2 g/d × 7 d	Doxycycline; ampicillin
Bartonella henselae (PIDJ 1998;17:447)	Cat-scratch disease	Azithromycin	Ciprofloxacin, sulfa-trimethoprim; gentamicin; rifampin
Bartonella henselae and *B. quintana* (NEJM 1997;337:1876)	Bacillary angiomatosis Trench fever Peliosis hepatis, osteomyelitis, endocarditis	Erythromycin 500 mg po qid × 2–4 mo Erythromycin plus rifampin IV	Doxycycline 100 mg po q12h; azithromycin Doxycycline + rifampin IV
Bordetella pertussis	Pertussis	Erythromycin 2g/d × 14 days	Sulfa-trimethoprim; clarithromycin; azithromycin

Continued

Organism	Usual disease	Preferred agent(s)	Alternatives (in random order)
Borrelia burgdorferi (see p 209)	Lyme disease, erythema migrans	Doxycycline 200 mg/d × 10 d (Ann Intern Med 2003;138:697) Amoxicillin or cefuroxime axetil	Penicillin G po or IV; cefotaxime; ceftriaxone; azithromycin; clarithromycin
	Lyme disease-late	Ceftriaxone	Penicillin G IV
	Prophylaxis	Doxycycline 200 mg × 1 within 72 hrs (NEJM 2001;345:79)	
Borrelia recurrentis (Ann Intern Med 1985;102:397)	Louse-borne relapsing fever	Tetracycline (0.5 g 3 1)	Erythromycin (0.5 g 3 1)
	Tick borne relapsing fever	Doxycycline (200 mg/d 3 5–10 d)	Erythromycin (0.5 g qid 3 5–10 d)
Brucella (Ann Intern Med 1992;117:25; CID 1992;15:582)	Brucellosis	Doxycycline (200 mg/d) 3 6 wks 1 streptomycin (1 g/d IM) or gentamicin × 3 wks	Doxycycline (200 mg/d) 1 rifampin (600–900 mg/d) 3 6 wks; sulfa-trimethoprim + gentamicin
	Brucella meningitis, endocarditis	Doxycycline + rifampin + sulfa-trimethoprim × months	
Burkholderia cepacia (Pseudomonas cepacia) (AAC 1999;43:213)	Septicemia Pneumonia	Sulfa-trimethoprim	Ceftazidime, impenem/meropenem; chloramphenicol
Burkholderia mallei	Glanders	Tetracycline + streptomycin	Streptomycin + chloramphenicol; impenem
Burkholderia pseudomallei (Pseudomonas pseudomallei) (CID 1999;29:381)	Melioidosis Septicemia	Ceftazidime (120 mg/kg/d up to 6 g/d by continuous infusion (AAC 39:2356, 1995) ± TMP-SMX (40 mg/kg/d trimethoprim) (CID 2001;33:29)	Sulfa-trimethoprim + chloramphenicol + doxycycline; impenem/meropenem; Note: TMP-SMX resistance in Thailand
	Localized	TMP-SMX; amoxicillin-clavulanate	Tetracycline; chloramphenicol; sulfisoxazole

Continued

21

Organism	Usual disease	Preferred agent(s)	Alternatives (in random order)
Calymmatobacterium granulomatis (MMWR 2002;51 RR-6)	Granuloma inguinale Donovanosis	Doxycycline 200 mg/d ≥ 21 days TMP-SMX 1 DS/d × ≥ 21 days	Ciprofloxacin 750 mg bid ≥ 21 days; erythromycin 500 mg bid × ≥ 21 days; cipro + gentamicin
Campylobacter fetus	Septicemia, vascular infections, meningitis	Imipenem; 3rd gen cephalosporin	Gentamicin; imipenem/meropenem
Campylobacter jejuni (CID 2001;32:331)	Diarrhea (see p 268)	Erythromycin 500 mg bid × 5 d or azithromycin	Tetracycline (4); fluoroquinolone (6)
Capnocytophaga canimorus (CDC group DF-2) (AAC 1988;32:78)	Dog and cat bites	Amoxicillin; Penicillin G	Doxycycline; amoxicillin-clavulanate; fluoroquinolone (6); macrolides (8); cefotaxime, ceftizoxime or ceftriaxone, imipenem/meropenem; vancomycin, clindamycin
	Bacteremia (asplenia)	Clindamycin; penicillin	Cephalosporins (3rd generation) (5); imipenem/meropenem; fluoroquinolones (6); beta-lactam-BLI (7)
Capnocytophaga ochracea (CDC group DF-1) (JID 1985;151:140)	Periodontal disease	Clindamycin; amoxicillin-clavulanic acid; erythromycin; doxycycline	
	Bactermia in neutropenic host	Clindamycin; imipenem/ meropenem/ertapenem	Beta-lactam-BLI (7); fluoroquinolone (6)
Cardiobacterium sp.	Endocarditis	Penicillin ± aminoglycoside	Cephalosporin (5) ± aminoglycoside (1)
Cat-scratch disease, (see *Bartonella henselae*)			
Chlamydia pneumoniae (now classified as Chlamydophila pneumoniae	Pneumonia (see p 255)	Doxycycline, erythromycin or clarithromycin × 10–14 d; Telithromycin × 7–10 d; azithromycin 3–5 d	Fluoroquinolone (6) × 10–14 d
Chlamydia psittaci	Psittacosis (see p 255)	Doxycycline	Chloramphenicol

Continued

Organism	Usual disease	Preferred agent(s)	Alternatives (in random order)
Chlamydia trachomatis (see pp 293–294) (MMWR 2002;51:RR-6)	Urethritis, cervicitis, PID, epididymitis, urethral syndrome	Doxycycline (200 mg/d × 7 d); azithromycin (1 g po × 1)	Erythromycin (500 mg qid × 7d); ofloxacillin (300 mg bid × 7d); amoxicillin
	Lymphogranuloma venereum	Doxycycline 200 mg/d × 21 d	Erythromycin 500 mg qid × 21 d
	Trachoma	Azithromycin 20 mg/kg × 1 (CID 1997;24:363)	Doxycycline 200 mg/d (oral + topical) × 14 d; a sulfonamide (oral + topical)
	Inclusion conjunctivitis	Erythromycin (oral or IV)	Sulfonamide
Citrobacter diversus	Urinary tract infections, pneumonia	Cephalosporin (2nd, 3rd gen) (5); cefepime; sulfa-trimethoprim	Fluoroquinolone (6); imipenem/ meropenem; aztreonam
Citrobacter freundii	Urinary tract infection, wound infection, septicemia, pneumonia	Imipenem/meropenem; fluoroquinolone (6); sulfa-trimethoprim	Cefepime; antipseudomonad penicillins; aztreonam; tigecycline ceftriaxone; ceftazidine amikacin; ertapenem
Clostridium difficile (NEJM 2002; 346:334)	Antibiotic-associated colitis and diarrhea (see p 268)	Metronidazole 250 mg po qid × 10 d	Vancomycin 125 mg po qid × 10 d or vancomycin 500 mg by nasogastric or rectal tube (patients unable to take po drugs)
Clostridium sp.	Gas gangrene Sepsis	Penicillin G (all systemic clostridial infections) + Clindamycin (JID 1987;155:220)	Chloramphenicol; metronidazole; ampicillin; clindamycin; imipenem/meropenem
	Tetanus	Metronidazole (Lancet 1989;2:1216) + tetanus toxoid + tetanus Immune globulin (500 IU IV)	Penicillin; cephalosporins; imipenem; macrolides; tetracycline
	Botulism	Penicillin + A/B or E equine antitoxin (10 mL IV) (available from the CDC at 404-639-3670)	

Continued

Organism	Usual disease	Preferred agent(s)	Alternatives (in random order)
Corynebacterium diphtheriae	Diphtheria	Erythromycin (250–500 mg qid) or penicillin (IM or po) × 14 d + antitoxin (20,000–40,000 units IM for pharyngeal disease ≤ 48 hrs; 80,000–120,000 units IV/IM for severe disease) (available from CDC at 404-639-3670)	Clindamycin; tetracycline (4)
Corynebacterium jeikeium (CDC group JK)	Septicemia	Vancomycin	Penicillin G + gentamicin; daptomycin; fluoroquinolone (6); macrolide (8)
Corynebacterium minutissimum	Erythrasma	Erythromycin	
Corynebacterium ulcerans	Pharyngitis	Erythromycin	
Coxiella burnetii (MMWR 2002;51:924)	Q fever	Doxycycline (200 mg/d × 2–3 wks)	Chloramphenicol; fluoroquinolone (6)
	Q fever endocarditis	Doxycycline (100 mg bid + hydroxychloroquine 200 mg tid × 18 mo–4 yr) (Arch Intern Med 1999;159:167)	Doxycycline + rifampin or fluoroquinolone (6) × 2 yrs.
Dysgonic fermenter type-2 (DF-2)	See Capnocytophaga canimoris		

Continued

Organism	Usual disease	Preferred agent(s)	Alternatives (in random order)
Ehrlichia chaffeensis E. phagocytophia (Now reclassified as Anaplasma phagocytophilum) (Emerg Infect Dis 1996;2:18; AAC 1997;41:76)	Ehrlichiosis–human monocyte ehrlichiosis (EMH) and human granulocyte ehrlichiosis (HGE)	Doxycycline (100 mg bid po or IV × 7–14 days)	Rifampin; fluoroquinolones (AAC 1997;41:76)
Ehrlichia chaffeensis	Monocytotrophic ehrlichiosis	Doxycycline	Chloramphenicol
Eikenella corrodens (AAC 1988;32:1143)	Oral infections, bite wounds	Ampicillin; amoxicillin	Tetracycline (4); amoxicillin-clavulanic acid; ampicillin-sulbactam; ceftriaxone; azithromycin; fluoroquinolone (6);
Enterobacter aerogenes, E. cloacae (JAMA 2003;298:885)	Sepsis, pneumonia, wound infections	imipenem/meropenem; cefepime; aminoglycoside (1);	Tigecycline; fluoroquinolone (6); aminoglycoside; sulfa-trimethoprim; aztreonam; cefotaxime, ceftriaxone; pip-tazo
	Urinary tract infection	Sulfa-trimethoprim Cephalosporin (3rd generation) (5)	Antipseudomonad penicillin (2); aminoglycoside; fluoroquinolone (6); imipenem; tigecycline
	Urinary tract infection	Ampicillin/amoxicillin	Nitrofurantoin; fosfonomycin; fluoroquinolone (6)
	Wound infections, intra-abdominal sepsis, bacteremia	Ampicillin ± aminoglycoside (1)	Vancomycin; daptomycin; linezolid; penicillin ± aminoglycoside (1); imipenem (E. faecalis); tigecycline
Enterococcus (E. faecalis and E. faecium) (Vancomycin sensitive)	Endocarditis	Penicillin G/ampicillin + gentamicin or streptomycin	Vancomycin + gentamicin or streptomycin; daptomycin

Continued

25

Organism	Usual disease	Preferred agent(s)	Alternatives (in random order)
Enterococcus faecium (vancomycin-resistant)	Urinary tract infection	Nitrofurantoin; fosfonomycin	Tigecycline
	Bacteremia and other systemic infections	Linezolid; daptomycin	Some strains sensitive to chloramphenicol, tetracycline, or fluoroquinolones; clinical results are variable (CID 1995;20:1137)
	Endocarditis	Daptomycin	
Erysipelothrix rhusiopathiae (AAC 1990;34:2038)	Localized cutaneous (erysipeloid)	Amoxicillin; fluoroquinolone (6)	Clindamycin; imipenem
	Endocarditis/disseminated	Penicillin 12–20 mil units/d × 4–6 wks	Cephalosporins—1st generation (5); fluoroquinolone
E. coli (JAMA 2003;289:885)	Septicemia, intra-abdominal sepsis, wound infection	Cephalosporin (3rd gen) (5) Ampicillin (if sensitive) Sulfa-trimethoprim (if sensitive)	Imipenem/meropenem/ertapenem; fluoroquinolone (6); cefepime; cephalosporin (1st or 2nd gen) (5); aztreonam; antipseudomonad penicillin (2); beta-lactam-BLI (7); tigecycline; aminoglyocide
	Urinary tract infection	TMP-SMX (if sensitive); fluoroquinolone	Cephalosporin (5); imipenem/ meropenem; tigecycline
	Diarrhea ETEC (travelers' diarrhea (see p 272)	Ciprofloxacin (500 mg bid × 3d); TMP-SMX (DS bid × 3d) (CID 2001;32:331); rifaximin (200 mg tid × 3d)	
Francisella tularensis (CID 1994;19:42)	Tularemia	Streptomycin (1 g 1M bid × 10 days); gentamicin (5 mg/kg/d × 10 days)	Tetracycline (4); chloramphenicol; ciprofloxacin × ≧ 14 days

Continued

Organism	Usual disease	Preferred agent(s)	Alternatives (in random order)
Fusobacterium	Oral/dental/pulmonary infection, liver abscess, female genital tract	Penicillin G; metronidazole; clindamycin; amoxicillin-clavulanate	Cefoxitin/Betalactam BLI (7) imipenem/meropenem/ertapenem Betalactam BLI (7)
Gardnerella vaginalis (MMWR 2002;51:RR-6) (see p 300)	Bacterial vaginosis	Metronidazole (500 mg bid × 7 d)	Clindamycin 2% 5 g topical qd × 7; metronidazole gel 0.75% 5 g bid × 5 d Metronidazole (2 g po × 1); clindamycin (300 mg po bid × 7 d)
Haemophilus aphrophilus	Sepsis, endocarditis	Penicillin G + aminoglycoside (1)	Cephalosporin (3rd gen) (5) + aminoglycoside (1)
H. ducreyi (MMWR 2002;51:RR-1)	Chancroid (see p 293)	Ceftriaxone (250 mg IM × 1) Erythromycin (500 mg qid × 7 d) Azithromycin (1 g po × 1)	Ciprofloxacin
H. influenzae (AAC 1997;41:292)	Meningitis (see p 234) Epiglottis, pneumonia (see p 253); arthritis; cellulitis	Cefotaxime; ceftriaxone	Cefuroxime (not meningitis); Meropenem; chloramphenicol
	Otitis, sinusitis, exacerbations of chronic bronchitis	Sulfa-trimethoprim; azithromycin Cephalosporin (2nd or 3rd gen); clarithromycin	Tetracycline (4); beta-lactamase-BLT (7); fluoroquinolone (6)
	Pneumonia, acute sinusitis, acute bacterial exacerbations of chronic bronchitis	Telithromycin; azithromycin; cephalosporin (2nd + 3rd gen); clarithromycin	Fluoroquinolone; beta-lactamase-BLT

Continued

27

Organism	Usual disease	Preferred agent(s)	Alternatives (in random order)
Hafnia alvei (see Enterobacter)			
Helicobacter pylori (Med Lett 1997;39:1 Ann Intern Med 1997;157:87 BMJ 2001;232:1047; NEJM 2002;347:1175) Med Letter Treatment Guidelines 2004;2:9 (see p 267)	Peptic ulcer disease	Omeprazole (20 g) + clarithromycin (500 mg bid) + either metronidazole (500 mg tid) or amoxicillin (1 gm bid) × 14 d	Bismuth subsalicylate (2 tabs bid) + tetracycline (500 mg qid) + metronidazole (500 mg tid) + omeprazole (20 mg bid) × 14 d Omeprazole + amoxicillin (1 g bid), + clarithromycin (500 mg bid) × 1 wk Alternative proton pump inhibitors: lansoprazole (Prevacid), pantoprazole (Protonix), esomeprazole (Nexium) rabeprazole (Aciphex)
Kingella sp.	Endocarditis	Penicillin + aminoglycoside	Cephalosporin (5) + aminoglycoside (1)
	Septic arthritis	Penicillin; cephalosporin	TMP-SMX; doxycycline; macrolides (8); fluoroquinolone (6)
Klebsiella pneumoniae K. oxytoca (JAMA 2003;289:885)	Septicemia, nosocomial pneumonia, intra-abdominal sepsis, urinary tract infection	Cephalosporin (3rd gen) (5) Imipenem/meropenem/ertapenem beta-lactam-BLI (7); cefepime; fluoroquinolone (6)	Aminoglycoside (1); sulfa-trimethoprim; tigecycline; aztreonam
Legionella sp (J Resp Dis 2002;23:229)	Legionnaires' disease (see p 247)	Gatifloxacin, moxifloxacin, or levofloxacin × 7–10 d Azithromycin × 5–7 d	Erythromycin; doxycycline; clarithromycin; sulfa-trimethoprim

Continued

Organism	Usual disease	Preferred agent(s)	Alternatives (in random order)
Leptospira spp (CID 1995;21:1)	Leptospirosis Mild disease	Doxycycline 200 mg/d Amoxicillin 500 mg qid	
	Serious disease	Penicillin G 1.5 mil units q6h Ampicillin 0.5–1 g IV q6h	
Leuconostoc (AAC 1990;34:543)	Bacteremia Wound infection	Penicillin/ampicillin	Erythromycin; aminoglycosides (1); clindamycin
Listeria monocytogenes (JCM 2003;41:483)	Meningitis (see p 234) Septicemia	Ampicillin or penicillin ± gentamicin	Sulfa-trimethoprim
Moraxella catarrhalis (Branhamella catarrhalis) (AAC 1996;40:2884)	Otitis, sinusitis, pneumonitis	Sulfa-trimethoprim; cephalosporin (2nd or 3rd gen) (5); amoxicillin-clavulanate macrolides (8)	Doxycycline; fluoroquinolone (6)
	Acute bacterial exacerbations of chronic bronchitis	Telithromycin, azithromycin; cephalosporin (2nd + 3rd gen); clarithromycin	Doxycycline; fluoroquinolone (6)
Morganella morganii	Bacteremia, pneumonia, urinary tract infection, wound infection	Fluoroquinolone (6); imipenem/ meropenem; cephalosporin (3rd gen) (5); cefepime	Sulfa-trimethoprim; aztreonam; antipseudomonad penicillin (2); aminoglycoside (1); beta-lactam-BLI
Mycobacterium abscessus	Cutaneous pulmonary	Amikacin + cefoxitin or imipenem	Clarithromycin ± clofazimine

Continued

Organism	Usual disease	Preferred agent(s)	Alternatives (in random order)
M. avium-intracellulare (see p 163)	Pulmonary infection	Clarithromycin or azithromycin, Ethambutol, ± rifabutin or ciprofloxacin (6)	Azithromycin; amikacin; ciprofloxacin/ ofloxacin/levofloxacin; streptomycin
	Disseminated infection (AIDS)	Clarithromycin + ethambutol ± rifabutin or ciprofloxacin (6)	Ethionamide; cycloserine; rifampin/rifabutin; amikacin
M. chelonae (see p 163)	Skin and soft tissue	Tobramycin + cefoxitin or imipenem	Clofazimine or clarithromycin, then sulfonamide, rifampin, doxycycline, or erythromycin
M. fortuitum (see p 163)	Soft tissue and wound infections Pulmonary	Amikacin + clarithromycin × 2–4 wk, then clarithromycin, ciprofloxacin, or doxycycline	Cefoxitin, rifampin, sulfonamides, ethambutol, linezolid, doxycycline
M. genavense (AIDS) (see p 164)	Disseminated disease	Clarithromycin + other agents	INH; ethambutol; rifampin; ciprofloxacin; pyrazinamide
M. haemophilum (AIDS) (see p 163)	Disseminated disease (skin, bone, gut, nodes) Pulmonary	Rifampin or rifabutin + amikacin + ciprofloxacin	Cycloserine
M. kansasii (see p 162)	Pulmonary infection	INH + rifampin ± ethambutol or streptomycin	Clarithromycin; azithromycin; ethionamide; cycloserine
M. leprae	Paucibacillary	Rifampin 600 mg/mo (supervised) plus dapsone 100 mg/d	Rifampin 600 mg/d plus dapsone 100 mg/d for 12 mo
	Multibacillary	Rifampin 600 mg/mo (supervised) + dapsone 100 mg/d + clofazimine 100 mg/mo (supervised) or 50 mg/d	Rifampin 600 mg/d plus dapsone 100 mg/d ± clofazimine 50 mg/d × ≥24 mo

Continued

Organism	Usual disease	Preferred agent(s)	Alternatives (in random order)
M. marinum (see p 163)	Soft tissue infections	Minocycline	Clarithromycin; rifampin, sulfa-trimethoprim doxycycline
M. tuberculosis (see pp 154)	Tuberculosis	INH + rifampin + pyrazinamide + ethambutol or streptomycin	Capreomycin, kanamycin or amikacin; gatifloxacin or moxifloxacin Ethionamide; PAS
M. ulcerans (see p 163)	Pulmonary	Rifampin + ethambutol Amikacin + sulfa-trimethoprim	
Mycoplasma hominis (CID 1996;23:671)	Genital tract infections	Doxycycline 200 mg/d × 7 d	
Mycoplasma pneumoniae	Pneumonia (see p 255)	Erythromycin, clarithromycin (× 7–10 d) azithromycin (× 3–5 d) doxycycline × 10–14 d; telithromycin × 7–10 d; azithromycin 3–5 d	Fluoroquinolones (6) × 7-10 d
Neisseria gonorrhoeae (see pp 285–286) (MMWR 2002;51:RR-6)	Genital tract infections	Ceftriaxone (125 mg IM × 1); ciprofloxacin (500 mg × 1); gatifloxacin (400 mg × 1) ofloxacin (400 mg × 1) (each with doxycycline or azithromycin)	Spectinomycin (2 g IM × 1); azithromycin (2 g po × 1); cefoxitin 2 g IM probenecid 1 g po
	Disseminated gonococcal infection	Ceftriaxone 1 g IV or IM/d until asymptomatic 24–48 hr, then oral Rx to complete 1 wk	Cefotaxime 1 g IV q8h

Continued

31

Organism	Usual disease	Preferred agent(s)	Alternatives (in random order)
N. meningitidis (see p 233)	Meningitis bacteremia, pericarditis, pneumonia	Penicillin G (up to 24 mil units/d IV) × 10–14 d	Ampicillin; cefotaxime; ceftriaxone; chloramphenicol; sulfa-trimethoprim
	Prophylaxis	Ciprofloxacin (500 mg × 1)	Rifampin (600 mg bid × 2 d) Ceftriaxone (250 mg IM × 1)
Nocardia asteroides (Clin Microbiol Rev 1994;7:357)	Nocardiosis: pulmonary infection, abscesses—skin, lung, brain	Sulfonamide (usually sulfadiazine or sulfisoxazole) (3–6 g/d) Sulfa-trimethoprim (5–10 mg/kg/d trimethoprim po or IV up to 15 mg/kg/d)	Minocycline ± sulfonamide Amikacin ± imipenem/meropenem/ ertapenem; ceftriaxone, linezolid, or sulfa-trimethoprim Imipenem + cefotaxime or sulfa-trimethoprim Cycloserine
Pasteurella multocida (AAC 1988; 32:213)	Animal bite wound	Penicillin G; ampicillin; amoxicillin	Tetracycline (4); fluoroquinolones; Cephalosporins (2nd and 3rd gen) (5) Amoxicillin-clavulanic acid; macrolides; tigecycline
	Septicemia, septic arthritis/osteomyelitis	Penicillin G	Cephalosporins (3rd gen) (5); beta-lactam-BLI (7); imipenem/meropenem; tigecycline
Peptostreptococcus	Oral/dental/pulmonary infection; intra-abdominal sepsis; gynecologic infection	Penicillin G; ampicillin; amoxicillin; clindamycin	Cephalosporin (1st gen) (5); chloramphenicol; macrolides (8); moxifloxacin, gatifloxacin; vancomycin; imipenem/ meropenem/ertapenem; tigecycline

Continued

Organism	Usual disease	Preferred agent(s)	Alternatives (in random order)
Plesiomonas shigelloides (CID 2001;51:331)	Diarrhea (usually not treated) (see p 273) Extra-intestinal infection	Sulfa-trimethoprim (I DS bid × 3 d) Fluoroquinolone (6) × 3 d Cephalosporin (3rd gen) (3) Aminoglycoside (1)	Aztreonam; sulfa-trimethoprim; imipenem/meropenem; fluoroquinolone (6)
Propionibacterium acnes	Acne	Tetracycline (4)	Clindamycin (topical); clindamycin
Proteus mirabilis (JCM 2002;40:1549)	Septicemia, urinary tract infection, intra-abdominal sepsis, wound infection	Ampicillin Cephalosporins (1st, 2nd, 3rd generation) (5)	Aminoglycosides (1); sulfa-trimethoprim; tetracycline Antipseudomonad penicillin (2); aztreonam; fluoroquinolone (6); beta-lactam-BLI (7)
Proteus vulgaris and other indole + proteus: M. morganii + P. rettgeri	Septicemia Urinary tract infection	Cephalosporin (3rd gen) (5) Imipenem/meropenem/ ertapenem; beta-lactam-BLI (7)	Aminoglycoside (1); sulfa-trimethoprim; antipseudomonad penicillin (2); cefepime; aztreonam; fluoroquinolone (6)
Providencia	Septicemia Urinary tract infection	Cephalosporin (3rd gen) (5) Imipenem/meropenem/ ertapenem	Aminoglycoside (1); aztreonam; cefepime; ticarcillin-clavulanate; sulfa-trimethoprim; pip-tazo fluoroquinolone (6)
Pseudomonas aeruginosa (JAMA 2003;289:885)	Septicemia, pneumonia Intra-abdominal sepsis	Aminoglycoside (tobramycin) Pip-tazo or Ticar-clav + aminoglycoside	Ciprofloxacin (6); ceftazidime; cefepime; imipenem/meropenem; aztreonam; each ± tobramycin or amikacin
	Urinary tract infections	Ciprofloxacin;	Imipenem/meropenem; antipseudomonal penicillin (2) ceftazidime; cefepime; cefoperazone; aztreonam; pip-tazo; ticar-clav; aminoglycoside

Continued

Organism	Usual disease	Preferred agent(s)	Alternatives (in random order)
P. cepacia (see *Burkholderia cepecia*)			
Rhodococcus equi (CID 2002;34:1379)	Localized + immunocompetent	2 oral agents: rifampin, erythromycin, or ciprofloxacin	
	Disseminated, severe, or immunosuppressed	2 parenteral agents: vancomycin, + erythromycin imipenem/ meropenem/ertapenem, amikacin rifampin	
Rickettsia spp (MMWR 2000;49:888)	Rocky Mountain spotted fever, Q fever, tick-bite fever, murine typhus, scrub typhus, typhus, trench fever	Doxycycline (100 mg po or IV bid × 7 days)	Chloramphenicol (2 g/d × 7 d) fluoroquinolone (6)
Rochalimaea quintana and *R. henselae* (see *Bartonella henselae* and *B. quintana*)			
Salmonella typhi (AAC 1999;43:1441; CID 2001;32:331)	Typhoid fever (see p 270)	Ceftriaxone 1–2 g/d × 10–14 d Ciprofloxacin 500 mg bid × 10 d If severely ill: Steroids (RID 1991;13:85)	Ampicillin/amoxicillin (preferred if sensitive); chloramphenicol (4 g IV/d); sulfa-trimethoprim (1 DS bid); azithromycin
	Carriers (see p 274) (Lancet 1987;2:162)	Ciprofloxacin (× 4–6 wks) Amoxicillin (× 6 wks) TMP-SMX (× 6 wks)	

34

Organism	Usual disease	Preferred agent(s)	Alternatives (in random order)
Salmonella sp. (other) (CID 2001;32:331)	Gastroenteritis (See indications p 271)	Ciprofloxacin (500 mg bid × 5–7 d) Ceftriaxone (100 mg/kg/d × 5–7 d) TMP-SMX (1 DS bid × 5–7 d)	Ofloxacin and norfloxacin
	Bacteremia	Ceftriaxone or fluoroquinolone (IV × 7–14 d)	
	Endovascular infection	Ceftriaxone, ampicillin, or ciprofloxacin (IV × 6 wks ± surgery)	
	Carrier	As for S. typhi (above)	
Serratia marcescens	Septicemia, urinary tract infection, pneumonia	Imipenem/meropenem/ertapenem	Cephalosporin (3rd gen) (5) ± gentamicin; imipenem/ meropenem; fluoroquinolone (6); antipseudomonad penicillin (2) + amikacin; aztreonam; pip/tazobactam; Ticar/sulbactam; tigecycline
Shigella spp (CID 2001;32:331)	Colitis (see p 271)	Sulfa-trimethoprim (1 DS bid × 3 d) Ciprofloxacin 500 mg bid × 3 d)	Fluoroquinolone (6); azithromycin
Spirillum minus	Rat-bite fever	Penicillin G (IV × 5–7 d) then amoxicillin × 7 days	Tetracycline (4); streptomycin Possibly effective: clindamycin; erythromycin; ceftriaxone
Staphylococcus aureus Methicillin-sensitive	Septicemia, pneumonia, cellulitis, wound infection	Penicillinase-resistant penicillin (3)	Cephalosporins (1st gen) (5); cefepime; imipenem/meropenem vancomycin; sulfa-trimethoprim; macrolide (8); beta-lactam-BLI (7); fluoroquinolone (6) (increasing resistance); clindamycin; tigecycline

Continued

35

Organism	Usual disease	Preferred agent(s)	Alternatives (in random order)
Staphylococcus aureus Methicillin-sensitive (*continued*)	Acute sinusitis	Telithromycin; amoxicillin; cephalosporin (2nd + 3rd gen)	Sulfa-trimethoprim; macrolide; clindamycin
Methicillin-resistant	As above	Vancomycin ± rifampin or gentamicin	Daptomycin (except pneumonia); linezolid Community-acquired MRSA are often sensitive to clindamycin, fluoroquinolones, TMP-SMX
Vancomycin-intermediate sensitive *S. aureus* (NEJM 1999;340:493)	As above	Vancomycin *plus* oxacillin, nafcillin, cefazolin, or cefotaxime (NEJM 1999;340:517); linezolid; daptomycin (except pneumonia)	Quinupristin-dalfopristin
Vancomycin-resistant *S. aureus* (NEJM 2003;348:1342; MMWR 2002;51:565)	As above	Linezolid; daptomycin (except pneumonia)	Quinupristin-dalfopristin; some strains sensitive to tetracycline, TMP-SMX, chloramphenicol
S. saprophyticus	Urinary tract infections	Sulfa-trimethoprim Ampicillin/amoxicillin Fluoroquinolone (6)	Cephalosporins (5); tetracycline (4); tigecycline
S. epidermidis Methicillin-sensitive	Septicemia Infected prosthetic devices	Oxacillin/nafcillin Cephalosporin (1st gen) (5)	Beta-lactam-BLI (7); fluoroquinolone (6); imipenem/meropenem/ertapenem; vancomycin; tigecycline
Methicillin-resistant	Septicemia Infected prosthetic devices	Vancomycin ± gentamicin or rifampin	Daptomycin; linezolid; (possibly effective—chloramphenicol, rifampin, tetracycline); tigecycline
Stenotrophomonas maltophilia (*Xanthomonas maltophilia*)	Septicemia, pneumonia, UTI	Sulfa-trimethoprim; tigecycline	Ceftazidime; fluoroquinolone (6); minocycline

Continued

Organism	Usual disease	Preferred agent(s)	Alternatives (in random order)
Streptobacillus moniliformis	Rat-bite fever Haverhill fever	Penicillin G IV × 5–7 d, then amoxicillin × 7 d	Tetracycline (4); erythromycin; clindamycin; streptomycin
Streptococcus, groups B, C, G; S. bovis, S. milleri, S. viridans, anaerobic streptococci (Peptostreptococcus) and penicillin-sensitive strains of S. pneumoniae (S. pyogenes—see pp 241, 245) (CID 2002;35:113)	Pharyngitis Soft tissue infection Pneumonia (see p 253) Abscesses	Penicillin G or V (if penicillin-resistant S. pneumoniae—see below)	Cephalosporin (1st gen) cefuroxime, cefotaxime, ceftriaxone; Erythromycin, clarithromycin, azithromycin Vancomycin; clindamycin; tigecycline
S. pneumoniae	Endocarditis	Penicillin G ± streptomycin or gentamicin	Cephalosporin: Parenteral—see above vancomycin
S. iniae	Bacteremia, cellulitis	Penicillin, clindamycin	Beta-lactams
S. pneumoniae (see p 253)	Meningitis (see p 233) Ocular infections	Vancomycin + cefotaxime or ceftriaxone	Cefotaxime; ceftriaxone (activity variable)
S. pneumoniae Penicillin-sensitive (MIC ≤ 1.0 µg/mL)	Pneumonia (see p 253)	Penicillin G; amoxicillin; cefotaxime or ceftriaxone	Telithromycin;† macrolides (8); cephalosporins—cefpodoxime, ceftibutin, cefprozil; fluoroquinolone (6); clindamycin; doxycycline; pip-tazobactam; sulfa-trimethoprim
	Meningitis	Penicillin; ceftriaxone; cefotaxime	Vancomycin, chloramphenicol

Continued

37

Organism	Usual disease	Preferred agent(s)	Alternatives (in random order)
Penicillin-intermediate sensitive (MIC 2 μg/mL)	Pneumonia	As for penicillin-sensitive strains (see previous page) OR telithromycin,† fluoroquinolone	Most active beta-lactams—amoxicillin; cefotaxime; ceftriaxone; ceftibutin; cefpodoxime Other options—vancomycin; clindamycin; beta-lactam-BLI's (7)—but not ticarcillin
	Meningitis	Vancomycin	
Penicillin-resistant (MIC ≥ 4.0 μg/mL)	Pneumonia	Telithromycin;† fluoroquinolone (6); vancomycin; linezolid	
	Meningitis	Vancomycin;† ceftriaxone or cefotaxime	
S. pyogenes	Pharyngitis (CID 2002;35:113)	Penicillin V 500 mg bid × 10 d Benzathine penicillin 1.2 mil units IM × 1	Erythromycin 250 mg po tid × 10 d
	Soft tissue	Penicillin; amoxicillin	
	Toxic shock syndrome	Clindamycin + penicillin + IVIG	
Treponema pallidum	Syphilis (see pp 286–289)	Penicillin G	Tetracycline (4); ceftriaxone
Tropheryma whippelii (Lancet 2003;361:231)	Whipple's disease	Induction: ceftriaxone (2 g IV/d) or penicillin (1.2 mil units/d) + strep (1 g/d) × 2 wks Maintenance: TMP-SMX (1 DS/d) or doxycycline/minocycline (200 mg/d × 1 yr)	

Continued

Organism	Usual disease	Preferred agent(s)	Alternatives (in random order)
Ureaplasma urealyticum	Genital tract infection	Doxycycline (200 mg/d × 7 d)	Macrolides (8); a tetracycline; ofloxacillin
Vibrio cholerae (CID 2001;32:331)	Cholera (see p 271)	Doxycycline (300 mg × 1); tetracycline (500 mg qid × 3 d)	Fluoroquinolone-single dose
Vibrio parahaemolyticus (CID 2001;32:331)	Diarrhea (usually not treated) (see p 272)	Tetracycline (4) Fluoroquinolone (6)	
Vibrio vulnificus (CID 2003;37:272)	Septicemia Wound infection Gastroenteritis	Tetracycline (4)	Cefotaxime/Ceftriaxone Ciprofloxacin
Xanthomonas maltophilia (see Stenotrophomonas maltophilia)			
Yersinia enterocolitica (CID 2001;32:331)	Enterocolitis and mesenteric adenitis (usually not treated)	Sulfa-trimethoprim; gentamicin; fluoroquinolone (6); doxycycline	Cephalosporin (3rd gen) (5)
	Septicemia	Aminoglycoside (gentamicin)	Chloramphenicol; ciprofloxacin; sulfa-trimethoprim
Yersinia pestis (JAMA 2000;283:2281)	Plague treatment	Streptomycin; gentamicin	Chloramphenicol; tetracycline (4); ciprofloxacin; sulfa-trimethoprim
	Prevention	Doxycycline Ciprofloxacin	Chloramphenicol; sulfa-trimethoprim

Continued

Organism	Usual disease	Preferred agent(s)	Alternatives (in random order)
Yersinia pseudo-tuberculosis	Mesenteric adenitis (usually not treated) Septicemia	Aminoglycoside (1) Ampicillin	Sulfa-trimethoprim; tetracycline (4)

1. Aminoglycosides: gentamicin, tobramycin, amikacin, netilimicin. Netilmicin is no longer available in the U.S.

2. Antipseudomonad penicillin: ticarcillin, piperacillin.

3. Penicillinase-resistant penicillins: nafcillin, oxacillin, methicillin, cloxacillin, dicloxacillin.

4. Tetracycline: Tetracycline, doxycycline, minocycline.

5. Cephalosporins and miscellaneous beta-lactams

    1st generation: Cefadroxil,* cefazolin, cephalexin,* cephapirin, cephradine*

    2nd generation: Cefaclor,* cefaclor ER, cefamandole, cefonanide, cefotetan, cefoxitin, cefuroxime,* cefprozil,* loracarbef*

    3rd generation: Cefotaxime, ceftizoxime, ceftazidime, cefoperazone, ceftriaxone, moxalactam, cefixime,* cefpodoxime,* cefdinir,* cefditoren,* ceftibuten*

    4th generation: Cefepime

    Cephamycins: Cefoxitin, cefotetan

    Monobactam: Aztreonam

    Carbapenem: Imipenem, meropenem, ertapenem

    Carbacephem: Loracarbef*

6. Fluoroquinolones: Norfloxacin, ciprofloxacin, ofloxacin, lomefloxacin, levofloxacin, trovafloxacin, gatifloxacin, gemifloxacin, and moxifloxacin. Systemic infections are usually treated with ciprofloxacin, ofloxacin, levofloxacin, gatifloxacin, or moxifloxacin; all may be used for urinary tract infections. With regard to spectrum: *P. aeruginosa*—ciprofloxacin and levofloxacin; *Mycobacterium*—ciprofloxacin, levofloxacin, gatifloxacin, moxifloxacin, or ofloxacin; *C. trachomatis*—ofloxacin; *S. pneumoniae*—levofloxacin; gatifloxacin, or moxifloxacin, or gemifloxacin; anaerobes—gatifloxacin and moxifloxacin are most active; ciprofloxacin and levofloxacin are least active.

7. Beta-lactam-beta-lactamase inhibitor. Amoxicillin + clavulanate (Augmentin), ticarcillin + clavulanate (Timentin), ampicillin + sulbactam (Unasyn), and piperacillin + tazobactam (Zosyn).

8. Macrolides: Erythromycin, clarithromycin, azithromycin, dirithromycin.

*Oral cephalosporins; cefuroxime has both oral and parenteral formulations.

†Telithromycin is also active agent against multi-drug resistant *Streptococcus pneumoniae.*

ANTIMICROBIAL DOSING REGIMENS IN RENAL FAILURE

A. GENERAL PRINCIPLES

1. Initial dose is not modified in renal failure.
2. Adjustments in subsequent doses for renally excreted drugs may be accomplished by *a*) giving the usual maintenance dose at extended intervals, usually three half-lives (extended interval method); *b*) giving reduced doses at the usual intervals (dose reduction method); or *c*) a combination of each.
3. Adjustments in dose are usually based on creatinine clearance that may be estimated by the Cockcroft-Gault equation (Nephron 16:31, 1976).

$$\text{Male: } \frac{\text{weight (kg)} \times (140 \text{ minus age in yr})}{72 \times \text{serum creatinine (mg/dL)}}$$

Female: Above value $\times$ 0.85

Pitfalls and notations with calculations follow.

a. **Elderly patient:** Serum creatinine may be deceptively low (with danger of overdosing) because of reduced muscle mass.
b. **Pregnancy, ascites, and other causes of volume expansion:** GFR may be increased (with danger of underdosing) in third trimester of pregnancy and patients with normal renal function who receive massive parenteral fluids.
c. **Obese patients:** Use lean body weight.
d. **Renal failure:** Formulas assume stable renal function; for patients with anuria or oliguria assume creatine clearance (CCr) of 5–8 mL/min.

B. AMINOGLYCOSIDE DOSING

1. GUIDELINES OF THE JOHNS HOPKINS HOSPITAL CLINICAL PHARMACOLOGY DEPARTMENT

Agent	Loading dose, regardless of renal function[b,c]	Subsequent doses (before level measurements)		Therapeutic levels (1 hr after start of infusion over 20–30 min)
		CCr > 70 mL/min	CCr < 70 mL/min[d]	
Gentamicin[a]	2 mg/kg	1.7–2 mg/kg/8 h	0.03 × CCr = mg/kg/8 h	5–10 µg/mL
Tobramycin[a]	2 mg/kg	1.7–2 mg/kg/8 h	0.03 × CCr = mg/kg/8 h	5–10 µg/mL
Amikacin[a]	8 mg/kg	7.5–8 mg/kg/8 h	0.12 × CCr = mg/kg/8 h	20–40 µg/mL

[a]Doses for gentamicin and tobramycin should be written in multiples of 5 mg; doses of amikacin and kanamycin should be written in multiples of 25 mg.
[b]Seriously ill patients with sepsis often need higher loading doses to achieve rapid therapeutic levels despite third spacing, e.g., 3 mg/kg for gentamicin and tobramycin.
[c]Obese patients: use calculated lean body weight plus 40% of excess fat.
[d]Patients who are oliguric or anuric: use CCr of 5–8 mL/min.

2. MAYO CLINIC GUIDELINES (Mayo Clin Proc 47:519, 1999)

a. Initial dose: Gentamicin, tobramycin, netilmicin: 1.5–2 mg/kg; amikacin: 7.5–15 mg/kg. This is based on ideal body weight (IBW) calculated for males: 50 kg + 2.3 kg (height in inches – 60 inches), and for female patients: 45 kg + 2.3 kg (height in inches – 60 inches). For obese patients (> 30% above ideal body

weight) calculate dosing weight is IBW + 0.4 (actual weight in kg − IBW).
   b. Maintenance dose: Cockcroft-Gault equation.

   3. **MONITORING:** Measure peak levels at 1 hr after start of 20- to 30-min infusion. Goal with q8h dosing is 5–10 μg/mL for gentamicin and tobramycin or 20–40 μg/mL for amikacin; peak levels when using low doses of gentamicin or tobramycin for synergy vs staph, strep or enterococcus is 3 μg/mL. Monitor for nephrotoxicity with serum creatinine qd or qod. **Monitor for ototoxicity when feasible in patients treated >3 days with periodic Romberg's sign and with reading an eye chart after rapid head movements.**

ONCE DAILY AMINOGLYCOSIDES

Rationale: see Infect Dis Clin Pract 5:12, 1996; AAC 39:650, 1995; Eur J Clin Microbiol Infect Dis 14:1029, 1995; Ann Intern Med 124:717, 1996

Clinical trials: 24 published trials (Eur J Clin Microbiol Infect Dis 14:1029, 1995): Showed comparable results with once daily versus multiple daily doses for therapeutic response and toxicity.

Contraindication: Patients receiving aminoglycosides for synergy with beta-lactam agents for streptococcal endocarditis or enterococcal infections should receive standard thrice daily dosing regimens.

Monitoring: Some authorities suggest monitoring predose levels (18 hr) after second dose, which should show gentamicin or tobramycin levels 0.6–2.0 μg/mL and amikacin levels 2.5–5.0 μg/mL; higher levels should lead to dose reduction. All patients receiving aminoglycosides should be monitored for nephrotoxicity and ototoxicity (see above).

Regimen

   1. *Standard dose*
      Gentamicin and tobramycin: 5–6 mg/kg/d (some use 4–7 mg/kg/d)
      Amikacin and streptomycin: 15–20 mg/kg/d
   2. *Dose adjustment based on trough levels*
      Gentamicin and tobramycin: ≤0.5 μg/mL
      Amikacin: <5 μg/mL
   3. Dose adjustment based on renal function (Mayo Clin Proc 1999;47:519)

Creatinine clearance (mL/min)	Dose (mg/kg) q24h	
	Gentamicin tobramycin	Amikacin
>80	5.0	15.0
60–79	4.0	12.0
50	3.5	7.5
40	2.5	4.0
<30	Conventional dosing	

C. DRUG THERAPY DOSING GUIDELINES

(Adapted in part from Drug Information for the Health Care Professional, USP DI, 23rd Edition, 2003; Physicians' Desk Reference, 57th Edition, 2003)

Drug	Major excretory route	Half-life (hr)* Normal	Half-life (hr)* Anuria	Usual regimen Oral	Usual regimen Parenteral	Maintenance regimen renal failure GFR 50–80 mL/min	GFR 10–50 mL/min	GFR <10 mL/min
Acyclovir	Renal	2–2.5	20	200 mg 3–5×/d 400 mg bid 800 mg 5×/d —	5–10 mg/kg q8h	Usual Usual Usual Usual	Usual Usual 800 mg q8h 5–12 mg/kg q12–24h	200 mg q12h 200 mg q12h 800 mg q12h 2.5–6 mg/kg q24h
Adofovir	Renal	1.6 IC–16	↑	10 mg q24h	—	Usual	10 mg q48–72h	10 mg q wk
Albendazole	Hepatic	8	8	400–800 mg bid	—	Usual	Usual	Usual
Amantadine	Renal	15–20	170	100 mg bid	—	100–150 mg q day	100 mg 2–3 ×/wk	100–200 mg q wk
Amdinocillin	Renal	1	3.3	—	10 mg/kg/q4–6h	Usual	10 mg/kg q6h	10 mg/kg q8h
Amikacin	Renal	2	30	—	7.5 mg/kg	<<<<<<<	See pp 41–42	>>>>>>>
Amoxicillin	Renal	1	15–20	250–500 mg q8h	—	0.25–0.5 g q12h	0.25–0.5 g q12–24h	0.25–0.5 g q12–24h
Amoxicillin clavulanic acid	Renal	1	8–16	250–500 mg q8h	—	Usual	0.25–0.5 g q12h	0.25–0.5 g q24–36h
Amphotericin B	Nonrenal	15 days	15 days	—	0.3–1.4 mg/kg/d	Usual	Usual	Usual
Amphotericin B lipid complex	Nonrenal	7 days (ABLC)	1 day (ABCD)	—	5 mg/kg/d (ABCD) 3–4 mg/kg/d (ABLC)	Usual	Usual	Usual
Amphotericin B liposomal	Nonrenal	4–6 days	4–6 days	—	3–5 mg/kg/d	Usual	Usual	Usual
Ampicillin	Renal	1	8–12	0.25–0.5 g q6h	1–3 g q4–6h	Usual	1–2 g q8h	1–2 g IV q 12h

Continued

43

Drug	Major excretory route	Half-life (hr)* Normal	Half-life (hr)* Anuria	Usual regimen Oral	Usual regimen Parenteral	Maintenance regimen renal failure GFR 50–80 mL/min	Maintenance regimen renal failure GFR 10–50 mL/min	Maintenance regimen renal failure GFR <10 mL/min
Ampicillin-sulbactam	Renal	1	8–12	—	1–2 g q6h	1–2 g IV q8h	1–2 g q8h	1–2 g IV q12h
Atovaquone	Gut	70	70	750 mg bid susp		Usual	Usual	Usual
Atovaquone + proguanil	Urinary	70	?	1–4 tabs/day	—	Usual	Usual	Unknown
Azithromycin	Hepatic	68	68	250 mg/d	500 mg/d	Usual	No data—	"usual close probable"
Aztreonam	Renal	1.7–2	6–9	—	1–2 g q6h	1–2 g q8–12h	1–2 g q12–18h	1–2 g q24h
Bacampicillin	Renal	1	8–12	0.4–0.8 g q12h	—	Usual	Usual	Usual
Capreomycin	Renal	4–6	50–100	1 g day 2×/wk	—	Usual	7.5 mg/kg q 1–2 days	7.5 mg/kg 2×/wk
Carbenicillin	Renal	1	13–16	0.5–1 g q6h	—	Usual	0.5–1 g q8h	Avoid
Caspofungin	Metabolized	9–11	9–11	—	70 mg d 1 50 mg qd	Usual	Usual	Usual
Cefaclor	Renal	0.75	2.8	0.25–0.5 g q8h	—	Usual	Usual	Usual
Cefadroxil	Renal	1.4	20–25	0.5–1 g q12–24h	—	Usual	0.5 g q12–24h	0.5 g q36h
Cefamandole	Renal	0.5–2.1	10	—	0.5–2 g q4–8h	Usual	1–2 g q8h	0.5–0.75 g q12h
Cefazolin	Renal	1.8	18–36	—	0.5–2 g q8h	0.5–1.5 g q8h	0.5–1 g q8–12h	0.25–0.75 g q18–24h
Cefdinir	Renal	1.7	?	300 mg bid	—	Usual	300 mg qd	300 mg qod
Cefditoren	Renal	1.4	4–5	200–400 mg bid	—	Usual	200 mg q12–24h	200 mg q24h Continued

Drug	Major excretory route	Half-life (hr)* Normal	Half-life (hr)* Anuria	Usual regimen Oral	Usual regimen Parenteral	Maintenance regimen renal failure GFR 50–80 mL/min	GFR 10–50 mL/min	GFR <10 mL/min
Cefepime	Renal	2	13	—	0.5–2 g q12h	0.5–2g q24h	0.5–1 g q24h	250–500 mg q24h
Cefixime	Renal (50%)	3–4	12	200 mg q12h	—	Usual	300 mg/d	200 mg/d
Cefmetazole	Renal	1.2	—	—	2 g q6–12h	1–2 g q12h	1–2 g q18–24h	1–2 g q48h
Cefonicid	Renal	4–5	50–60	—	0.5–2 g q24h	8–25 mg/kg q24h	4–8 mg/kg q24h	4 mg/kg q3–5d
Cefoperazone	Gut	1.9–2.5	2–2.5	—	1–2 g q6–12h	Usual	Usual	Usual
Cefotanide	Renal	3	20–40	—	0.5–1 g q12h	Usual	0.5–1 g q24h	0.5–1 g q48–72h
Cefotaxime	Renal	1.1	3	—	1–2 g q4–8h	Usual	1–2 g q6–12h	1–2 g q12h
Cefotetan	Renal	3–4	12–30	—	1–2 g q12h	Usual	1–2 g q24h	1–2 g q48h
Cefoxitin	Renal	0.7	13–22	—	1–2 g q6–8h	1–2 g q8–12h	1–2 g q12–24h	0.5–1 g q12–48h
Cefpodoxime	Renal	2.4	—	200–400 mg q12h	—	Usual q12h	200–400 mg q16–24h	200–400 mg q24–48h
Cefprozil	Renal	1.3	5–6	0.25–0.5 g q12h	—	Usual	0.25–0.5 g q24h	0.25 g q12–24h
Ceftazidime	Renal	0.9–1.7	15–25	—	1–2 g q8–12h	Usual	1 g q12–24h	0.5 g q24–48h
Ceftibutin	Renal	2.4	?	400 mg/d	—	Usual	200 mg/d	100 mg/d
Ceftizoxime	Renal	1.4–1.8	25–35	—	1–3 g q6–8h	0.5–1.5 g q8h	0.25–1 g q12h	0.25–0.5 g q24h

Continued

45

Drug	Major excretory route	Half-life (hr)* Normal	Half-life (hr)* Anuria	Usual regimen Oral	Usual regimen Parenteral	Maintenance regimen renal failure GFR 50–80 mL/min	GFR 10–50 mL/min	GFR <10 mL/min
Ceftriaxone	Renal and biliary	6–9	12–15	—	1–2 g q24h	Usual	Usual	Usual
Cefuroxime	Renal	1.3–1.7	20	—	0.75–1.5 g q8h	Usual	0.75–1.5 g q8–12h	0.75 g q24h
Cefuroxime axetil	Renal	1.2	20	250 mg q12h	—	Usual	Usual	250 mg q24h
Cephalexin	Renal	0.9	5–30	0.25–1 g q6h	—	Usual	0.25–1 g q8–12h	0.25–1 g q24–48h
Cephalothin	Renal	0.5–0.9	3–8	—	0.5–2 g q4–8h	Usual	1.0–1.5 g q6h	0.5 g q8h
Cephapirin	Renal	0.6–0.9	2.4	—	0.5–2 g q4–6h	0.5–2 g q6h	0.5–2 g q8h	0.5–2 g q12h
Cephradine	Renal	0.7–2	8–15	0.25–1 g q6h / —	— / 0.5–2 g q4–6h	Usual / 0.5–1 g q6h	0.5 g q6h / 0.5–1 g q6–24h	0.25 g q12h / 0.5–1 g q24–72h
Chloramphenicol	Hepatic	2.5	3–7	0.25–0.75 g q6h	0.25–1 g q6h	Usual	Usual	Usual
Chloroquine	Renal and metabolized	48–120	?	300–600 mg po qd	—	Usual	Usual	150–300 mg po qd
Cidofovir	Renal	17–65	↑	—	5 mg/kg q 2 wk	Usual	Contraindicated	Contraindicated
Cinoxacin	Renal	1.5	8.5	0.25–0.5 g q12h	—	0.25 g q8h	0.25 g q12h	0.25 g q24h
Ciprofloxacin	Renal and hepatic metabolism	4 / slight	5–10	0.25–0.75 g q12h / —	— / 400 mg q12h	Usual / Usual	0.25–0.5 g q12h / 0.4 g q18h	0.25–0.5 g q18h / 0.4 g q24h

Continued

Drug	Major excretory route	Half-life (hr)* Normal	Half-life (hr)* Anuria	Usual regimen Oral	Usual regimen Parenteral	Maintenance regimen renal failure GFR 50–80 mL/min	Maintenance regimen renal failure GFR 10–50 mL/min	Maintenance regimen renal failure GFR <10 mL/min
Clarithromycin	Hepatic and renal metabolism	4	2–3.5	250–500 mg q12h	—	Usual	Usual	250–500 mg q24h
Clindamycin	Hepatic	2–2.5	0.8	150–300 mg q6h	300–900 mg q6–8h	Usual	Usual	Usual
Cloxacillin	Renal	0.5	0.8	0.5–1 g q6h	—	Usual	Usual	Usual
Colistin	Renal	3–8	10–20	—	1.5 mg/kg q6–12h	2.5–3.8 mg/kg/d	1.5–2.5 mg/kg q24h	0.6 mg/kg q24h
Cyclacillin	Renal	0.6	—	0.5–1 g q6h	—	Usual	Usual	0.5–1 g q12h
Cycloserine	Renal	8–12	?	250–500 mg bid	—	Usual	250–500 mg qd	250 mg qd
Dapsone	Hepatic metabolism	30	Slight	50–100 mg/d	—	Usual	Usual	No data
Daptomycin	Renal	9.4	30	—	4 mg/kg/d	Usual	4 mg/kg q48h CrCl <30 mL/min	
Dicloxacillin	Renal	0.5–0.9	1–1.6	0.25–0.5 g q6h	—	Usual	Usual	Usual
Dirithromycin	Bile	30–44	30–44	500 mg/d	—	Usual	Usual	Usual
Doxycycline	Renal and gut	14–25	15–36	100 mg bid	100 mg bid	Usual	Usual	Usual
Enoxacin	Renal and hepatic	3–6	—	200–400 mg bid	—	Usual	1/2 usual dose	1/2 usual dose
Entecavir	Urine	128–149	↑	0.5–1 gm qd	—	Usual	0.25–0.5 mg qd	0.15–0.25 qd
Ertapenem	Renal and hepatic	4	?	—	1 g q24h	Usual	Usual	500 mg qd

Continued

Drug	Major excretory route	Half-life (hr)* Normal	Half-life (hr)* Anuria	Usual regimen Oral	Usual regimen Parenteral	Maintenance regimen renal failure GFR 50–80 mL/min	Maintenance regimen renal failure GFR 10–50 mL/min	Maintenance regimen renal failure GFR <10 mL/min
Erythromycin	Hepatic metabolism	1.2–1.6	4–6	0.25–0.5 g q6h	1 g q6h	Usual	Usual	Usual
Ethambutol	Renal	3–4	8	15–25 mg/kg q24h	—	15 mg/kg q24h	15 mg/kg q24–36h	15 mg/kg q48h
Ethionamide	Metabolized	4	9	0.5–1 g/d, 1–3 doses	—	Usual	Usual	5 mg/kg q48h
Famciclovir	Renal	2.3	13	125 mg q12h 500 mg q8h	— —	Usual Usual	125 mg q24h 500 mg q 12–24h	125 mg q48h 250 mg q48h
Fluconazole	Renal	20–50	100	100–200 mg/d	100–400 mg/d	Usual	50% usual dose	25–50% mg/d
Flucytosine	Renal	3–6	70	25 mg/kg q6h	—	Usual	25 mg/kg q12–24h	25 mg/kg q24hr
Foscarnet induction	Renal	3	8	—	60 mg/kg q8h	40–50 mg/kg q8h	20–30 mg/kg q8h	Contra-indicated (CrCl <20 mL/min)
maintenance					90 mg/kg qd	60–70 mg/kg qd	50–70 mg/kg qd	Contra-indicated (CrCl <20 mL/min)
Fosfomycin	Renal	—	—	3 gm × 1	—	Usual	No data	Not indicated

Continued

		Half-life (hr)*		Usual regimen		Maintenance regimen renal failure		
Drug	Major excretory route	Normal	Anuria	Oral	Parenteral	GFR 50–80 mL/min	GFR 10–50 mL/min	GFR <10 mL/min
Ganciclovir—induction doses (maintenance— 1/2 dose)	Renal	2.5–3.6	10	—	5 mg/kg q12h 5 mg/kg/d	2.5 mg/kg bid 2.5 mg/kg/d	2.5 mg/kg qd 1.2 mg/kg/d	1.25 mg/kg 3×/wk 0.6 mg/kg/3×/wk
Ganciclovir—oral	GI	3–7	10	1000 mg tid	—	500 mg tid	500 mg/d	500 mg 3×/wk
Gatifloxacin	Renal	8		400 mg qd	400 mg qd	Usual	200 mg qd	200 mg qd
Gemifloxacin	Renal	5–9	↑	320 mg qd	—	Usual	160 mg qd	160 mg qd
Gentamicin	Renal	2	48	—	1.7 mg/kg q8h	<<<<<<< See pp 41–42 >>>>>>>		
Griseofulvin microsize ultramicrosize	Hepatic metabolism Same	24 24	24 24	0.5–1 g qd 0.33–0.66 g qd	— —	Usual Usual	Usual Usual	Usual Usual
Imipenem- cilastatin	Renal	0.8–1	3.5	—	0.5–1 g q6h	0.5 g q6–8h	0.5 g q8–12h	0.25–0.5 mg q12h
Interferon alpha	Nonrenal	2–3	Same ?	—	3 mil units q3d (HCV) 30–35 mil units/wk (HCV)	Usual	Usual	Usual(?)
Isoniazid	Hepatic	0.5–4	2–10	300 mg q24h	300 mg q24h	Usual	Usual	Slow acety- lators 1/2 dose
Itraconazole	Hepatic	20–60	20–60	200–400 mg/d	200 mg/d	Usual	Usual	Contraindicated with CrCl < 30 due to accu- mulation of cyclodextrin
Ivermectin	Metabolized	16	16	12–18 mg × 1	—	Usual	Usual	Usual

Continued

Drug	Major excretory route	Half-life (hr)* Normal	Half-life (hr)* Anuria	Usual regimen Oral	Usual regimen Parenteral	Maintenance regimen renal failure GFR 50–80 mL/min	Maintenance regimen renal failure GFR 10–50 mL/min	Maintenance regimen renal failure GFR <10 mL/min
Kanamycin	Renal	2–3	27–30	—	7.5 mg/kg q12h	<<<<<<< See pp 41–42 >>>>>>>>		
Ketoconazole	Hepatic metabolism	1–4	1–4	200–400 mg q12–24h	—	Usual	Usual	Usual
Lamivudine	Renal	5–7 IC-12	↑	100 mg q24h (HBV)	—	Usual	100 mg × 1 50 mg q24h	35 mg × 1 then 15 mg qd
Levofloxacin	Renal	6.3	35	500–750 mg q24h	500 mg q24h	Usual	500–750 mg then 250 mg qd or 750 mg q48h	500–750 mg qd then 250–500 mg q48h
Linezolid	Nonrenal	5–7	5–7	600 mg bid	600 mg bid	Usual	Usual	Usual
Lomefloxacin	Renal	8	45	400 mg q24h	—	Usual	400 mg; then 200 mg qd	200 mg qd
Loracarbef	Renal	1	32	200–400 mg q12h	—	Usual	200–400 mg q24h	200–400 mg q3–5d
Mebendazole	Metabolized + GI	—	—	100 mg bid × 3d	—	Usual	Usual	Usual
Mefloquine	Hepatic	2–4 wk	2–4 wk	1250 mg × 1 250 mg q wk	—	Usual	Usual	Usual
Meropenem	Renal	1	↑	—	1 g q8h	Usual	0.5–1 gm q12h	500 mg q24h
Methenamine hippurate	Renal	3–6	?	1 g q12h	—	Usual	Avoid	Avoid
mandelate	Renal	3–6	?	1 g q6h	—	Usual	Avoid	Avoid
Methicillin	Renal (hepatic)	0.5	4	—	1–2 g q4–6h	1–2 g q6h	1–2 g q8h	1–2 g q12h
Metronidazole	Hepatic	6–14	8–15	0.25–0.75 g tid	0.5 g q6h	Usual	Usual	Usual

Continued

Drug	Major excretory route	Half-life (hr)* Normal	Half-life (hr)* Anuria	Usual regimen Oral	Usual regimen Parenteral	Maintenance regimen renal failure GFR 50–80 mL/min	Maintenance regimen renal failure GFR 10–50 mL/min	Maintenance regimen renal failure GFR <10 mL/min
Mezlocillin	Renal	1	1.5	—	3–4 g q4–6h	Usual	3 g q8h	2 g q8h
Micafungin	Metabolized	15	15	—	150 mg qd	Usual	Usual	Usual
Miconazole	Hepatic	0.5–1	0.5–1	—	0.4–1.2 g q8h	Usual	Usual	Usual
Minocycline	Hepatic and metabolized	11–26	17–30	100 mg q12h	100 mg q12h	Usual	Usual	Usual
Moxifloxacin	Metabolized	12	12	400 mg qd	400 mg qd	Usual	Usual	Usual
Nafcillin	Hepatic metabolism	0.5	1.2	0.5–1 g q6h	0.5–2 g q4–6h	Usual	Usual	Usual
Nalidixic acid	Renal and hepatic metabolism	1.5	21	1 g q6h	—	Usual	Usual	Avoid
Netilmicin	Renal	2.5	35	—	2.0 mg/kg q8h	<<<<<< See pp 41–42 >>>>>>		
Nitazoxamide	Metabolized	1–1.6	1–1.6	500 mg q6–12h	—	Usual	Usual	Usual
Nitrofurantoin	Renal	0.3	1	50–100 mg q6–8h	—	Usual	Avoid	Avoid
Norfloxacin	Renal and hepatic metabolism	3.5	8	400 mg bid	—	Usual	400 mg qd	400 mg qd
Nystatin	Not absorbed	—	—	0.4–1 mil units 3–5 ×/d	—	Usual	Usual	Usual
Ofloxacin	Renal	6	40	200–400 mg bid	200–400 mg q12h	Usual	200–400 mg qd	100–200 mg qd
Oseltamivir	Renal	6–10 hr	↑	75 mg bid	—	Usual	75 mg qd	Avoid

Continued

Drug	Major excretory route	Half-life (hr)* Normal	Half-life (hr)* Anuria	Usual regimen Oral	Usual regimen Parenteral	Maintenance regimen renal failure GFR 50–80 mL/min	GFR 10–50 mL/min	GFR <10 mL/min
Oxacillin	Renal	0.5	1	0.5–1 g q6h	1–3 g q6h	Usual	Usual	Usual
Peginterferon	Renal-30%	40	Slight ↑	—	180 mcg/kg SC q wk (Roche) 1.5 mcg/kg SC q wk (Schering)	Usual	Half dose(?)	Half dose(?)
Penicillin G crystalline procaine	Renal Renal	0.5 24	7–10 —	—	1–4 mil units q4–6h 0.6–1.2 mil units IM q12h	Usual Usual	Usual Usual	1/2 usual dose Usual
benzathine	Renal	10–15 days	—	—	0.6–1.2 mil units IM	Usual	Usual	Usual
Penicillin V	Renal	0.5–1.0	7–10	0.4–0.8 mil units q6h	—	Usual	Usual	Usual
Pentamidine	Non-renal	6	6–8	—	4 mg/kg q24h	Usual	4 mg/kg q24–36h	4 mg/kg q48h
Piperacillin	Renal	1	3	—	3–4 g q4–6h	Usual	3 g q8h	3 g q12h
Piperacillin + tazobactam	Renal	1	3	—	3/0.375 g q6h	Usual	2/0.25 g q6h	2/0.25 g q8h
Polymyxin B	Renal	6	48	—	7500–12,500 units/kg/d q12h	7500–12,500 units/kg/d q12h	5625–12,500 units/kg/d q12h	3750–6250 units/kg/d q12h
Praziquantel	Hepatic metabolism	0.8–1.5	?	10–25 mg/kg tid	—	Usual	Usual	Usual
Pyrazinamide	Metabolized	10–16	?	15–35 mg/kg/d	—	Usual	Usual	12–20 mg/kg/d
Pyrimethamine	Hepatic metabolism	1.5–5 days	?	25–75 mg/d	—	Usual	Usual	Usual
Quinacrine	Renal	5 days	—	100–200 mg q6–8h	—	Usual	?	?
Quinine	Hepatic metabolism	4–5	4–5	650 mg tid	7.5–10 mg/kg q8h	Usual	Usual	Usual

Continued

Drug	Major excretory route	Half-life (hr)* Normal	Half-life (hr)* Anuria	Usual regimen Oral	Usual regimen Parenteral	Maintenance regimen renal failure GFR 50–80 mL/min	Maintenance regimen renal failure GFR 10–50 mL/min	Maintenance regimen renal failure GFR <10 mL/min
Quinupristin/ dalfopristin	Hepatic metabolism	1.5	1.5	—	7.5 mg/kg q8–12h	Usual	Usual	Usual
Ribavirin	Hepatic	0.5–2 IC-40	Same	0.8–1.2 g/d	—	Usual	Not recommended	Not recommended
Rifampin	Hepatic	Early 2–5 Late 2	2–5	600 mg/d	600 mg/d	Usual	Usual	Usual or half dose
Rifapentine	Hepatic	16–19h	—	600 mg 2×/wk	—	Usual	Usual	
Rimantadine	Hepatic	24–30	48–60	100 mg bid	—	Usual	Usual	100 mg/d
Spectinomycin	Renal	1–3	?	—	2 g/d IM	Usual	Usual	
Streptomycin	Renal	2–5	100–110	—	500 mg q12h	15 mg/kg q24–72h	15 mg/kg q72–96h	7.5 mg/kg q72–96h
Sulfadiazine	Renal	8–17	22–34	0.5–1.5 g q4–6h	—	Usual	0.5–1.5 g q8–12h (½ dose)	0.5–1.5 g q12–24h (⅓ dose)
Sulfisoxazole	Renal	3–7	6–12	1–2 g q6h	—	Usual	1 g q8–12h	1 g q12–24h
Telithromycin	Hepatic	9.8 hr	↑ sl	800 mg qd	—	Usual	Usual	600 mg qd
						GFR <30 mL/min reduce dosage to 600 mg qd		
Tetracycline	Renal	8	50–100	0.25–0.5 g q6h	—	Usual	Use doxycycline	
Thiobendazole	Metabolized urine	—	—	50 mg/kg/d × 2	—	Usual	Caution	Caution
Ticarcillin	Renal	1–1.5	16	—	3 g q4h	Usual	2–3 g q6–8h	2 g q12h

Continued

53

Drug	Major excretory route	Half-life (hr)* Normal	Half-life (hr)* Anuria	Usual regimen Oral	Usual regimen Parenteral	Maintenance regimen renal failure GFR 50–80 mL/min	Maintenance regimen renal failure GFR 10–50 mL/min	Maintenance regimen renal failure GFR <10 mL/min
Ticarcillin + clavulanic acid	Renal	1–1.5	16	—	3 g q4–6h	Usual	2–3 g q6–8h	2 g q12h
Tigecycline	Renal & hepatic	42	42	—	100 mg, then 50 mg qd	Usual	Usual	Usual
Tobramycin	Renal	2.5	56	—	1.7 mg/kg q8h	<<<<<< See pp 41–42 >>>>>>>		
Trimethoprim	Renal	8–15	T:24	100 mg q12h	—	Usual	100 mg q24h	Avoid
Trimethoprim-sulfamethoxazole	Renal	T:8–15 S:7–12	T:24 S:22–50	2–4 tabs/d or 1–2 DS/d	3–5 mg/kg q6–12h	Usual	Half dose 3–5 mg/kg q12–24h	½–⅓ standard dose ⅓–½ standard dose
Trimetrexate	Metabolized	11	No data	—	45 mg/m²/d	Usual	No data	No data
Valacyclovir	Renal	2.5–3.3	14	1000 mg tid 500 mg bid	—	Usual	1 g q 12–24 hr 500 mg q 12–24 h	500 mg qd 500 mg qd
Valganciclovir	Renal	4 IC-18	20	900 mg bid × 3 wks 900 mg qd	—	Usual	½ dose	450 mg qod × 3 wks 450 mg biw
Vancomycin	Renal	6–8	200–250	0.125–0.5 g q6h	15 mg/kg q12h	Usual 1 gm q 12–24h	Usual 1 gm q 3d	0.125 g po q6h 0.5–1 gm q 3d
Voriconazole	Hepatic	—	—	200 mg q12h	6 mg/kg q12h × 2, then 4 mg/kg q12h	Usual	po-usual IV-not recommended	po-usual IV-not recommended
Zanamivir	Renal	3	18	10 mg bid inhaled	—	Usual	No data	No data

*Half life in serum.

IC = intracellular half life.

D. ANTIMICROBIAL DOSING REGIMENS DURING DIALYSIS

(Adapted from Principles and Practice of Infectious Diseases, 4th Edition, Churchill Livingstone, New York:1995:506–519; American Hospital Formulary Service 2004)

Drug	Hemodialysis	Peritoneal dialysis
Acyclovir	2.5–5.0 mg/kg/d dose postdialysis	2.5 mg/kg/d
Adofovir	10 mg q7d	—
Albendazole	Usual dose	—
Amdinocillin	No extra dose	—
Amikacin	2.5–3.75 mg/kg postdialysis	Loading dose predialysis 9–20 mg/L dialysate*
Amoxicillin	0.25 g postdialysis	250 mg q12h
Amoxicillin + clavulanic acid	0.50 g (amoxicillin) + 0.125 (CA) halfway through dialysis and another dose at end	Usual regimen
Amphotericin B	Usual regimen	Usual regimen
Amphotericin lipid forms	Usual regimen	Usual regimen
Ampicillin	Usual dose; give postdialysis	250 mg q12h
Ampicillin + sulbactam	1 gm q12h & 2 g ampicillin postdialysis	Usual regimen
Atovaquone	Usual regimen	Usual regimen
Azithromycin	Usual regimen	Usual regimen
Aztreonam	1/8 initial dose (60–250 mg) postdialysis	1–2 gm loading dose, then 250–500 q8h
Carbenicillin	0.75–2.0 g postdialysis	2 g 6–12h
Caspofungin	Usual regimen	Usual regimen
Cefaclor	500 mg dose postdialysis	Usual regimen
Cefadroxil	0.5–1.0 g postdialysis	0.5 g/d
Cefamandole	Repeat dose postdialysis	0.5–1.0 g q12h
Cefazolin	1 gm postdialysis	0.5 g q12h
Cefdinir	300 mg plus 300 mg postdialysis	—
Cefditoren	200 mg qd + dose postdialysis	—
Cefepime	1–2 gm postdialysis	1–2 gm q48h
Cefoperazone	Schedule dose postdialysis	Usual regimen
Cefotaxime	1–2 gm qd + 1 gm postdialysis	0.5–2 g/d

Continued

Drug	Hemodialysis	Peritoneal dialysis
Cefotetan	1/4 usual dose q24h on non-dialysis days and 1/2 dose on dialysis days	1 g/d
Cefoxitin	1–2 g postdialysis	1 g/d
Cefpodoxime	200–400 mg 3×/wk	200–400 mg q24h
Cefprozil	250–500 mg postdialysis	0.25 g q12–24h
Ceftazidime	1 g loading 1 g postdialysis	0.5–1.0 g loading, then 0.5 g/d or 250 mg in each 2 L dialysate
Ceftibutin	400 mg postdialysis	100–200 mg qd
Ceftizoxime	1 gm postdialysis	1 g/d
Ceftriaxone	1–2 gm qd; No extra dose	Usual regimen
Cefuroxime	750 mg postdialysis	750 mg/d
Cephalexin	0.25–1.0 g postdialysis	250 mg po tid
Cephalothin	Supplemental dose postdialysis	Option to add ≤6 mg/dL to dialysate
Cephradine	250 mg at start, then 250 mg at 12 & 36–48 hrs postdialysis	0.5–1 gm q6–24h; 0.5 gm po q6h
Chloramphenicol	500 mg postdialysis	Usual dose
Cidofovir	Dose postdialysis	Usual dose
Ciprofloxacin	250–500 mg q24h postdialysis	250–500 mg/d
Clarithromycin	500 mg postdialysis	Usual dose
Clindamycin	Usual regimen	Usual regimen
Clofazimine	Usual regimen	Usual regimen
Clotrizamine	Usual regimen	Usual regimen
Cloxacillin	Usual regimen	Usual regimen
Colistimathate	No supplemental dose	—
Daptomycin	4 mg/kg q48h	4 mg/kg q48h
Dicloxacillin	Usual regimen	Usual regimen
Doxycycline	Usual regimen	Usual regimen
Entecavir	0.5 mg qd postdialysis 1.0 lamivudine resistant	1.0 mg qd lamivudine resistant
Ertapenem	500 mg qd 150 mg supplement postdialysis	1 gm qd
Erythromycin	Usual regimen	Usual regimen
Ethambutol	15–20 mg/kg/d postdialysis 3 ×/wk	15 mg/kg/48 hrs

Continued

Drug	Hemodialysis	Peritoneal dialysis
Famciclovir	250 mg (zoster) or 125 mg (genital herpes) q48h + dose postdialysis	—
Fluconazole	200 mg postdialysis	25–50% usual dose
Flucytosine	dose postdialysis	0.5–1.0 g/d
Foscarnet	60 mg/kg postdialysis	Contraindicated
Ganciclovir—IV	1.25 mg/kg postdialysis given postdialysis on dialysis days	?
Gatifloxacin	200 mg qd	200 mg qd
Gentamicin	1.0–1.7 mg/kg postdialysis	Loading dose predialysis, 2–4 mg/L dialysate*
Griseofluvin	Usual dose	Usual dose
Imipenem + cilastatin	0.25 gm IV q12h + 0.25 gm postdialysis	250 mg IV q12h
Interferon	Usual	Usual
Isoniazid	Daily dose postdialysis	Daily dose postdialysis or 1/2 usual dose is slow acetylator
Itraconazole	Usual regimen	100 mg q12–24h
Kanamycin	4–5 mg/kg postdialysis	3.75 mg/kg/d
Ketoconazole	Usual regimen	Usual regimen
Lamivudine	25–50 mg/d dose postdialysis	25–50 mg/d
Levofloxacin	500–750 mg, then 250–500 mg q48h	500–750 mg, then 250–500 mg q48h
Linezolid	Usual dose; give postdialysis on dialysis days	Usual dose
Loracarbef	Additional dose postdialysis	0.2–0.4 q3–5 days
Mebendazole	Usual regimen	Usual regimen
Mefloquine	Usual regimen	Usual regimen
Meropenem	Additional dose postdialysis	0.5 g IV q24h
Metronidazole	Usual regimen	Usual regimen
Mezlocillin	2–3 g postdialysis then 3–4 g q12h	3 g q12h
Minocycline	Usual regimen	Usual regimen
Moxalactam	1–2 g postdialysis	1–2 g/d
Moxifloxacin	Usual regimen	Usual regimen
Nafcillin	Usual regimen	Usual regimen

Continued

Drug	Hemodialysis	Peritoneal dialysis
Netilmicin	2 mg/kg postdialysis	Loading dose predialysis 3–5 mg/L dialysate*
Ofloxacin	200 mg, then 100 mg q24h	100–200 mg q24h
Oxacillin	Usual regimen	Usual regimen
Paromomycin	Usual regimen	Usual regimen
Peginterferon	—	—
Penicillin G	500,000 units postdialysis	—
Penicillin V	0.5–2 mU IV q4–6h + 500,000 units postdialysis	0.5–2 mU IV q4–6h
Pentamidine	Usual regimen	Usual regimen
Piperacillin	2 gm q8h + 1 gm postdialysis	2 gm q8h
Piperacillin—tazobactam	2/0.25 g q8h + 0.75 gm postdialysis	2.25 g q8h
Praziquantel	Usual regimen	—
Pyrazinamide	Usual dose postdialysis	Avoid—no data
Quinidine	Usual regimen + 100–200 mg postdialysis	Not known
Quinine	Usual regimen, dose postdialysis on dialysis days	—
Quinupristin—dalfopristin	Usual regimen	Usual regimen
Ribavirin	Not recommended	—
Rifamixin	Usual regimen	Usual regimen
Rifampin	300–600 mg qd	300–600 mg qd
Rifapentine	Usual regimen	Usual regimen
Streptomycin	12–15 mg/kg 2–3 ×/wk	20–40 mg/L dialysate
Sulfadiazine	Dose postdialysis	—
Sulfamethoxazole	1 gm qd; dose postdialysis on dialysis days	1 gm q24h
Sulfisoxazole	1 gm q12h, supplement 2 gm postdialysis	1 gm q8h
Telithromycin	600 mg postdialysis on dialysis days	No data
Tetracycline	Use doxycycline	Use doxycycline
Ticarcillin	3 g postdialysis, then 2 g q12h	3.1 gm q12h
Ticarcillin + clavulanic acid	2 gm q12h plus 3.1, then 2 g q12h	3 g (ticarcillin) q12h

Continued

Drug	Hemodialysis	Peritoneal dialysis
Tiglycycline	Usual regimen	Usual regimen
Tobramycin	1.0–1.7 mg/kg postdialysis; monitor levels and redose for < 2 mcg/mL	Loading dose predialysis, 2–4 mg/L dialysate*
Trimethoprim-sulfa	4–5 mg/kg (as trimethoprim) postdialysis	0.16/0.8 g q48h
Valacyclovir	500 mg postdialysis only	500 mg qd
Valganciclovir	Not recommended	—
Vancomycin	1–2 g/wk	0.5–1.0 g/wk
Vidarabine	Scheduled dose postdialysis	
Voriconazole	IV-not recommended po-standard dose postdialysis	IV-not recommended po-standard dose

* Aminoglycosides given for prolonged periods to patients receiving continuous peritoneal dialysis have been associated with high rates of ototoxicity. Monitor level after loading dose, and follow for symptoms of ototoxicity with periodic Romberg's sign and reading after rapid head movement.

Use of Antimicrobial Agents in Hepatic Disease

Many antimicrobial agents are metabolized by the liver and/or excreted via the biliary tract. Nevertheless, few require dose modifications in hepatic disease; with few exceptions, doses are usually modified only if there is concurrent renal failure and/or the liver disease is either acute or is associated with severe hepatic failure as indicated by ascites or jaundice. The following recommendations are adapted from *Drug Information for the Health Care Professional*, USP DI, 21st Edition, 2001.

Agent: Recommended Dose Modification

Adofovir: Standard dose

Aztreonam: Some recommend a dose reduction of 20–25%.

Caspofungin: Usual maintenance dose of 50 mg/d is reduced to 35 mg/d with moderate hepatic disease; no data for severe hepatic disease.

Cefoperazone: Maximum dose is 4 g/d; if higher, monitor levels; with coexisting renal impairment maximum dose is 1–2 g/d.

Ceftriaxone: Maximum daily dose of 2 g with severe hepatic and renal impairment.

Chlarithromycin: May require decrease in dose with hepatic and renal dysfunction.

Chloramphenicol: Use with caution with renal and/or hepatic failure; monitor serum levels to achieve levels of 5–20 μg/mL.

Chloroquin: 30–50% decrease in dose

Clindamycen: Dose reduction recommended only for severe hepatic failure.

Daptomycin: No dose adjustment.

Entecavir: No dose reduction

Fluoroquinolones: Use standard dose except with trovafloxacin (see below).

Griseofulvin: May need dose reduction

Isoniazid: Use with caution and monitor hepatic function for mild-moderate hepatic disease; acute liver disease or history of INH-associated hepatic injury is contraindication to INH.

Itraconazole: Two-fold increase in half-life with cirrhosis; give with caution.

Linezolid: No dose adjustment.

Metronidazole: Modify dose for severe hepatic failure, although specific guidelines are not provided; peak serum levels with 500 mg doses are 10–20 μg/mL.

Mezlocillin: Reduce dose by 50% or double the dosing interval.

Nafcillin: Metabolized by liver and largely eliminated in bile; nevertheless, dose modifications are suggested only for combined hepatic and renal failure.

Penicillin G.: Dose reduction for hepatic failure only when accompanied by renal failure.

Peginterferon: Standard dose

Ribavirin: AUC is unchanged wih severe hepatic failure.

Rifampin: Induces hepatic enzymes responsible for inactivating methadone, corticosteroids, oral anti-diabetic agents, digitalis, quinidine, cyclosporine, oral anticoagulants, estrogens, oral contraceptives, and chloramphenicol. Concurrent use of these drugs with rifampin and use in patients with prior liver disease require careful review.

Rimantadine: Severe hepatitis disease use 100 mg/d (half dose).

Telithromycin: No dose adjustment.

Thiabendazole: Use with caution.

<u>Ticarcillin:</u> For patients with hepatic dysfunction and creatinine clearance <10 mL/min, give 2 g/d IV in one or two doses.

<u>Ticarcillin/clavulanate:</u> For patients with hepatic dysfunction and creatinine clearance <10 mL/min give usual loading dose (3.1 g) followed by 2 g once daily.

<u>Voriconazole:</u> Mild to moderate hepatic insufficiency—6 mg/kg IV q12h × 2, then 2 mg/kg IV q12h (Standard loading dose, then half dose).

ADVERSE REACTIONS TO ANTIMICROBIAL AGENTS

A. Adverse Reactions by Class

Adapted from Medical Letter Handbook of Antimicrobial Therapy, Revised Edition 2000:5–200

Drug	Frequent	Occasional	Rare
Acyclovir (Zovirax)	Irritation at infusion site	Rash—nausea and vomiting; diarrhea; renal toxicity (especially with rapid IV infusion, prior renal disease, and nephrotoxic drugs); dizziness; abnormal liver function tests; itching; headache Topical—local reaction	CNS (especially with high dose in renal failure)—agitation, encephalopathy, lethargy, tremor, transient hemiparesis, disorientation, seizures, hallucinations, anemia, hypotension, neutropenia
Adofovir		Asthenia, GI intolerance (nausea, vomiting, diarrhea, abdominal pain), headache, pruritus, rash	Nephrotoxicity; lactic acidosis
Albendazole		Diarrhea, abdominal pain	Leukopenia, alopecia, increased transaminase levels
Amantadine (Symmetrel)	Insomnia, lethargy, dizziness, inability to concentrate (10–15% of adults receiving 200 mg/d)	GI intolerance especially nausea (5–10%), rash, depression, confusion, livedo reticularis	CNS—lethargy, tremor, confusion, obtundation, delirium, psychosis, visual hallucinations, paranoia, mania, seizures (primarily in elderly renal failure and/ or seizure disorder), heart failure, eczematoid dermatitis, photosensitivity, oculogyric episodes, orthostatic hypotension, peripheral edema, bone marrow suppression, sudden loss of vision, urinary retention
Aminoglycosides Tobramycin Gentamicin Amikacin Netilmicin Kanamycin	Renal failure—related to dose, duration, hepatic function, prior renal function, concurrent nephrotoxic drugs, hydration status, hypotension, increased trough levels, and advanced age (Am J Med 1987;83:1091) (monitor creatinine 3–7×/wk and output). Nephrotoxicity is usually reversible	Vestibular and auditory damage: related to dose and duration, only risk is advanced age (AAC 1987;31:1383) —note dizziness, vertigo, roaring, tinnitis, high tone hearing loss; ototoxicity is irreversible	Fever, rash, blurred vision, neuromuscular blockage especially with myasthenia or Parkinson's—may be reversible with calcium salts, paresthesias, hypotension, allergic reactions—usually caused by sulfites in some preparations

Continued

Drug	Frequent	Occasional	Rare
Aminosalicylic acid (PAS)	GI intolerance	Liver damage; allergic reactions, thyroid enlargement, hepatotoxicity	Acidosis, vasculitis, hypoglycemia (diabetes), hypokalemia, encephalopathy, decreased prothrombin activity, myalgias, renal damage, gastric hemorrhage
Amoxicillin + clavulanic acid	Similar to amoxicillin—see penicillins		
Amphotericin B (Fungizone)	Fever (maximal at 1 hr) and chills (at 2 hr)—prevent/reduce with hydrocortisone, ibuprofen, ASA, acetaminophen, meperidine Renal tubular acidosis—dose dependent and usually reversible in absence of prior renal damage and dose <3 g, reduce with hydration and sodium supplementations Hypokalemia Anemia (treat severe anemia with erythropoietin) Phlebitis and pain at injection site (add 1,000 units heparin to infusions)	Hypomagnesemia, nausea, vomiting, metallic taste, headache	Hypotension, rash, pruritus, blurred vision, peripheral neuropathy, convulsions, hemorrhagic gastroenteritis, arrhythmias, diabetes insipidus, hearing loss, pulmonary edema, anaphylaxis, acute hepatic failure, eosinophilia, leukopenia, thrombocytopenia, delirium (especially with intrathecal use)
Amphotericin B lipid complex and liposomal (Amphotec, Abelcet, AmBisome)	Chills and fever during infusion; infusion-related side effects and nephrotoxicity are significantly less compared with amphotericin B (Amphotec > Abelcet > AmBisome) (CID 2000;31:1155) Dose-related nephrotoxicity (substantially less than with amphotericin B; Abelcet > Amphotec > AmBisome)	GI intolerance, electrolyte abnormalities	Hypotension, anaphylaxis

Continued

Drug	Frequent	Occasional	Rare
Ampicillin + sulbactam (Unasyn)	Similar to those for ampicillin alone—see penicillins		
Atovaquone (Mepron)	Rash—20%; rash requiring discontinuation—4%; GI intolerance—20%; diarrhea—20%	Nausea, vomiting, mild diarrhea; headache in comparative trial for PCP—9% required discontinuation because of side effects vs 24% with sulfatrimetho- prim; 7% vs 21% with IV pentamidine	Fever, elevated aminotransferases (generally mild), abdominal pain
Atovaquone + proguanil (Malarone)	Abdominal pain—20%, nausea—12%, vomiting—20%, headache—10%, diarrhea—8%	Dizziness—5%, increased transaminases	
Azithromycin (Zithromax)		GI intolerance (4%), diarrhea, nausea, abdominal pain, vaginitis	Reversible hearing loss (more common with 500 mg × 30–90 days); erythema multiforme; increased transaminase; C. difficile colitis
Aztreonam (Azactam)	Eosinophilia	Phlebitis at infusion site, rash, diarrhea, nausea, eosinophilia, abnormal liver function tests	Thrombocytopenia, colitis, hypotension, unusual taste, seizures, chills
Bacitracin			Rash, blood dyscrasia
Bithionol (Bitin)	Photosensitivity, vomiting; diarrhea, abdominal pain, urticaria		Leukopenia, toxic hepatitis
Capreomycin	Renal damage (tubular necrosis especially in patients with prior renal damage): increased creatinine, proteinuria, cylindruria—monitor UA and creatinine weekly	Ototoxicity (vestibular > auditory—should assess vestibular function before and during treatment); electrolyte abnormalities; pain, induration, sterile abscesses at injection sites	Allergic reactions, leukopenia, leukocytosis, neuromuscular blockage (large IV doses— reversed with neostigmine), hypersensitivity reactions, hepatitis?
Caspofungin	Nausea, vomiting		Histamine-mediated adverse drug reaction with rash, face swelling, pruritis; fever; increased alkaline phosphotase; hypokalemia; proteinuria

Continued

Drug	Frequent	Occasional	Rare
Ceftibutin	—	GI intolerance—4%, headache, diarrhea, rash pruritis; 2% in clinical trial discontinued drug due to ADR	*C. difficile*-associated diarrhea, colitis
Cephalosporins	Phlebitis at infusion sites; diarrhea (especially cefoperazone and cefixime); pain at IM injection sites (less with cefazolin)	Allergic reactions (anaphylaxis rare), diarrhea and *C. difficile* colitis, hypoprothrombinemia (cefamandole, cefoperazone, moxalactam), platelet dysfunction (moxalactam), eosinophilia, positive Coombs' test Serum sickness (especially prolonged parenteral use of cefaclor), cholelithiasis (ceftriaxone)	Hemolytic anemia, interstitial nephritis (cephalothin), hepatic dysfunction, convulsions (high dose with renal failure), neutropenia, thrombocytopenia, confusion, disorientation, hallucinations
Chloramphenicol (Chloromycetin)		GI intolerance (oral), marrow suppression (dose related)	Fatal aplastic anemia (1:40,000), fever, allergic reactions, peripheral neuropathy, optic neuritis, *C. difficile* colitis
Chloroquine (Aralen)		Visual disturbances (related to dose and duration of treatment with ≥100 g as used for rheumatoid arthritis), GI intolerance, pruritus, weight loss, alopecia	CNS—headache, confusion, dizziness, extraocular muscle palsies, psychosis, peripheral neuropathy, cardiac toxicity, hemolysis (G6PD deficiency), marrow suppression, exacerbate psoriasis, eczema and other rashes, photophobia, myalgias, hematemesis
Cidofovir	Nephropathy—dose dependent: Reduce with IV hydration and probenecid; monitor creatinine and urinalysis. Report renal failure to Gilead: 800-GILEAD-5 or the FDA: 800-FDA-1088. Probenecid: Chills, fever, headache, rash, nausea in 30–50%	GI intolerance, neutropenia, metabolic acidosis	Uveitis, ocular hypotony

Continued

Drug	Frequent	Occasional	Rare
Ciprofloxacin (Cipro)	See quinolones		
Clarithromycin (Biaxin)		GI intolerance (4%), diarrhea	Headache, transaminase elevation, *C. difficile* colitis, reversible dose-related hearing loss
Clindamycin (Cleocin)	Diarrhea (frequency of *C. difficile* toxin is 5% for all clindamycin recipients and 15–25% for those with clindamycin-associated diarrhea)	Rash, *C. difficile* colitis, GI intolerance (oral)	Blood dyscrasias, hepatic damage, neutropenia, neuromuscular blockade, eosinophilia, fever, metallic taste, phlebitis at IV infusion sites, esophageal ulceration
Colistimethate (Coly-Mycin)	See polymyxins		
Cycloserine (Seromycin)	CNS—anxiety, confusion, depression, somnolence, disorientation, head-ache, hallucinations, tremor, hyper-reflexia, increased CSF protein, and pressure (dose related and reversible) (contraindicated in active alcoholics; twitching and seizures prevented with large doses of pyridoxine—100 mg tid)	Liver damage, malabsorption, peripheral neuropathy, folate deficiency, anemia	Coma, seizures (contraindicated in epileptics), hypersensitivity reactions, heart failure, arrhythmias
Dapsone	Rash, fever, nausea, anorexia, neutropenia—sufficiently severe to require discontinuation in 30–40% of HIV infected patients	Blood dyscrasias (methemoglobinemia and sulfahemoglobinemia ± G6PD deficiency)—warn patient to observe for cyanosis and dark urine; nephrotic syndrome; blurred vision; photosensitivity, tinnitis; insomnia; irritability; headache (transient)	Hypoalbuminemia, epidermal necrolysis, optic atrophy, agranulocytosis, peripheral neuropathy, aplastic anemia, "sulfone syndrome" (fever, exfoliative dermatitis, jaundice, adenopathy, methemo-globinemia, and anemia—treat with steroids), renal papillary necrosis
Daptomycin (Cubicin)		Dose related elevated CPK with or without symptoms or myopathy (reversible)	Elevated transaminases; neuropathy
Diethylcarbamazine citrate (Hetrazan)	Severe allergic or febrile reactions in patient with microfilaria in blood or skin, GI intolerance		Encephalopathy

Continued

Drug	Frequent	Occasional	Rare
Diloxanide (Furamide)	Flatulence, diarrhea, nausea		Dizziness, diplopia, headache, urticaria
Dirithromycin	GI intolerance, abdominal pain, nausea	—	—
Eflornithine (DFMO, Ornidyl)	Anemia, leukopenia	Diarrhea, thrombocytopenia, seizures	Hearing loss
Emetine	Arrhythmias, precordial pain, muscle weakness, phlebitis	Diarrhea, vomiting; neuropathy, heart failure; headache, dyspnea	
Entecavir	Exacerbation of hepatitis when entecavir (or lamivudine or tenofovir) is discontinued	—	Headache, nausea, dizziness, fatigue (< 1%)
Ertapenem		Nausea, vomiting, diarrhea; increased ALT; seizures in 0.5%	
Erythromycins	GI intolerance (related to oral doses); phlebitis (IV)	Diarrhea, stomatitis, cholestatic hepatitis (especially estolate-reversible), generalized rash	Allergic reactions, *C. difficile* colitis, hemolytic anemia, reversible ototoxicity (especially high dose and renal failure), QT prolongation with drug induced torsades de pointes especially in women (JAMA 280:1774, 1998), hypothermia, aggravation of myasthenia gravis
Ethambutol (Myambutol)		Optic neuritis (decreased acuity, reduced color discrimination, constricted fields, scotomata—dose related and infrequent with 15 mg/kg), GI intolerance, confusion, precipitation of acute gout	Hypersensitivity reactions, peripheral neuropathy, thrombocytopenia, toxic epidermal necrolysis, lichenoid skin rash
Ethionamide (Trecator)	GI intolerance (CNS effect)	Allergic reactions, peripheral neuropathy (prevented with pyridoxine), reversible liver damage (9%) with jaundice (1–3%)—monitor transaminase q2–4 wk, gynecomastia, menstrual irregularity	Optic neuritis, gouty arthritis, hypothyroidism, impotence, poor diabetic control, rash, hypotension

Continued

Drug	Frequent	Occasional	Rare
Famciclovir (Famvir)			Headache, nausea, fatigue
Fluconazole (Diflucan)	GI intolerance (bloating, nausea, vomiting, pain, anorexia, weight loss) dose related: 8–11% with 400 mg/d, 30% with >400 mg/d. Reversible alopecia in 10–20% receiving ≥400 mg/d × 3 mo (Ann Intern Med 123:354, 1995)	Transaminase elevations to ≥ 8 × normal (1%), headache, rash, diarrhea, prolonged prothrombin time with warfarin	Hepatic necrosis, Stevens-Johnson syndrome, thrombocytopenia, anaphylaxis, possible seizures
Flucytosine (Ancobon) Note: Levels should be <100 μg/mL	GI intolerance—nausea, vomiting, diarrhea	Marrow suppression with leukopenia or thrombocytopenia (dose related, especially with renal failure, serum concentration >100 μg/mL, or concurrent amphotericin); confusion; rash; hepatitis (dose related); enterocolitis; headache; photosensitivity reaction	Hallucinations, eosinophilia, blood dyscrasias with agranulocytosis and pancytopenia, fatal hepatitis, anaphylaxis, anemia
Fluoroquinolones— see quinolones			
Foscarnet (Foscavir)	Renal failure (usually reversible; 30% get creatinine >2 mg/dL; monitor serum creatinine 1–3 ×/wk and discontinue if creatinine >2.9 mg/dL)	Mineral and electrolyte changes—reduced calcium, magnesium, phosphorus, ionized calcium, potassium—monitor serum electrolytes 1–2 ×/wk and monitor for symptoms of paresthesias; seizures (10%); fever; GI intolerance; anemia; genital ulceration; neuropathy	Marrow suppression, arrhythmias, nephrogenic diabetes insipidus, hypertension
Fosfomycin	—	Diarrhea (10%), headache, vaginitis, nausea	Angioedema, aplastic anemia, cholestatic jaundice, hepatic necrosis, toxic megacolon
Furazolidone (Furoxone)	GI intolerance	Allergic reactions, pulmonary infiltrates, headache, fever	Hemolytic anemia (G6PD deficiency), hypotension, polyneuropathy, hypoglycemia, agranulocytosis, disulfiram reaction with alcohol

Continued

Drug	Frequent	Occasional	Rare
Ganciclovir—IV (Cytovene)	Neutropenia (ANC <500/mm³ in 15–20%, usually early in treatment and responds within 3–7 days to drug holiday or to G-CSF/GM-CSF); thrombocytopenia (platelet count <20,000/mm³ in 10%, reversible). Monitor CBC 2–3×/wk and discontinue with ANC <500–750/mm³ or platelet count <25,000/mm³	Anemia; fever; rash; CNS—headache, seizures, confusion; changes in mental status; abnormal liver function tests (2–3%)	CNS—psychosis, delirium, confusion, agitation; neuropathy; impaired reproductive function (?); hematuria; renal failure; nausea; vomiting; GI bleeding or perforation; myocardiopathy; hypotension; ataxia; coma; somnolence; alopecia; prutitis; urticaria
Griseofulvin (Fulvicin)	Headache (often resolves with continued treatment)	Photosensitivity	GI disturbances, allergic reactions, paresthesias, exacerbation of lupus or leprosy, liver damage, lymphadenopathy, blood dyscrasias, thrush, transient hearing loss, fatigue, dizziness, insomnia, psychosis
Halofantrine (Halfan)		Diarrhea, abdominal pain	
Imipenem + cilastatin (Primaxin)		Phlebitis at infusion sites, allergic reactions, nausea, vomiting and diarrhea, eosinophilia, hepatotoxicity (transient), drug fever, transient hypotension during infusion, seizures (increased rates with high doses, renal failure, elderly patient, prior seizure disorder)	Myoclonus, C. difficile colitis, bone marrow suppression, renal toxicity
Interferon alfa (Roferon A, Intron)	Flu-like illness (80% with >5 mil units/d); fever; fatigue; anorexia; headache; myalgias Depression GI intolerance with nausea, vomiting, and pain or diarrhea (20–65%) Toxic effects start within 6 hr and last 2–12 hr; pretreat with NSAIDs	Marrow suppression—leukopenia, anemia ± thrombocytopenia (3–70%, dose related, usually transient and well tolerated); neuropsychiatric effects—psychosis, confusion, somnolence; anxiety; hepatitis—dose related in up to 40% receiving high doses; alopecia (8%); rash; activation of lupus; proteinuria	Edema, arrhythmias, cardiomyopathy, renal failure, hearing loss, pulmonary infiltrates. Some patients with hepatitis B have increased risk of decompensation with decreasing albumin levels, prolonged prothrombin time, and increased ALT; delirium, obtundation

Continued

69

Drug	Frequent	Occasional	Rare
Iodoquinol		Rash, acne, GI intolerance—nausea, diarrhea, cramps	Optic atrophy, vision loss, peripheral neuropathy (with use for months), iodine sensitivity
Isoniazid (INH)	Hepatitis—age related <20 yr—nil; 35–6%; 45–11%; 55–18%. Rate of symptomatic hepatitis + transaminase levels ≥5× ULN among patients taking INH prophylaxis by current guidelines is only 0.1% (Ann Intern Med 281:1014, 1999). Patient should be warned of symptoms, and drug should be discontinued if transaminase levels are ≥3–5 × normal limit	Allergic reactions; fever; peripheral neuropathy (reduced with pyridoxine) especially with alcoholism, diabetes, pregnancy, malnutrition, glossitis	CNS—optic neuritis, psychosis, agitation, depression, hallucination, paranoia, convulsions; toxic encephalopathy; twitching; coma; blood dyscrasias; hyperglycemia; lupus-like syndrome; keratitis; pellagra-like rash; B-6 and folate deficiency; chronic liver injury
Itraconazole (Sporanox)		Headache; GI intolerance—nausea (10%), vomiting, rash (8%), high dose (600 mg/day)—hypokalemia, adrenal insufficiency, impotence, gynecomastia, leg edema	Hepatitis (1/1000), toxic epidural necrolysis, hypertension
Ivermectin (Stromectol)			Mazzotti reaction in onchocerciasis with hypotension, fever, pruritus, bone and joint pain
IVIG		Hypotension, flushing, fever, chills, headache	Renal failure, hemolysis, aseptic meningitis, hyponatremia, anaphylaxis
Ketoconazole (Nizoral)	GI intolerance (dose related; take with food or at hs to improve tolerance) Temporary increase in transaminase levels (2–5%)	Endocrine—decreased steroid and testosterone synthesis with impotence, gynecomastia, oligospermia, reduced libido; menstrual abnormalities (prolonged use and dose related, usually ≥600 mg/d); headache; somnolence; dizziness; asthenia; pruritus; rash; abdominal pain; photophobia	Abrupt and fulminant hepatitis (1:15,000), rare cases of fetal hepatic necrosis, anaphylaxis, lethargy, arthralgias, fever, marrow suppression, hypothyroidism (genetically determined), hallucinations, thrombocytopenia

Continued

Drug	Frequent	Occasional	Rare
Lamivudine	Exacerbation of hepatitis B when drug is discontinued (as with tenofovir or entecavir)	—	Nausea
Linezolid		Neutropenia, thrombocytopenia, anemia—monitor CBC weekly (see MedWatch—www.fda.gov/medwatch/feedback.htm); diarrhea, nausea, headache	Fever, thrush, rash, dizziness
Mebendazole (Vermox)		Diarrhea, abdominal pain	Leukopenia, agranulocytosis, hypospermia
Mefloquine (Lariam)	Vertigo, light-headedness, nausea, nightmares, headache, visual disturbances (dose related), decreased fine motor function	Psychosis and panic attacks, seizures; disorientation (dose related—rare at doses used for prophylaxis); GI intolerance; dizziness	Prolonged cardiac conduction, hypotension, seizures, coma
Melarsoprol (Mel B)	Heart damage, hypertension, colic, encephalopathy, vomiting	Peripheral neuropathy	Shock
Meropenem		Diarrhea (5%), nausea, headache, rash	Anaphylaxis, seizures (especially with CNS disorders or renal failure), thrombocytopenia, pseudomembranous colitis
Methenamine (Mandelamine)		GI intolerance, dysuria (reduced dose or acidification)	Allergic reactions, edema, tinnitus, muscle cramps
Metronidazole (Flagyl)	GI intolerance, metallic taste, headache	Peripheral neuropathy (prolonged use—reversible), phlebitis at injection sites, disulfiram-like reaction with alcohol, insomnia, stomatitis	Seizures, ataxic encephalitis, *C. difficile* colitis, leukopenia, dysuria, pancreatitis, allergic reactions, mutagenic in Ames test (significance in ?), depression, uncontrolled crying, hallucinations, agitation, *C. difficile* colitis
Micafungin (Mycamine)	—	GI intolerance, elevated hepatic enzymes	Rash, pruritis, face swelling and flushing (histamine release)

Continued

Drug	Frequent	Occasional / Rare
Miconazole (Monistat)	Phlebitis at injection sites; chills; pruritus; rash; dizziness; blurred vision; hyperlipidemia; nausea; vomiting; hyponatremia; hyperlipidemia; irritation with topical use	Marrow suppression—anemia and thrombocytopenia, renal damage, anaphylaxis, hypotension, thrombocytosis, psychosis, cardiac arrhythmias or cardiac arrest with initial dose
Nalidixic acid (NegGram)	See quinolones	
Niclosamide (Niclocide)	Nausea, abdominal pain	
Nifurtimox (Lampit)	GI intolerance, loss of memory, sleep disorders, paresthesias, weakness, polyneuritis	Seizures, fever, pulmonary infiltrates
Nitazoxanide (Alinia)	Abdominal pain and nausea (give with food), headache	Allergic reaction, fever, rash, pruritis
Nitrofurantoin (Macrodantin)	GI intolerance	Hypersensitivity reactions, pulmonary infiltrates (acute, subacute, or chronic ± fever, eosinophilia, rash, or lupus-like reaction)	Peripheral neuropathy, hepatitis, hemolytic anemia (G6PD deficiency), lactic acidosis, parotitis, pancreatitis, pulmonary fibrosis, cholestatic jaundice, trigeminal neuralgia
Nitrofurazone	Local irritation	Allergic reactions, contact dermatitis, renal failure with wound dressing in severe burn patients
Nystatin (Mycostatin)	GI intolerance	Allergic reactions
Ofloxacin (Floxin)	See quinolones	
Ornidazole	Dizziness, headache, GI intolerance	Reversible peripheral neuropathy
Oseltamivir	Dizziness, headache, fatigue, insomnia; Nausea, vomiting (nausea usually resolves in 1–2 days and reduced with food)	

Continued

Drug	Frequent	Occasional	Rare
Oxamniquine (Vansil)		Headache, fever, dizziness, somnolence, GI intolerance, hepatitis, insomnia, EEG changes, ECG changes, orange discoloration of urine	Seizures, neuropsychiatric disturbances
Paromomycin (Humatin)	GI intolerance		Ototoxicity and nephrotoxicity (especially with GI absorption plus renal failure)
Peginterferon	See interferon. Side effect profile is identical.		
Penicillins	Hypersensitivity reactions, rash (especially ampicillin and amoxicillin), diarrhea (especially ampicillin)	GI intolerance (oral agents), fever, Coombs' test positive, phlebitis at infusion sites and sterile abscesses at IM sites, Jarisch-Herxheimer reaction (syphilis or other spirochetal infections)	Anaphylaxis; leukopenia; thrombocytopenia; *C. difficile* colitis (especially ampicillin); hepatic damage; renal damage; CNS—seizures, twitching (high doses in patients with renal failure); hyperkalemia (penicillin G infusion); abnormal platelet aggregation with bleeding diathesis (carbenicillin, ticarcillin, piperacillin, nafcillin); thrombocytopenia (methicillin, mezlocillin); sodium overload (ticarcillin, nafcillin); GI bleeding (dicloxacillin)
Pentamidine (Pentam NebuPent)	Nephrotoxicity—in 25%, usually reversible with discontinuation (IV Pentam) Aerosol administration—cough (30%), pretreat with albuterol, 2 puffs	Hypotension (administer IV over 60 min); hypoglycemia (5–10%, usually occurs after day 5 of treatment including past treatment, may last days or weeks, treat with IV glucose); diabetes mellitus, may be insulin dependent; cardiotoxicity; delirium; rash (including Stevens-Johnson syndrome); marrow suppression (common in AIDS patients); GI intolerance with nausea, vomiting, abdominal pain, anorexia, and/or bad taste Aerosol administration—asthma reaction (2–5%)	Hepatotoxicity, leukopenia, thrombocytopenia, pancreatitis, toxic epidermal necrolysis, fever

Continued

73

Drug	Frequent	Occasional	Rare
Polymyxins (Aerosporin)	Pain and phlebitis at injection sites, neurotoxicity (ataxia, paresthesias), nephrotoxicity, dizziness, drowsiness, facial flushing		Allergic reactions, neuromuscular blockade—sometimes reversed with IV CaCl (not neostigmine)
Praziquantel (Biltricide)	Malaise, headache, dizziness	Sedation, abdominal pain, fever, sweating, fatigue	Pruritis, rash
Primaquine		Hemolytic anemia (G6PD deficiency); warm patient to observe for dark urine and cyanosis, or screen for G6PD deficiency; GI intolerance	Headache, pruritus, neutropenia, CNS symptoms, hypertension, arrhythmias, disturbed visual accommodation
Pyrazinamide	Non-gouty polyarthralgia, asymptomatic hyperuricemia	Hepatitis (dose related, frequency not increased when given with INH or rifampin, rarely serious), GI intolerance, gout (treated with allopurinol and probenecid)	Rash, fever, porphyria, photosensitivity
Pyrimethamine (Daraprim)		Folic acid deficiency with megaloblastic anemia and pancytopenia (dose related and reversed with leucovorin), allergic reactions, GI intolerance (nausea, anorexia, vomiting)	CNS—ataxia, tremors, headache, malaise, seizures (dose related), fatigue
Quinacrine (Atabrine)	Dizziness, headache, vomiting, diarrhea	Yellow staining of skin, psychosis, blood dyscrasias, rash, insomnia	Hepatic necrosis, seizures, exfoliative dermatitis, ocular effects like chloroquine
Quinine		GI intolerance, cinchonism (tinnitus, headache, visual disturbances), hemolytic anemia (G6PD deficiency)	Arrhythmias, hypotension with rapid IV infusion, hypoglycemia, hepatitis, thrombocytopenia

Continued

Drug	Frequent	Occasional	Rare
Quinolones Ciprofloxacin Enoxacin Gatifloxacin Gemifloxacin Levofloxacin Lomefloxacin Moxifloxacin Nalidixic acid Norfloxacin Ofloxacin Trovafloxacin	Animal studies show arthropathies in weight-bearing joints of immature animals; significance in humans is unknown Contraindicated during pregnancy and in persons <18 yr Gemifloxacin—high rate of apparently inconsequential rash especially with persons < 40 years, women and courses > 7 days	GI intolerance; CNS—headache, malaise, insomnia, restlessness, dizziness; allergic reactions; diarrhea; photosensitivity (especially lomefloxacin and naladixic acid); increased hepatic enzymes; tendon rupture (especially Achilles—over 100 cases reported); prolonged QT interval (rare, but important, especially when combined with other drugs that can cause this)	Papilledema; nystagmus; visual disturbances; diarrhea; C. difficile colitis; marrow suppression; photosensitivity; anaphylaxis; serum sickness; seizures; toxic psychosis; CNS stimulation—tremors, restlessness, insomnia, delirium, psychosis, confusion, hallucinations; encephalopathy with coma; interstitial nephritis; prolonged bleeding time; vasculitis Hepatotoxicity—trovafloxacin implicated in 14 cases of liver failure resulting in liver transplantation or death, which led to revised indications that generally limit the drug to hospital use for patients with infections that cannot be managed with alternative antibiotics
Quinupristin–dalfopristin	Arthralgias and myalgias Hyperbilirubinemia	Phlebitis at IV infusion sites, rash, nausea, headache, transaminase increase	Colitis
Ribavirin + interferon (see interferon)	Hemolytic anemia in wk 1–4; dose related	Cough, dyspnea, fatigue, headache, insomnia, GI intolerance	
Rifabutin (Mycobutin)	Orange discoloration of urine, tears (contact lens), sweat (see drug interactions) Uveitis with eye pain, photophobia, redness, and blurred vision—usually high doses (600 mg/d or concurrent use of fluconazole or clarithromycin); usually responsive to topical corticosteroids plus mydriatics (NEJM 330:438, 1994) Major concern is drug interactions because rifabutin accelerates cytochrome P-450 (see drug interactions)	Hepatitis, GI intolerance, allergic reactions	Dose-related polyarthralgias, thrombotic thrombocytopenic purpura, hemolysis, myositis, confusion, seizures

Continued

Drug	Frequent	Occasional	Rare
Rifampin (Rifadin)	Orange discoloration of urine, tears (contact lens), sweat Major concerns are drug interactions because rifampin accelerates cytochrome P-450	Hepatitis—usually cholestatic changes during first month (frequency not increased when given with INH); jaundice (usually reversible with dose reduction and/or continued use); GI intolerance; hypersensitivity reactions; accelerated metabolism of steroids so increase steroid requirement in adrenal insufficiency; may require alternative to oral contraceptives; contraindicated for concurrent use with protease inhibitors (see drug interactions); flu-like syndrome with intermittent use characterized by dyspnea, wheezing	Thrombocytopenia, leukopenia, hemolytic anemia, eosinophilia, renal damage, proximal myopathy, hyperuricemia, anaphylaxis, renal damage, acute organic brain syndrome, C. difficile colitis
Rifaximin (Xifaxin)	—	—	Antibiotic-associated diarrhea
Rimantadine (Flumadine)	—	GI intolerance (3–8%); CNS—light head-edness, insomnia, reduced concentration, nervousness (4–8%, about half the rate with amantadine)	Seizures (primarily in patients with seizure disorder)
Sodium stibogluconate (Pentostam)	Muscle pain, joint stiffness, nausea, T-wave flattening, increased hepatic enzymes	Weakness, colic, hepatic damage, bradycardia, leukopenia	Diarrhea, rash, pruritus, hemolytic anemia, cardiac damage, renal damage, shock, sudden death
Spectinomycin (Trobicin)	—	Pain at injection site, urticaria, fever, insomnia, dizziness, nausea, headache	Anaphylaxis, fever, anemia, renal failure and abnormal liver function test (multiple doses)
Sulfonamides	Allergic reactions—rash, pruritus, fever (appears to be dose related, usually within 7–10 days of initial dose), cross reactions noted between sulfonamides including thiazide diuretics and oral hypoglycemics	Periarteritis nodosum, lupus, Stevens-Johnson syndrome, serum sickness; crystalluria with renal damage, urolithiasis and oliguria (prevent with increasing urine pH, hydration, and use of sulfonamide-sulfonamide combinations); GI intolerance; photosensitivity; hepatitis	Myocarditis, psychosis, confusion, euphoria, disorientation, neuropathy, dizziness, depression, hemolytic anemia (G6PD deficiency), marrow suppression, agranulocytosis

Continued

Drug	Frequent	Occasional	Rare
Suramin	GI intolerance, pruritis, photophobia, hyperesthesia	Peripheral neuropathy, renal damage, blood dyscrasias, optic atrophy	
Telithromycin		GI intolerance—nausea, vomiting, diarrhea; dysgeusia; headache; dizziness	Elevated transaminases (reversible), *C. difficile* colitis; exacerbation of myasthenia gravis; potential to prolong QTc interval (similar to clarithromycin) Blurred vision—most commonly after first or second dose and lasting hours—reversible
Terbinafine		GI intolerance—diarrhea, dyspepsia, abdominal pain; rash; taste perversion; hepatitis; pruritis	Anaphylaxis, neutropenia
Tetracyclines Demeclocycline Doxycycline Minocycline Tetracycline	GI intolerance (dose related); stains and deforms teeth in children up to 8 yr; vertigo (minocycline); negative nitrogen balance and increased azotemia with renal failure (except doxycycline; vaginitis)	Hepatotoxicity (dose related, esp pregnant women); esophageal ulcerations; diarrhea; candidiasis (thrush and vaginitis); photosensitivity (esp demeclocycline and doxycycline); phlebitis with IV treatment and pain with IM injection	Malabsorption, allergic reactions, visual disturbances, aggravation of myasthenia (reversed with Ca^{++}), hemolytic anemia, *C. difficile* colitis, increased intracranial pressure, hemolytic anemia, papilledema
Thiabendazole (Mintezol)	Nausea, vomiting, vertigo	Rash, hallucinations, olfactory disturbances, leukopenia	Stevens-Johnson syndrome, shock, tinnitis, cholestasis, seizures, angioneurotic edema
Ticarcillin + clavulanic acid (Timentin)	Similar to those for ticarcillin alone	See penicillins	
Tigecycline (Tygacil)	Nausea, diarrhea, vomiting, abdominal pain (5–25%)	Hyperbilirubinemia Potential for tooth discoloration in children and offspring of pregnant women	*C. difficile*-associated colitis
Trifluridine (Viroptic)		Burning at application site	Palpebral edema, hypersensitivity reactions, epithelial keratopathy

Continued

Drug	Frequent	Occasional	Rare
Trimethoprim	GI intolerance (dose related), rash, pruritis	Marrow suppression—megaloblastic anemia, neutropenia, thrombocytopenia (hematologic toxicity increased with folate depletion and high doses—treat with leucovorin, 3–15 mg/d × 3 days); reversible hyperkalemia (dose related); photosensitivity	Pancytopenia; erythema multiforme, Stevens-Johnson syndrome, TEN
Trimethoprim-sulfamethoxazole (see sulfonamides and trimethoprim) (Bactrim, Septra)	Fever, leukopenia, rash, and/or GI intolerance in 25–50% of HIV-infected persons; dose related and most tolerate readmministration of lower dose after 2 wk discontinuation; reactions noted above for sulfonamides and trimethoprim	Candida vaginitis, thrush (AIDS patients); anemia; thrombocytopenia, renal failure; hemolytic anemia with G6PD deficiency; hepatitis including cholestatic jaundice	Ataxia, apathy, ankle clonus, erythema multiforme, Stevens-Johnson syndrome, C. difficile-associated colitis, pancreatitis, hepatic necrosis
Trimetrexate	Marrow suppression with neutropenia and thrombocytopenia. Must give with folinic acid (leucovorin) 20–40 mg/m² q6h). Must monitor CBC, renal function, and liver function, tests ≥2 times a week	Hepatotoxicity with increased trans-aminase levels (3%), rash (3%); GI toxicity (1%), stomatitis, nephrotoxicity	Seizures— ? relation, anaphylaxis
Tryparsamide	Nausea, vomiting	Impaired vision, optic atrophy, fever, allergic reactions, rash, tinnitus	
Valacyclovir (Valtrex)			GI intolerance—nausea, vomiting, diarrhea, headache, constipation
Valganciclovir (Valtrex)	Neutropenia; anemia; contraindicated with ANC < 500 or Hgb < 8 g/dL GI intolerance	Thrombocytopenia; confusion; headache; fever; abnormal LFTs, rash	

Continued

Drug	Frequent	Occasional	Rare
Vancomycin (Vancocin)	Phlebitis at injection sites	"Red-man syndrome" (flushing over chest and face) ± hypotension and pruritis (infusion >60 min; may be reversed or prevented with anti-histamine); fever; eosinophilia; allergic reactions with rash	Anaphylaxis, ototoxicity and nephrotoxicity (dose related), peripheral neuropathy, marrow suppression
Voricmazole (Valtrex)	Visual disturbances in 20% (blurring, color distortion, etc)—usually treat through; D/C in < 1%	Increased LFTs D/C for hepatotoxicity in 4–8%; hallucination in 4%; rash in 6%	
Zanamivir		Bronchospasm or reduced expiratory flow rate especially in patients with asthma or chronic lung disease; should have rapidly acting broncho-dilator available in susceptible patients	Dizziness

B. **Penicillin Allergy**—Guidelines based primarily on recommendations of the
   Joint Council of Allergy, Asthma and Immunology (J Allergy Clin Immunol
   1998;101:S465–S528 See also: Ann Intern Med 2004;141:16; Allergy Asthma
   Proc 2005;26:59; Mayo Clin Proc 2005;80:405; Curr Allergy Asthma Rep
   2005;5:9) and the CDC recommendations for penicillin skin testing (MMWR
   2002;51:RR-6)

1. **Classification of Penicillin Hypersensitivity Reactions** (JAMA 2001;285:2498)

Type	Mechanism	Clinical expression
I	IgE	Urticaria, angioedema, anaphylaxis,* laryngeal edema, asthma frequency—0.02%, mortality—10%
II	Cytotoxic Ab of IgG class	Hemolytic anemia
III	Immune complexes IgG and IgM Ab	Serum sickness
IV	Cell-mediated	Contact dermatitis
Idiopathic	Unknown	Maculopapular rash (common), interstitial nephritis, drug fever, eosinophilia, exfoliative dermatitis, Stevens-Johnson syndrome

*Anaphylaxis is defined as an immediate systemic reaction due to IgE. Anaphylactoid reactions mimic anaphylaxis but are not caused by IgE.

2. **Cross Reactions Among Beta-lactam Agents** (J Allergy Clin Immunol 1998;
   101:S465; Ann Intern Med 2004;141:16)
   - Allergy to one penicillin indicates allergy to all.
   - Allergy to penicillins may indicate allergy to cephalosporins and carbapenems
     (imipenem, meropenem, etc.); it is generally considered safe to give cephalo-
     sporins to patients with non–IgE-mediated reactions to penicillins such as macu-
     lopapular rashes. The risk of an allergic reaction to a cephalosporin in a patient
     with penicillin allergy is <10%; it is greater with first generation cephalosporins
     than second or third generation agents. Penicillin skin testing is a valid method to
     test safety of cephalosporins in penicillin-allergic patients.
   - If a cephalosporin is needed, the recommendation is skin test with cefuroxime or
     ceftriaxone; if negative, cefuroxime or ceftriaxone may be given as low dose
     challenge (1% usual dose, followed by 10% usual dose at 1 hour later and then full
     dose 1 hour later) (Ann Intern Med 2004;141:16).
   - There are rare cross reactions with aztreonam.
   - Ampicillin and amoxicillin cause morbilliform rashes in 5–13% of patients; these do
     not constitute a reaction meriting skin testing unless the reaction is urticarial or
     anaphylactic.
   - Serum sickness to cefaclor is caused by a hereditary defect in metabolism and
     does not indicate risk with other beta-lactams (Immunol Allergy Clin N. Am 1998;
     189:745).

3. **Skin Testing**
   This is considered a safe, rapid, and effective method to exclude an IgE-mediated
   response with ≥97% assurance (MMWR 1993;42(RR-14):45; Allergy Asthma Proc.
   2005;26:59)
   a. **The indication is a patient who has a history of an allergic reaction** to
      penicillin or a cephalosporin and who needs penicillin. Morbilliform rashes to
      amoxicillin or ampicillin do not count as a positive history. The test may be used
      for the penicillin allergic patient who requires a cephalosporin as well.

b. **Patients with a history of severe reactions during the past year** should be tested in a monitored setting in which treatment for anaphylaxis is possible. Antigens should be diluted 100-fold.

c. **Patients with a history of penicillin allergy** and a negative skin test should receive penicillin 250 mg po and be observed for 1 hr before treatment with therapeutic doses.

Those with a positive skin test should be desensitized.

d. **Penicillin allergy skin testing:** Patient should not have taken antihistamines in the previous 48 hr.

    (1) <u>Reagents</u> (Ann Allergy Asthma Immunol 1999;83:665; MMWR 2002;51: RR-6)
- Major determinants:

    Benzylpenicilloyl-polylysine (Pre-Pen, Taylor Co Decatur IL) as conjugated of benzylpenicillin with poly-L-lysine in concentration of 6 $\times$ 10^{-5} mEq penicilloyl moieties.

- Minor determinants:

    Freshly diluted aqueous penicillin G.

- Positive control (histamine 1 mg/mL).

- Negative control (buffered saline solution).

    Dilute the antigens 100-fold for preliminary testing if there has been an immediate generalized reaction within the past year.

    (2) <u>Procedure</u>

    <u>Epicutaneous (scratch or prick) test</u>: apply one drop of material to volar forearm and pierce epidermis with a 26-gauge needle without drawing blood; observe for 20 min. A wheal of $\geq$4 mm is a positive test. If there is no wheal $\geq$4 mm or systemic reaction, proceed to intradermal test. With a positive scratch test, the subsequent intradermal test should be performed with the corresponding reagent diluted 10^2–10^4 fold.

    <u>Intradermal test</u>: Inject 0.02 mL intradermally raising a 2- to 3-mm wheal using a 27-gauge short-bevelled needle; observe for 20 min. A wheal of 2 mm larger than original wheal is positive.

    (3) <u>Interpretation</u>

    For test to be interpretable, negative (saline) control must elicit no reaction, and positive (histamine) control must elicit a positive reaction.

    <u>Positive test</u>: A wheal >2 mm in mean diameter to any penicillin reagent; erythema must be present. A positive history and a positive skin test gives a 50% chance of an immediate reaction if penicillin is given (J Allergy Clin Immunol 1998;101:S465)

    <u>Negative test</u>: Wheals at site of penicillin reagents are equivalent to negative control. A negative test to major and minor determinants gives a 97–99% probability of no immediate reaction if penicillin is given (J Allergy Clin Immunol 1998;101:S465)

    <u>Indeterminate</u>: All other results.

Epicutaneous test	Histamine	Diluent	Conclusion
Neg	Pos	Neg	Do epidermal test; wheal 2 mm larger than original wheal at 15–20 min is positive
Neg	Neg	Neg	False negative. No conclusion.
Pos	Pos	Neg	Avoid penicillin or desensitize

From Ann Intern Med 1987;107:204; JAMA 1993;270:2456

e. **Experience with test** (JAMA 1993;270:2456)
   Test results in 4977 patients with indication for penicillin therapy
   - Results by history of penicillin reaction

Positive history	55*/776 (7.1%)
Negative history	73/4201 (1.7%)
Total	128/4977 (2.6%)

   *History of urticaria—34/274 (12.4%), rash—7/166 (4%), other or uncertain—5/284 (1.7%)

   - Reaction pattern with 128 positives

Positive—major determinants	96 (75%)
Positive—minor determinants	13 (10%)
Positive—both	19 (15%)

   - Results with penicillin given to 596 patients with positive history and negative skin test

Anaphylaxis	2/596 (0.3%)
Urticaria	15/596 (2.5%)
Rash/pruritis	13/596 (2.1%)

f. **Experience with cephalosporins**
   - Literature review of 15,987 patients who received first or second generation cephalosporins showed reactions in 8.1% with a history of penicillin reaction versus 1.9% without this history (Arch Intern Med 1992;152:930).
   - A review of 9388 patients with a history of penicillin allergy showed 2 cases of anaphylaxis (0.02%) with cephalosporin treatment.
   - The rate of cephalosporin reactions with a positive penicillin skin test is 6/135 (4.4%) compared to 2/351 (0.6%) in those with a negative skin test (NEJM 2001;345:804).
   - Patients with an allergic reaction to a cephalosporin should not receive the same agent again, but other cephalosporins with different side chains may not cause cross reactions. Animal studies suggest side-chain specific antibodies may dominate the immune response to cephalosporins (Biochem 1971;123:183; Ann Intern Med 1987;107:204).
   - With need for cephalosporin—skin test and give graded challenge if negative—1% standard dose; 10% standard dose 1 hour later and then full dose 1 hour later. Best data are with cefuroxime and ceftriaxone (Ann Intern Med 2004;141:16)

4. **Testing without Minor Determinant**
   If the full battery of skin test reagents is unavailable (minor determinant is difficult to obtain), testing should be performed with major determinant (Pre-Pen, Taylor Pharmaceutical Co, Decatur, IL) and penicillin G (benzylpenicillin G 6000 units/mL). This testing detects 90–97% of allergic patients; because lack of minor determinants misses 3–10% of allergic patients, caution is necessary. Patients at high risk of anaphylaxis (history of penicillin-induced anaphylaxis, urticaria, asthma etc should be tested with a 100-fold dilution of test reagents before testing full strength. A 10-fold dilution is suggested for other types of immediate, generalized reactions within the past year. Test methods are described above using the epicutaneous (scratch) test followed by the intradermal test.

5. **Penicillin Desensitization** (MMWR 2002;51:RR-6))
   a. **Penicillin desensitization should be performed in a hospital** because IgE-mediated reactions can occur, although they are rare. Desensitization may be done po or IV, although oral administration is often considered safer, simpler, and easier. Desensitization requires about 4 hr, after which the first dose is given.

b. Parenteral desensitization: Give 1 unit penicillin IV, and then double the dose at 15-min intervals or increase the dose 10-fold at 20- to 30-min intervals.

c. Oral desensitization protocol (NEJM 1985;312:1229):

Dose[a]	Penicillin V suspension (units/mL)	Amount[b] mL	units	Cumulative dose (units)
1	1000	0.1	100	100
2	1000	0.2	200	300
3	1000	0.4	400	700
4	1000	0.8	800	1500
5	1000	1.6	1600	3100
6	1000	3.2	3200	6300
7	1000	6.4	6400	12,700
8	10,000	1.2	12,000	24,700
9	10,000	2.4	24,000	48,700
10	10,000	4.8	48,000	96,700
11	80,000	1.0	80,000	176,700
12	80,000	2.0	160,000	336,700
13	80,000	4.0	320,000	656,700
14	80,000	8.0	640,000	1,296,700

Observation period: 30 min before parenteral administration of penicillin.

[a]Interval between doses, 15 min; elapsed time, 3 hr and 45 min; cumulative dose, 1.3 mil units.

[b]Specific amount of drug was diluted in approximately 30 mL of water and then given po.

6. **Management of Allergic Reactions**
   - Medical facilities should have a protocol for dealing with allergic reactions, especially anaphylaxis. Supplies include oxygen, aqueous epinephrine, injectable antihistamine, IV steroids, airway intubation suppliers, and IV access supplies.
   - <u>Epinephrine</u>: IgE-mediated reactions
   - <u>Antihistamines</u>: Accelerated and late urticaria, maculopapular rashes
   - <u>Glucocorticoids</u>: Severe urticaria, prolonged systemic anaphylaxis, serum sickness, contact dermatitis, exfoliative and bullous skin reactions, interstitial nephritis, pulmonary and hepatic reactions

7. **Anaphylactic Shock**

	Epinephrine dose
Initial treatment	
SC (preferred) or IM: Repeat every 20–30 min prn up to 3×	0.3–0.5 mL (1:1000)
Severe shock or inadequate response to IM or SC: IV administration	3–5 mL at 5- to 10-min intervals (1:10,000)

DRUG INTERACTIONS

(Adapted from Medical Letter Handbook of Adverse Drug Interactions, 2000 and Drug Information for the Health Care Professional, USP DI, 21st Edition, 2001

Drug	Effect of interaction
Acyclovir	
Narcotics	Increased meperidine level
Probenecid	Possible increased acyclovir level
Adofovir	
Ibuprofen	Adofovir AUC increases 23%
Amantadine	
Anticholinergics	Hallucination, confusion, nightmares
Thiazide diuretics	Increased amantadine toxicity with hydrochlorothiazide-triamterene combination
Trimethoprim–sulfamethoxazole	Amantadine toxicity with delirium
Aminoglycosides	
Amphotericin	Increased nephrotoxicity
Bumetanide	Ototoxicity
Cephalosporins	Increased nephrotoxicity
Cisplatin	Increased nephrotoxicity—avoid
Cyclosporine	Increased nephrotoxicity—avoid
Enflurane	Increased nephrotoxicity—avoid
Ethacrynic acid	Increased ototoxicity—avoid
Furosemide	Increased oto- and nephrotoxicity—avoid
Gallium	Increased nephrotoxicity
MgSO$_4$	Increased neuromuscular blockage
Malathion	Possible respiratory depression
Methotrexate	Possible decreased methotrexate activity with oral aminoglycosides
Neuromuscular blocking agents	Increased neuromuscular blockade
Vancomycin	Increased nephrotoxicity and possible increased ototoxicity
Aminosalicylic acid (PAS)	
Anticoagulants, oral	Increased hypoprothrombinemia
Digitalis	Decreased digoxin level
Probenecid	Increased PAS toxicity
Rifampin	Decreased rifampin effectiveness (give as separate doses by 8–12 hr)
Amphotericin B	
Aminoglycosides	Increased nephrotoxicity
Capreomycin	Increased nephrotoxicity
Cisplatin	Increased nephrotoxicity
Corticosteroids	Increased hypokalemia

Continued

Drug	Effect of interaction
Cyclosporine	Increased nephrotoxicity (JID 29:106, 1994)—avoid
Digitalis	Increased cardiotoxicity due to hypokalemia—monitor K^+
Diuretics	Increased hypokalemia
Leukocyte transfusions	Acute pulmonary toxicity
Methoxyflurane	Increased nephrotoxicity
Pentamidine	Increased nephrotoxicity
Skeletal muscle relaxants	Increased effect of relaxants
Vancomycin	Increased nephrotoxicity

Atovaquone	
AZT	Increased AZT levels (Clin Pharmacol Ther 59:14, 1996)
Food (fat)	Increased absorption (should be taken with meals)
Metoclopramide	Decreased atovaquone levels
Rifampin and rifabutin	Decreased atovaquone levels
Sulfa-trimethoprim	Slight decrease in TMP-SMX levels
Tetracycline	Decreased atovaquone levels (40%)—avoid

Azithromycin	
Antacids with Mg^{++} or Al^{++}	Area under curve does not change peak level
Coumadin	Increased prothrombin time
Food	Tablets: No effect
	Oral suspension: Absorption increases, but area under curve is unchanged
Theophylline	Increased theophylline levels (Pharmacotherapy 17:827, 1997)

Capreomycin	
Aminoglycosides	Increased oto- and nephrotoxicity—avoid
Theophylline	Increased theophylline effect and toxicity

Caspofungin	
Cyclosporine	Increases levels of caspofungin 35%—avoid or monitor LFTs
Dexamethasone	May decrease caspofungin levels
Efavireniz	May decrease caspofungin levels
Nelfinavir	May decrease caspofungin levels
Nevirapine	May decrease caspofungin levels
Phenytoin	May decrease caspofungin levels
Rifampin	May decrease caspofungin levels
Tacrolimus	May decrease caspofungin levels

Cephalosporins	
Alcohol	Disulfiram-like reaction for those with tetrazole-thiomethyl side chain: Cefamandole, cefoperazone, cefotetan
Aminoglycosides	Possibly increased nephrotoxicity
Antacids with Al^{++} or Mg^{++} or H_2 blockers	Reduced absorption of cefdinir and cefditoren, take ≥2 hr apart
Contraceptives	Decreased contraceptive effect; mechanism unknown—two case reports (Br J Clin Pharmacol 25:527, 1988)
Cyclosporine	Increased cyclosporine levels with ceftriaxone (Nephron 59:681, 1991)

Continued

Drug	Effect of interaction
Ethacrynic acid	Increased nephrotoxicity
Food	Most oral agents are unaffected; oral cefuroxime absorption promoted
Furosemide	Increased nephrotoxicity
Probenecid	Increased concentrations of most cephalosporins

Chloramphenicol

Drug	Effect of interaction
Anticoagulants, oral	Increased hypoprothrombinemia
Chlorpropamide	Increased chlorpropamide activity
Dicumarol	Increased dicumarol activity
Phenobarbital	Decreased concentrations of chloramphenicol
Phenytoin	Increased phenytoin activity
Rifampin	Decreased chloramphenicol levels (NEJM 312:788, 1985)
Tolbutamide	Increased tolbutamide activity

Cidofovir

Drug	Effect of interaction
Nephrotoxic drugs	Promotes nephrotoxicity—must avoid concurrent use of aminoglycosides, amphotericin B, foscarnet, IV pentamidine, and nonsteroidal anti-inflammatory agents —avoid all
Probenecid	Reduces nephrotoxicity of cidofovir and must be given before cidofovir infusion. Probenecid increases levels of acetaminophen, acyclovir, aminosalicylic acid, barbiturates, beta-lactam antibiotics, benzodiazepines, bumetanide, clofibrate, methotrexate, furosemide, and theophylline

Ciprofloxacin (see fluoroquinolones)

Clarithromycin

Drug	Effect of interaction
Carbamazepine	Increased carbamazepine levels and possible reduction in clarithromycin effect (Ann Pharmacother 28:1197, 1994)—avoid
Cisapride	Ventricular arrhythmias—avoid
Disopyramide	Increased disopyramide levels with cardiac arrhythmia (Lancet 349:326, 1997)—avoid
Pimozide	Increased pimozide levels with cardiac toxicity (Clin Pharmacol Ther 59:189, 1996)
Rifabutin	Increased rifabutin levels with uveitis (Genitourin Med 72:419, 1996)
Seldane	Ventricular arrhythmias—avoid
Theophylline	Elevated theophylline levels

Clindamycin

Drug	Effect of interaction
Antiperistaltic agents (Lomotil, loperamide)	Increased risk and severity of *C. difficile* colitis

Cycloserine

Drug	Effect of interaction
Alcohol	Increased alcohol effect or convulsions; warn patients
Ethionamide	Increased CNS toxicity

Continued

Drug	Effect of interaction
Isoniazid	CNS toxicity, dizziness, drowsiness
Phenytoin	Increased phenytoin effect (toxicity)

Dapsone

Coumadin	Increased prothrombin time
ddI	Decreased levels of dapsone
Primaquine	Increased hemolysis with G6PD deficiency
Probenecid	Increased dapsone levels
Pyrimethamine	Increased marrow toxicity (monitor CBC)
Rifampin	Decreased levels of dapsone
Saquinavir	Increased levels of dapsone
Trimethoprim	Increased levels of both drugs

Daptomycin

HMG-CoA reductase inhibitors (statins)	Caution with concurrent use since both may cause myopathy—recommend temporary discontinuation of statins

Ertapenem

Dextrose	Incompatible—do not infuse in dextrose
Probenecid	Increased ertapenem AUC 25%

Erythromycins (inhibit cytochrome P-450)

Anticoagulants, oral	Increased hypoprothrombinemia
Carbamazepine	Increased carbamazepine toxicity
Cisapride (Propulsid)	Ventricular arrhythmias—avoid
Corticosteroids	Increased methylprednisolone levels
Cyclosporine	Increased cyclosporine toxicity (nephrotoxicity)
Digoxin	Increased digitalis levels
Disopyramide*	Increased disopyramide levels—avoid
Entecavir	None known
Ergot alkaloids	Increased ergot levels
Felodipine	Increased felodipine levels (Clin Pharmacol Ther 60:25, 1996)
Phenytoin	Possible decreased phenytoin levels
Quinidine	Increased quinidine levels with cardiac toxicity (Pharmacotherapy 117:626, 1997)
Seldane	Ventricular arrhythmias—avoid
Tacrolimus	Increased tacrolimus levels (Lancet 344:825, 1994)
Theophylline	Increased theophylline levels (Pharmacotherapy 17:827, 1997)
Triazolam	Increased triazolam toxicity
Valproate	Increased valproate levels (Ann Intern Med 116:877, 1992)

Ethionamide

Cycloserine	Increased CNS toxicity
Isoniazid	Increased CNS toxicity

Famciclovir

Cimetidine	Increased penciclovir levels
Digoxin	Increased digoxin levels
Probenecid	Increased penciclovir levels
Theophylline	Increased penciclovir levels

Continued

Drug	Effect of interaction
Fluconazole (inhibits cytochrome P-450)	
Alprazolam	Increased sedation
Atovaquone	Increased atovaquone levels
Benzodiazepines	Increased benzodiazepine levels
Caffeine	Possible caffeine toxicity
Cisapride (Propulsid)	Ventricular arrhythmias—avoid
Clarithromycin	Increased clarithromycin levels
Contraceptive	Decreased contraceptive effect—three cases reported
Coumadin	Increased prothrombin time
Cyclosporine	Increased cyclosporine nephrotoxicity
Midazolam	Increased sedation
Nortriptyline	Increased sedation, cardiac arrythmias
Phenytoin	Increased phenytoin levels
Rifabutin	Increased rifabutin levels with possible uveitis—avoid
Rifampin	Reduced fluconazole absorption
Saquinavir	Increased saquinavir levels
Seldane	Ventricular arrhythmias—avoid
Sulfonylureas	Increased levels with hypoglycemia
Tacrolimus	Increased nephrotoxicity
Theophylline	Increased levels of theophylline
Triazolam	Increased sedation
Zidovudine	Increased levels of zidovudine (JID 169:1103, 1994)
Fluoroquinolones (ciprofloxacin, norfloxacin, ofloxacin, levofloxacin, trovafloxacin, gatifloxacin, moxifloxacin, gemifloxacin, lomefloxacin)	
Antacids	Decreased fluoroquinolone absorption with Mg^{++}, Ca^{++}, or Al^{++} containing antacids or sucralfate; give antacid > 2 hr after fluoroquinolone
Anticoagulants, oral	Increased hypoprothrombinemia
Caffeine	Increased caffeine effect; significance?; not noted with ofloxacin, sparfloxacin, levofloxacin
Cyclosporine	Possible increased nephrotoxicity
Diazepam	Increased diazepam levels with ciprofloxacin (Eur J Clin Pharmacol 44:365, 1993)
Food	Decreased absorption of norfloxacin and ciprofloxacin: Take 1–2 hr before or after meal
Food (dairy products)	Decreased absorption
Foscarnet	Possible seizures with ciprofloxacin (Ann Pharmacother 28:869, 1994)
Iron	Decreased fluoroquinolone absorption—give quinolone >2 hr before or ≥6 hr after iron
Nonsteroidal anti-inflammatory agents	Possible seizures and increased epileptogenic potential of theophylline, opiates, tricyclics, and neuroleptics
Pentoxifylline	Headaches with ciprofloxacin
Phenytoin	Possible decrease in phenytoin level
Probenecid	Increased fluoroquinolone levels

Continued

Drug	Effect of interaction
Theophylline	Increased theophylline toxicity—especially ciprofloxacin and enoxacin; not noted with ofloxacin, levofloxacin, or sparfloxacin
Zinc	Decreased fluoroquinoline absorption
Foscarnet	
Aminoglycosides	Increased renal toxicity
Amphotericin B	Increased renal toxicity
Pentamidine	Increased hypocalcemia
Ganciclovir	
AZT (Retrovir)	Increased leukopenia: Must monitor CBC and discontinue or give G-CSF
Imipenem	Increased frequency of seizures (?)
Myelosuppressing drugs: TMP-SMX, AZT, azathioprine, pyrimethamine, flucytosine, interferon, doxorubicin, vinblastine, vincristine	Increased leukopenia
Probenecid	Increased ganciclovir levels
Griseofulvin	
Alcohol	Possibly potentiates effect of alcohol
Anticoagulant, oral	Decreased anticoagulant effect
Aspirin	Decreased aspirin effect
Contraceptive	Decreased contraceptive effect
Cyclosporine	Possible decreased cyclosporine effect
Food	Fat increases absorption
Phenobarbital	Decreased griseofulvin levels
Theophylline	Decreased theophylline effect
Imipenem	
Ganciclovir	Increased frequency of seizures—avoid
Probenecid	Increased imipenem levels
Isoniazid	
Alcohol	Increased hepatitis; decreased INH effect in some
Antacids	Decreased INH with Al^{++} containing antacids
Anticoagulants, oral	Possible increased hypoprothrombinemia
Benzodiazepines	Increased effects of benzodiazepines
Carbamazepine	Increased toxicity of both drugs (NEJM 307:1325, 1982)—avoid
Cycloserine	Increased CNS toxicity, dizziness, drowsiness
Diazepam	Increased diazepam levels—reduce diazepam dose
Disulfiram	Psychotic episodes, ataxia (Am J Psychol 125:1725, 1969)—avoid
Enflurane	Possible nephrotoxicity—avoid
Ethionamide	Increased CNS toxicity
Food	Decreased absorption INH

Continued

Drug	Effect of interaction
Itraconazole	Decreased itraconazole levels
Ketoconazole	Decreased ketoconazole levels—avoid
Phenytoin	Increased phenytoin toxicity
Rifampin, rifabutin	Possible increased hepatic toxicity
Theophylline	Increased theophylline levels
Tyramine (foods and fluids rich in tyramine)	Palpitations, sweating, urticaria, headache, vomiting, and hypertension with consumption of cheese, wine, some fish (rare reaction to monoamine-rich foods) (Lancet 2:671, 1985)
Vincristine	Increased neurotoxicity

Itraconazole (inhibits cytochrome P-450)

Drug	Effect of interaction
Alprazolam	Increased sedation—avoid
Antacids	Decreased itraconazole absorption
Astemizole	Ventricular arrhythmias—avoid
Carbamazepine (Tegretol)	Decreased itraconazole levels
Cisapride	Ventricular arrhythmias—avoid
Contraceptives	Decreased contraceptive effect
Coumadin	Increased hypoprothrombinemia
Cyclosporine	Increased cyclosporine levels with nephrotoxicity
ddI	Reduced itraconazole absorption
Digoxin	Increased digoxin levels
Felodipine	Increased felodipine with edema
Food	Increased itraconazole absorption: Give with meal
H_2 antagonists, antacids, omeprazole	Decreased itraconazole absorption—avoid
Hypoglycemics, oral	Severe hypoglycemia
INH	Decreased itraconazole levels
Loratadine	Increased loratadine levels with cardiac arrhythmia
Lovastatin	Large increase in lovastatin levels with possible rhabdomyolysis (NEJM 333:664, 1995)
Midazolam	Increased midazolam levels—avoid
Nifedipine	Increased nifedipine with edema
Phenobarbital	Decreased itraconazole levels
Phenytoin	Decreased itraconazole levels
Protease inhibitors	Increased level of saquinavir and indinavir
Rifampin, rifabutin	Decreased itraconazole levels (CID 18:266, 1994)
Seldane (terfenadine)	Ventricular arrhythmias—avoid
Tacrolimus	Increased tacrolimus levels—monitor levels
Triazolam	Increased triazolam effect—avoid
Sucralfate	Decreased itraconazole absorption
Sulfonylureas	Increased sulfonylurea with hypoglycemia

Ketoconazole (inhibits cytochrome P-450)

Drug	Effect of interaction
Alcohol	Possible disulfiram-like reaction
Alprazolam	Increased alprazolam with increased sedation
Anticoagulants, oral	Increased hypoprothrombinemia
Astemizole	Increased astemizole levels—avoid

Continued

Drug	Effect of interaction
Chlordiazepoxide	Increased chlordiazepoxide toxicity
Cisapride (Propulsid)	Ventricular arrhythmias—avoid
Contraceptives	Decreased contraceptive effect
Corticosteroids	Increased methylprednisolone levels
Cyclosporine	Increased cyclosporine levels
ddI	Decreased ketoconazole level—give ≥2 hr apart
Food	Decreased absorption: take 1–2 hr before or after meal
H_2 antagonists, antacids, omeprazole	Decreased ketoconazole effect; use sucralfate or antacids given 2 hr before
Hypoglycemics, oral	Severe hypoglycemia
Indinavir	Increase indinavir levels 70%
Isoniazid	Decreased ketoconazole levels (NEJM 311:1681, 1984) —avoid
Loratadine (Claritin)	Increased loratadine levels
Midazolam	Increased midazolam levels—avoid
Phenobarbital	Reduced ketoconazole levels
Phenytoin	Altered metabolism of both drugs; increased phenytoin levels and decreased ketoconazole levels
Rifampin, rifabutin	Decreased levels of both drugs—avoid
Ritonavir	Increased ritonavir levels
Saquinavir	Increased saquinavir levels by 150% (often desired)
Seldane (terfenadine)	Ventricular arrhythmias—avoid
Sucralfate	Possible decreased ketoconazole effect
Tacrolimus	Possible tacrolimus toxicity
Theophylline	Increased theophylline levels
Triazolam	Increased triazolam toxicity—avoid
Linezolid	
Phenylpropanolamine	Risk of hypertension
Pseudoephedrine	Risk of hypertension
Tyramine > 100 mg/d	Risk of hypertension
Mebendazole	
Phenytoin and carbamazepine	Decreased mebendazole concentrations; clinically significant only for extraintestinal helminthic infections
Mefloquine	
Beta-adenergic blockers	Increased risk of cardiac toxicity including cardiac arrest —avoid
Chloroquine	Increased risk of seizures
Halofantrine	QT prolongation—avoid
Quinidine	Increased risk of cardiac toxicity including cardiac arrest —avoid
Quinine	Increased risk of cardiac toxicity including cardiac arrest —avoid
Meropenem	
probenecid	Increases meropenem levels 40%—avoid

Continued

Drug	Effect of Interaction
Metronidazole	
Alcohol	Disulfiram-like reaction (flushing, headache, nausea $\pm$ vomiting, and chest/abdominal pain)
Anticoagulants, oral	Increased hypoprothrombinemia
Barbiturates	Decreased metronidazole effect with phenobarbital
Cimetidine	Possible increased metronidazole toxicity—avoid
Corticosteroids	Decreased metronidazole levels
Disulfiram	Organic brain syndrome (NEJM 280:1482, 1969)—avoid
Fluorouracil	Transient neutropenia
Food	Food often reduces gastric irritation
Lithium	Lithium toxicity—monitor lithium levels (JAMA 257:3365, 1987)
Phenobarbital	Decreased metronidazole levels—double metronidazole dose if phenobarbital is essential (NEJM 305:529, 1983)
Miconazole	
Aminoglycosides	Possible decreased tobramycin levels
Anticoagulant, oral	Increased hypoprothrombinemia
Hypoglycemics	Severe hypoglycemia with sulfonylurea
Phenytoin	Increased phenytoin toxicity
Nalidixic acid	
Anticoagulants, oral	Increased hypoprothrombinemia
Nitrofurantoin	
Antacids	Possible decreased nitrofurantoin effect; give 6 hr apart
Food	Increases absorption
Probenecid	Decreased nitrofurantoin effect (for UTIs)
Nitazoxanide	None known; caution with oral anticoagulant
Anticoagulant (oral)	Caution—may increase anticoagulant effect
Oseltamivir	
probenecid	Increases levels of oseltamivir
Penicillins	
Allopurinol	Increased frequency of rash with ampicillin
Anticoagulants, oral	Decreased anticoagulant effect with nafcillin and dicloxacillin
Cephalosporins	Increased cefotaxime toxicity with mezlocillin + renal failure
Contraceptives	Possible decreased contraceptive effect with ampicillin or oxacillin
Cyclosporine	Decreased cyclosporine effect with nafcillin and increased cyclosporine toxicity with ticarcillin
Food	Decreased absorption of oral ampicillin, cloxacillin, oxacillin, dicloxacillin, and penicillin G
Lithium	Hypernatremia with ticarcillin
Methotrexate	Possible increased methotrexate toxicity
Probenecid	Increased concentrations of penicillins

Continued

Drug	Effect of interaction
Pentamidine	
Aminoglycosides	Increased nephrotoxicity
Amphotericin B	Increased nephrotoxicity
Capreomycin	Increased nephrotoxicity
Foscarnet	Increased nephrotoxicity
Piperazine	
chlorpromazine	Possibly induces seizures
Polymyxin or colistimethate	
Aminoglycoside	Increased nephrotoxicity; increased neuromuscular blockade
Neuromuscular blocking agents	Increased neuromuscular blockade
Vancomycin	Increased nephrotoxicity
Pyrazinamide	
allopurinol	Failure to decrease hyperuricemia—avoid
Pyrimethamine	
Antacids	Possible decreased pyrimethamine absorption
Dapsone	Agranulocytosis reported
Kaolin	Possible decreased pyrimethamine absorption
Phenothiazines	Possible chlorpromazine toxicity
Quinolones (see fluoroquinolones)	
Quinupristin-dalfopristin (inhibits cytochrome P-450 3A4) (Synercid)	
Cyclosporine	Increased cyclosporine levels—63% (monitor cyclosporine levels)
Midazolam	Increased midazolam levels—33%
Nifedipine	Increased nifedipine levels
Terfenadine	Increased terfenadine levels—44%
(other drugs metabolized by cytochrome P-450 3A4: Astemizole, diazepam, verapamil, diltiazem, lovastatin, cisapride, protease inhibitors, carbamazepine quinidine)	
Ribavirin	
ddI	Increased intracellular ddI with risk of pancreatitis, neuropathy, or lactic acidosis—avoid
AZT, 3TC, ABC	Possible in vitro antagonism; significance not known
Rifabutin: Presumed to be identical to rifampin except for clarithromycin and fluconazole, both of which increase rifabutin levels and increase risk of uveitis. Effect on cytochrome P-450 is somewhat less than rifampin. Rifabutin should not be given concurrently with saquinavir; dose with indinavir should be reduced by 50%	
Rifampin (induces cytochrome P-450)	
Aminosalicylic acid (PAS)	Decreased effectiveness of rifampin; give in separate doses by 8–12 hr
Amprenavir	Reduced amprenavir levels
Anticoagulants	Decreased hypoprothrombinemia

Continued

Drug	Effect of interaction
Atovaquone	Decreased atovaquone levels
Barbiturates	Decreased barbiturate levels
Beta-adrenergic blockers	Decreased beta-blocker levels
Chloramphenicol	Decreased chloramphenicol levels
Clofazimine	Reduced rifampin levels
Clofibrate	Decreased clofibrate levels
Contraceptives	Decreased contraceptive levels (JAMA 227:608, 1974)
Corticosteroids	Decreased corticosteroid levels (Arch Intern Med 154:1521, 1994); if used together—increase corticosteroid dose
Cyclosporine	Decreased cyclosporine levels—avoid
Dapsone	Decreased dapsone effect (not significant with treatment of leprosy)
Delavirdine	Reduced delavirdine levels
Diazepam	Decreased diazepam levels
Digitalis	Decreased digitalis levels
Disopyramide	Decreased disopyramide levels—avoid
Doxycycline	Decreased doxycycline levels
Efavirenz	Efavirenz can be used with rifampin in standard doses for both drugs
Estrogens	Decreased estrogen effect—use alternative method of birth control
Fluconazole	Decreased fluconazole levels
Food	Decreased absorption
Haloperidol	Decreased haloperidol levels
Hypoglycemics	Decreased hypoglycemic effect of sulfonylurea
Isoniazid	Increased hepatotoxicity
Ketoconazole*	Decreased effect of ketoconazole and rifampin—avoid
Methadone	Methadone withdrawal symptoms
Mexiletine	Decreased antiarrhythmic levels
Nevirapine*	Combination not recommended
Nifedipine	Decreased antihypertensive effect
Nisoldipine	Decreased nisoldipine antihypersensitive effect
Phenytoin	Decreased phenytoin levels
Progestins	Decreased norethindrone levels
Protease inhibitors	Ritonavir and ritonavir + saquinavir can be used with standard doses; other protease inhibitors should be avoided
Quinidine	Decreased quinidine levels
Theophyllines	Decreased theophylline levels
Triazolam	Decreased triazolam levels (Br J Clin Pharmacol 42:249, 1997)
Trimethoprim	Decreased trimethoprim levels
Trimetrexate	Decreased trimetrexate levels
Verapamil	Decreased verapamil levels

Continued

Drug	Effect of interaction
Rifaximin	Induces P450 (CYP 3A4) in vitro but no apparent effect in vivo (minimal absorption)

Sulfonamides

Drug	Effect of interaction
Anticoagulants, oral	Increased hypoprothrombinemia
Barbiturates	Increased thiopental levels
Digoxin	Decreased digoxin levels with sulfasalazine
Food	Decreased absorption
Hypoglycemics	Increased hypoglycemic effect of sulfonylurea
Methotrexate	Possible increased methotrexate toxicity
Monoamine oxidase inhibitors	Possible increased phenelzine toxicity with sulfisoxazole
Phenytoin	Increased phenytoin levels except with sulfisoxazole

Telithromycin (inhibitor of P450 (CYP 3A4)

Drug	Effect of interaction
Anticoagulants (oral)	Potentiation of anticoagulation—monitor INR
Atorvastatin	Increased atorvastitin levels with risk of myopathy
Cisapride	Prolonged QTc interval—Avoid
Digoxin	Increased digoxin levels
Itraconazole	Increased telithromycin levels
Ketoconazole	Increased telithromycin levels
Lovastatin	Increased lovastatin levels with risk of myopathy
Metoprolol	Increased AUC of metoprolol
Midazolam	Increased midazolam levels, monitor and adjust dose if necessary
Pimozide	Prolonged QTc interval—Avoid
Rifampin	Decreased AUC of telithromycin
Simvastatin	Increased simvastatin levels with risk of myopathy
Sotalol	Decreased AUC of sotalol
Theophylline	Increased GI intolerance

Tetracyclines

Drug	Effect of interaction
Alcohol	Decreased doxycycline effect in alcoholics
Antacids	Decreased tetracycline effect with antacids containing Ca^{++}, Al^{++}, Mg^{++}, and $NaHCO_3$ (give 3 hr apart)—avoid
Anticoagulants, oral	Increased hypoprothrombinemia
Antidepressants, tricyclic	Localized hemosiderosis with amitriptyline—avoid
Antidiarrheal agents	Agents containing kaolin and pectin or bismuth subsalicylate decrease tetracycline effect
Barbiturates	Decreased doxycycline effect (Br Med J 2:470, 1974)—avoid
Bismuth subsalicylate, Pepto-Bismol	Decreased tetracycline effect
Carbamazepine (Tegretol)	Decreased doxycycline effect—avoid
Contraceptives, oral	Decreased contraceptive effect—avoid
Digoxin	Increased digoxin level (10% of population)

Continued

Drug	Effect of interaction
Food (dairy products)	Decreased absorption (except doxycycline)
Iron, oral	Decreased tetracycline effect (except with doxycycline) and decreased iron effect; give 3 hr before
Laxatives	Agents containing Mg^{++} decrease tetracycline effect
Lithium	Increased lithium toxicity—monitor levels (J Clin Psychopharmacol 17:59, 1997)
Methotrexate	Possible increased methotrexate toxicity
Methoxyflurane anesthesia, Penthrane	Possibly lethal nephrotoxicity
Milk	Decreased absorption of tetracycline. Does not apply to doxycycline or minocycline—avoid
Molindone	Decreased tetracycline levels
Phenformin	Decreased doxycycline levels—avoid
Phenytoin	Decreased doxycycline levels
Rifampin	Possible decreased doxycycline levels
Theophylline	Possible increased theophylline toxicity
Zinc	Decreased tetracycline levels—avoid
Thiabendazole	
Theophyllines	Increased theophylline toxicity
Trimethoprim	
Amantadine	Increased levels of both drugs
Azathioprine	Leukopenia
Contraceptives	Decreased contraceptive effect—two case reports (Br J Clin Pharmacol 25:527, 1988)
Cyclosporine	Increased nephrotoxicity
Dapsone	Increased levels of both drugs; increased methemoglobinemia
Digoxin	Possible increased digitalis levels
Phenytoin	Increased phenytoin levels
Rifampin	Decreased trimethroprim levels
Thiazide diuretics	Possible increased hyponatremia with concomitant use of amiloride with thiazide diuretics
Trimethoprim-sulfamethoxazole	See trimethoprim
Amantadine	Amantadine toxicity with delirium (Am J Med Sci 298:410, 1992)
Anticoagulants, oral	Increased hypoprothrombinemia
Atovaquone	Slight decrease in TMP-SMX levels
Contraceptives	Decreased contraceptive effect—five case reports (Br J Clin Pharmacol 25:527, 1988)
Mercaptopurine	Decreased mercaptopurine activity—avoid
Methotrexate	Megaloblastic anemia—avoid
Paromomycin	Increased nephrotoxicity
Phenytoin	Increased phenytoin toxicity
Procainamide	Increased procainamide levels

Continued

Drug	Effect of interaction
Tricyclic antidepressants	Recurrence of depression
	Possible imipramine toxicity
	Desipramine toxicity
Trimetrexate	
Acetaminophen	Increased trimetrexate levels
AZT	Increased bone marrow suppression
Cimetidine	Increased trimetrexate levels
Erythromycin	Increased trimetrexate levels
Fluconazole	Increased trimetrexate levels
Ketoconazole	Increased trimetrexate levels
Rifampin, rifabutin	Decreased trimetrexate levels
Valacyclovir	
Cimetidine	Increased acyclovir levels
Probenecid	Increased acyclovir levels
Valganciclovir	
Myelosuppressive drugs	Increased risk of anemia, neutropenia, and thrombo-cytopenia
Probenecid	Increased ganciclovir levels
Vancomycin	
Aminoglycosides	Increased nephrotoxicity and possible increased ototoxicity
Amphotericin B	Increased nephrotoxicity
Cisplatin	Increased nephrotoxicity
Digoxin	Possible decreased digoxin effect
Neuromuscular blocking agents	Increased succinylcholine and vecuronium effect
Paromomycin	Increased nephrotoxicity
Polymyxin	Increased nephrotoxicity
Voriconazole (Drugs that induce cytochrome P-450 enzymatic activity reduce voriconazole activity; drugs that inhibit cytochrome P-450 increase toxicity. Voriconazole inhibits cytochrome P-450 enzymes)	
Astemizole	Risk ventricular arrhythmia—avoid
Barbiturates	Increase barbiturate levels—avoid long acting barbiturates
Benzodiazepines	Anticipated prolonged sedative effect—avoid midazolam, triazolam, and alprazolam
Calcium channel blockers	May increase calcium channel blocker level—monitor for toxicity
Cisapride	Risk ventricular arrhythmias—avoid
Cyclosporine	Risk nephrotoxicity—use half cyclosporine dose and monitor levels
Ergot	Risk ergotism
Pimozide	Risk ventricular arrhythmias—avoid
Quinidine	Risk ventricular arrhythmias—avoid

Continued

Drug	Effect of interaction
Rifampin	Reduce voriconazole levels—avoid
Rifabutin	Reduce voriconazole levels—avoid
Sirolimus	Risk sirolimus toxicity—avoid
Statins	Anticipated increase in statin levels—consider lower statin dose
Tacrolimus	Increase tacrolimus levels—reduce dose to $\frac{1}{3}$ and monitor
Warfarin	Increase prothrombin time 2×—monitor prothrombin time

PREVENTIVE TREATMENT

A. ADULT IMMUNIZATION SCHEDULE

MMWR 2004;53:Q1–4

Vaccine	19–49 yrs	50–64 yrs	>65 yrs
Tetanus, diphtheria	Booster dose every 10 yrs		
Influenza	Medical, occupational, or household contact indication	Annual dose	
Pneumovax	Medical indication		1 dose or revaccination at 5 yrs
Measles, rubella, Mumps	1 dose if no documented prior dose or other evidence of immunity		
Varicella	2 doses (0 and 4–8 wks) if susceptible (see below)		
Hepatitis A	2 doses (0, 6–12 mo) for indications (see below)		
Hepatitis B	3 doses (0, 4, and 6 mo) for indications (see below)		

Note: The only true contraindications to vaccinations are a history of severe allergic reaction after a prior dose or a vaccine constituent. Severely immunocompromised persons should not receive live virus vaccines. (MMWR 2002;51 RR-2:8)

Common mistakes which are not contraindications

1. Mild illness ± fever
2. Local reaction ± fever with prior vaccination
3. Current antimicrobial therapy
4. Convalescent phase of illness
5. Fever <40.5°C

B. VACCINES AVAILABLE IN UNITED STATES

MMWR 2002;51(RR-2)

Vaccine (Type)	Indications (adults)	Route and usual regimen[a] and cost
Anthrax vaccine adsorbed (AVA) (inactivated vaccine)	Military; persons considered high risk for inhalation anthrax	0.5 mL SC × 6 doses: 0, 2, 4 wks, then 6, 12 & 18 mo.
BCG (bacillus of Calmette-Guérin) (Live bacteria)	No longer advocated	Percutaneous of 0.2–0.3 mL
Cholera (Inactivated bacteria)	Not recommended by WHO, but sometimes required for international travel	0.5 mL SC × 2 >1 wk apart or intradermal 0.2 mL × 2

Continued

Vaccine (Type)	Indications (adults)	Route and usual regimen[a] and cost
DT (tetanus diphtheria) (Toxoids) Aventis 800-822-2463	Primary series if not given previously Booster q10 yrs Injury Travelers: If risk diphtheria high Pregnant women with last dose > 6 yrs	Primary series: 0.5 mL IM at 0, 1–2 mo & 6–12 mo. Boosters: 0.5 mL q10 yrs Injury $10/dose
DTP (diphtheria, tetanus, pertussis) (Toxoids and inactivated bacteria; Td or DT preferred for adults)		0.5 mL IM
eIPV (inactivated polio-virus vaccine) (Enhanced inactivated viruses of all three serotypes)	Travel to epidemic areas and immunocompromised patient or household contact Note: Polio is eradicated in Western hemisphere	0.5 mL SC × 1
Haemophilus influenzae B conjugate (HbCV) (Polysaccharide conjugated to protein)	Adult at risk—splenectomy	0.5 mL IM × 1
HB (hepatitis B) Inactive viral antigen (surface antigen) Recombivax HB (Merck) Energix (GSK) Twinrix (GSK) (See below)	All infants and children by age 18 yrs Increased risk: Public safety workers exposed to blood; health care workers; injection drug users; gay men; household/sex contacts pos for HBsAg; dialysis patients, hemophilia patients; multiple sex partners	Energix-B 20 mcg (1 mL) at 0, 1 and 6 mo or 0, 1, 2 & 6 mo (more rapid immunity) 2nd and 3d dose must be separated by > 2 mo for both vaccines Recombivax HB 10 mcg (1 mL) at 0, 1 & 6 mo; Recombivax HB 40 mcg (1 mL) at 0, 1 & 6 mo for dialysis pts and possibly other immuno-compromised pts. Onset protection = 1 mo post 3rd dose

Vaccine (Type)	Indications (adults)	Route and usual regimen[a] and cost
		Infant born to HBsAg pos mother: HBIG + HBV vaccine Recombivax HB $71/10 mcg and /40 mcg Energix B $55/20 mcg
Hepatitis A (Inactivated virus with 1440 ELISA units/mL) Havrix (SKB) VAQTA (Merck)	Travel to or work in endemic areas; gay men; injection drug users; chronic liver disease; HCV infection; persons with occupational risk (lab workers who handle HAV)	1 mL IM (deltoid mm) + booster dose at 6–12 mo Havrix—$59/dose VAQTA—$63/dose
Hepatitis A and B Twinrix (GSK) Bivalent vaccine with 720 ELISA units HAV Ag (Havrix) and 20 mcg HBsAg (Energix-B).	Indications for HAV and HBV vaccine including travelers who can receive two doses before travel	1 mL IM at 0, 1, and 6 mo Twinrix—$92/dose
• Trivalent vaccine 2005–6: $H_1N_1/B/H_3N_2$ (Fugian strain) (Inactivated vaccine) Wyeth 800 934-5556 Park Davis 800-543-2111 Cannaught	Persons >50 yrs Residence in chronic care facilities Chronic illness (heart, lung, diabetes, immunosupp., sickle cell; splenectomy) Pregnancy—2nd & 3d trim Health care workers Alaskan natives, American Indians Travelers to S. Hem April Sept (high risk patients) Anyone who wants vaccine if suppy adequate	0.1 mL IM deltoid Mid Oct–Nov $4/dose
• FluMist (Live attenuated: the same 3 viruses)	Immunocompetent pts aged 5–49 yrs	Nasal administration $27/dose

Continued

Vaccine (Type)	Indications (adults)	Route and usual regimen[a] and cost
Japanese B encephalitis (Inactivated JE virus)	Travel >1 mo in epidemic area	1 mL SC at days 0, 7, and 30
Measles (Live virus)	Unvaccinated adults born after 1956 without measles; unless pos serology or documented vaccination— highest priority are women of childbearing potential, health care workers, international. travelers	0.5 mL SC × 1 with second >1 mo after first
Meningococcal vaccine (Bacterial polysaccharides of serotypes A/C/Y/W-135) Aventist 800-822 2463	Outbreaks of *N. meningitidis* serotype C disease; offer to college freshman in dormitories. Travel to epidemic area primarily Sub Saharan Africa during epidemics	0.5 mL SC × 1 $81/dose
MMR (M, measles; M, mumps; r, rubella) (Live viruses)	Usual form for persons susceptible to two of these viruses No link to autism found by IOM (BMJ 2001;322:1083)	0.5 mL SC × 1 or 2 with >1 mo after first
Mumps (Live virus)	Unvaccinated adults born after 1956 without mumps	0.5 mL SC × 1
OPV (oral poliovirus vaccine) (Live viruses of all three serotypes)	All-IPV schedule recommended in U.S. at 2, 4, 6–18 mos, 4–6 y per CDC-2000	po × 1
Pertussis (Inactivated whole bacteria)		IM—Distributed by Biologic Products Program, Michigan Department of Public Health (phone: 517-335-8120)
Pertussis (acellular) diphtheria (toxoid) tetanus (toxoid) (Boostrix, GSK)	Adolescents 16–18 yrs (FDA) Possible benefit with adult booster q10 yrs (Ann Intern Med 2005;142:832)	0.5 ml IM deltoid (age 10–18 yrs)
Plague (Inactivated bacteria)	Selected travelers to epidemic areas	1.0 mL IM, then 0.2 mL at 1 mo and 4–7 mo

Continued

Vaccine (Type)	Indications (adults)	Route and usual regimen[a] and cost
Pneumococcal vaccine (Capsular polysaccharides of 23 serotypes)	Age >65 yrs, chronic disease (heart, lung, cirrhosis, renal diabetes), CSF leak, compromised host including HIV, ≥2 weeks before splenectomy Native Alaskans, American Indians, functional asplenia Revaccinate at 5 yrs if chronic renal disease, immunosuppression, vaccinated <65 yrs and now >65 yrs	0.5 mL SC or IM $16/dose
Prevnar (7 valent conjugate vaccine for children)		0.5 mL IM (peds only)
Rabies Cell culture vaccines HDCV: Imovax 800-822-2463 Rabies vaccine absorbed: RVA 517-327-1500 PCEV: Rab Abert 800-247-7668	Exposure to potentially rabid animal. In US—bats are most likely source even without known bite. Developing countries— dogs are most likely source. Low probability US—dogs, cats, skunks, racoons, foxes & other carnivores	Postexposure prophylaxis 1 mL IM days 0, 3, 7, 14 & 28 (PCEV given intradermally) $700/series Preexposure prophylaxis: 1 mL 1D (PCEC) IM (HDCV or RVA) day 0, 7, 21 or 28 (3 doses)
Rubella (Live virus)	Unvaccinated adults without rubella	0.5 mL SC × 1
Tetanus (Toxoid)	TD preferred	0.5 mL IM × 1 $5/dose
Typhoid • Oral live attenuated Ty21 Vivotif Berna	Travelers to endemic areas, microbiologists Travel to areas endemic areas for typhoid—Peru, India, Pakistan, Chile or outbreaks	Vivotif—1 cap qod × 4 (empty stomach) starting 2 wks before travel Continued risk Revaccination at 5 yrs $38.50/series
• Polysaccharide IM Vaccine: Typhim V1 Aventist	As above	Ty21a—0.5 mL IM × 1 Continued risk: Revaccination at 2 yrs $49/dose

Continued

Vaccine (Type)	Indications (adults)	Route and usual regimen[a] and cost
Varicella (Live attenuated virus)	Susceptible adults (negative history of chickenpox ± negative serology) and risk category: Health care workers, household contacts of immunosuppressed patient, persons living or working in high-risk area (schools, day care centers), nonpregnant women of childbearing age, or international travelers	Adults: 0.5 mL SC × 2 separated by 4–8 wk $65/dose
Yellow fever (attenuated 17 D strain)	Travel to epidemic areas	0.5 mL SC × 1 $62/dose

[a]Assumes childhood immunizations have been completed

[b]Dt, tetanus and diphtheria toxoids for use in children aged <7 yr. Td, tetanus and diphtheria toxoids for use in persons aged ≥7 yr. Td contains the same amount of tetanus toxoid as DPT or DT but a reduced dose of diphtheria toxoid.

C. RECOMMENDATIONS BY RISK CATEGORY

Adapted from Guide for Adult Immunization, American College of Physicians, 3rd Edition, Philadelphia 1994:1–218; MMWR 2002;51(RR-2)

Category/vaccine	Comments
AGE	
18–24 yr	
Td[a] (0.5 mL IM)	Booster every 10 yr at mid-decades (age 25, 35, 45, etc) or single dose at midlife (age 50) for those who completed primary series
	Primary series (3 doses) if uncertain history of complete series[a]
Measles[b] (MMR, 0.5 mL SC × 1 or 2)	Post-high school institutions should require two doses of live measles vaccine (separated by 1 mo); first dose preferably given before entry
	Adults born after 1976 should have 2 doses of MMR if there is no documented immunization or evidence of immunity
Rubella[c] (MMR, 0.5 mL SC × 1)	Especially susceptible females; pregnancy now or within 3 mo postvaccination is contraindication to vaccination
Influenza	Advocated for young adults at increased risk of exposure (military recruits, students in dorms, etc) Indications listed for 25–64 yr olds apply here
Pneumococcal Vaccine	Indications for 25–64 yr olds apply here as well

Continued

Category/vaccine	Comments
Meningococcus 0.5 mL SC × 1	Military—new recruits Offer to college students—especially freshmen who live in close quarters (JAMA 2001;286:720; CID 2002;35:1376)
25–64 yr	
Td[a]	Booster every 10 yr Primary series (3 doses) if uncertain history of complete series
Influenza	<u>Medical indication:</u> Chronic heart or lung disease, diabetes, renal failure, hemoglobinopathy, pregnancy, immunosuppression <u>Occupational:</u> Healthcare worker or employee in chronic care facility <u>Miscellaneous:</u> anyone who wishes the vaccine
Pneumococcal vaccine	<u>Medical indication:</u> Pulmonary disorder other than asthma, diabetes, liver disease, renal disease, immunosuppression, cochlear implants <u>Geographic indications:</u> Alaskan natives and some American Indians, residents of nursing homes
Mumps[c]	As above
Measles[b] (MMR, 0.5 mL SC × 1)	Persons born after 1957—need positive serology or proof of vaccination
Rubella[c] (MMR, 0.5 mL SC × 1)	Principally females ≤45 yr of childbearing potential; pregnancy now or within 3 mo after vaccination is contraindication to vaccination
≥65 yr	
Td[a]	Booster every 10 yr
Influenza (0.5 mL IM)	Annually, usually in October–November
Pneumococcal (23 valent, 0.5 mL IM or SC)	Single dose; efficacy for elderly established for preventing invasive pneumococcal infection (bacteremia and meningitis) but not for preventing pneumonia (NEJM 2003;348:1737; NEJM 2003;348:1747) Revaccinate if >65 yrs and vaccinated > 5 yrs previously when <65 yrs
PREGNANCY	All pregnant women should be screened for hepatitis B surface antigen (HBsAg) and rubella antibody Live virus vaccines[d] should be avoided unless specifically indicated. It is preferable to delay vaccines and toxoids until 2nd or 3rd trimester. Immune globulins are safe; most vaccines are a theoretical risk only
Td[a] (0.5 mL IM)	If not previously vaccinated—dose at 0, 4 wk (preferably second and third trimesters) and 6–12 mo; protection to infant is conferred by placental transfer of maternal antibody

Continued

Category/vaccine	Comments
Measles	Risk for premature labor and spontaneous abortion; exposed pregnant women who are susceptible[b] should receive immune globulin within 6 days and then MMR post-delivery at least 3 mo after immune globulin (MMR is contraindicated during pregnancy)
Mumps	No sequelae noted; immune globulin is of no value, and MMR is contraindicated
Rubella	Rubella during first 16 wk carries great risk, e.g., 15–20% rate of neonatal death and 20–50% incidence of congenital rubella syndrome; history of rubella is unreliable indicator of immunity. Women exposed during first 20 wk should have rubella serology and if not immune should be offered abortion. Inadvertent vaccine administration to 300 pregnant women showed no vaccine-associated malformations
Hepatitis A	Immune globulin preferably within 1 wk of exposure
Hepatitis B	All pregnant women should have prenatal screening for HBsAg; newborn infants of HBsAg carriers should receive HBIG and HBV vaccine; pregnant women who are HBsAg negative and at high risk should receive HBV vaccine
Inactivated polio vaccine (0.5 mL po)	Advised if exposure is imminent in women who completed the primary series more than 10 yr ago. Unimmunized women should receive two doses separated by 1–2 mo; unimmunized women at high risk who need immediate protection should receive oral live polio vaccine
Influenza Pneumococcal vaccine	Not routinely recommended, but can be given if there are other indications
Varicella (VZIG, 125 units/10 kg IM; maximum 625 units)	Varicella-zoster immune globulin (VZIG) may prevent or modify maternal infection

FAMILY MEMBER EXPOSURE

Recommendations apply to household contacts

H. influenzae type B	*H. influenzae* meningitis: Rifampin prophylaxis for all household contacts in households with another child <4 yr; contraindicated in pregnant women
Hepatitis A	Immune globulin within 2 wk of exposure
Hepatitis B	HBV vaccine (three doses) plus HBV immune globulin for those with intimate contact and no serologic evidence of prior infection

Continued

Category/vaccine	Comments
Influenza A and B	With exposure to influenza A unimmunized high-risk family members should receive prophylactic amantadine, rimantadine, or oseltamivir (×14 days) and vaccine; prevention of influenza B requires oseltamivir or zanamivir
Meningococcal infection	Rifampin, ciprofloxacin, or ceftriaxone for close contacts of meningococcal meningitis
Varicella-zoster	No treatment unless immunocompromised or pregnant: consider VZIG

RESIDENTS OF NURSING HOMES

Influenza (0.5 mL IM)	Annually for staff and residents; vaccination rates of 80% required to prevent outbreaks; for influenza A outbreaks consider prophylaxis with amantadine or rimantadine
Pneumococcal (23 valent, 0.5 mL IM)	Single dose, efficacy not clearly established in this population
Td[a] (0.5 mL IM)	Booster dose at mid-decades

RESIDENTS OF INSTITUTIONS FOR MENTALLY RETARDED

Hepatitis B	Screen all new admissions and long-term residents: HBV vaccine for susceptible residents (seroprevalence rates are 30–80%)

PRISON INMATES

Hepatitis B	As above

HOMELESS

Td[a]	Most will need primary series or booster
Measles, rubella, mumps	MMR 0.5 mL SC (young adults)
Influenza	Annual
Pneumococcal vaccine (0.5 mL IM)	Give × 1

HEALTH CARE WORKERS

Hepatitis B (1.0 mL IM × 3)	Personnel in contact with blood or blood products; serologic screening with vaccination only of seronegatives is optional; serologic studies show 5% are non-responders (negative for anti-HBs) even with repeat vaccinations
Influenza (0.5 mL IM)	Annual usually in October–November
Rubella (MMR, 0.5 mL SC)	Personnel who might transmit rubella to pregnant patients or other health care workers should have documented immunity or vaccination

Continued

Category/vaccine	Comments
Mumps (MMR, 0.5 mL SC)	Personnel with no documented history of mumps or vaccine should be vaccinated
Measles (MMR, 0.5 mL SC)	Personnel who do not have immunity[b] should be vaccinated; those vaccinated in or after 1957 should receive an additional dose, and those who are unvaccinated should receive two doses separated by at least 1 mo; during outbreak in medical setting vaccinate (or revaccinate) all health care workers with direct patient contact
Polio	Persons with incomplete primary series should receive inactivated polio vaccine
Varicella	Personnel with negative history of chickenpox and/or negative serology (5–10% of adults have negative serology)

IMMIGRANTS AND REFUGEES

Td[a]	Immunize if not previously done
Rubella, measles, mumps (MMR 0.5 mL SC)	Most have been vaccinated or had these conditions, although MMR is advocated except for pregnant women
Polio	Adults will usually be immune
Hepatitis B	Screen for HBsAg and vaccinate susceptible family members and sexual partners of carriers; screening is especially important for pregnant women

HOMOSEXUAL MEN

Hepatitis B Hepatitis A	Prevaccination serologic screening advocated because 30–80% have serologic evidence of HBV markers

IV DRUG ABUSERS

Hepatitis B Hepatitis A	As above; seroprevalence rates of HBV markers are 50–80%

IMMUNODEFICIENCY

HIV infection

Measles	Vaccine is contraindicated. Postexposure prophylaxis with immune globulin for AIDS patients with CD4 count <200/mm³: Immune globulin—0.5 mL/kg IM (15 mL maximum)
Pneumococcal vaccine (0.5 mL SC)	*Recommended for patients with CD4 count > 200/mm³. Revaccination at 5 yr*
Influenza (0.5 mL IM)	*Annual*

Continued

Category/vaccine	Comments
Hepatitis A	All with HCV co-infection, chronic liver disease, HBsAg pos, IDU and MSM, (if seronegative), to HAV
Hepatitis B	All who have negative screening anti-HBc or anti-HBs
Asplenia	
Pneumococcal vaccine (0.5 mL IM)	Recommended, preferably given ≥2 wk before elective splenectomy; revaccinate those who received the 14 valent vaccine and those vaccinated >5 yr previously
Meningococcal vaccine (0.5 mL SC)	Indicated
H. influenzae B conjugate (0.5 mL IM)	Consider
Renal failure	
Hepatitis B (1.0 mL IM × 3)	For patients whose renal disease is likely to result in dialysis or transplantation; double dose and periodic boosters advocated
Pneumococcal vaccine (0.5 mL SC)	Give × 1
Influenza (0.5 mL IM)	Annual
Bone marrow transplant recipients	At 12 mo post-transplant: Revaccinate with inactivated vaccines including Td, hepatitis B, eIVP, _H. influenza_ type B, Pneumovax, and influenza; at ≥ 24 mo—MMR if not immunosuppressed and no graft-vs-host disease (see Vaccine Adults, CDC 3:1).
Alcoholics	
Pneumococcal vaccine (0.5 mL SC)	Give × 1
DIABETES AND OTHER HIGH-RISK DISEASES	
Influenza (0.5 mL IM)	Annually from October to December
Pneumococcal vaccine (0.5 mL SC)	Give × 1
TRAVEL[a] (recommendations of Med Lett Guidelines 2004;2:33; CDC Health Information for	For travelers to developed countries (Canada, Europe, Japan, Australia, New Zealand) the risk of developing vaccine-preventable disease is no greater than for those traveling in the U.S. Each country has its own vaccine requirements

Continued

Category/vaccine	Comments
International Travel 2004)	Smallpox vaccination is no longer required and should not be given
Yellow fever (0.5 mL SC) (see MMWR 1990; 39(RR6)) Single dose ≥10 days before travel Booster q10 yrs	Recommended and usually required for endemic area: Tropical South America and most of Africa between 15° North and 15° South. (CID 2002;34:1369) Available only at sites designated by local or state health departments (see www2.ncid.cdc.gov/travel/ yellowfever) Some African countries require certification of vaccination by all incoming travelers; some countries in Africa, South America, or Asia require certification of vaccination by travelers traveling from or through endemic areas Contraindications: Age <4 mo and hypersensitivity to eggs. Relative contraindications are pregnancy, age 4–9 months and immunosuppression (HIV, leukemia, lymphoma, generalized malignancy, cancer chemo-therapy, chronic steroid use) (MMWR 2002;51 RR-17:1; MMWR 2002;51:989) ACIP reported 7 cases of multiple organ failure in recipients of 17D derived yellow fever vaccine; all became ill within 2–5 days of vaccination and six died (MMWR 2001;50:643) (http://www.cdc.gov/ncidod/dvbid/yellowfever/index.htm).
Cholera	Risk is very low. Oral vaccine (Dukoral) is available in Europe (Chiron) and Canada (Aventist). Not currently recommended but consider for travelers who work in refugee camps
Typhoid fever (Typhim V1— single dose at >2 wks before travel or Vivotif Berna—4 oral doses qod beginning at least 1 wk before travel)	Recommended for travel to rural areas of countries where typhoid fever is endemic or any area of an outbreak, primarily travelers outside the usual tourist routes in Latin America, Asia, and Africa Live oral vaccine—Vivotif (1 cap every other day × 4 starting at least 2 wk before travel)—is preferred over the parenteral killed bacterial vaccine because of comparable efficacy, longer protection, and better tolerance (Lancet 1990;336:891); available from Berna Prod (800-533-5899). New polysaccharide vaccine (Typhim Vi, Connaught 800-822-2463) is also effective and requires only one IM dose (J Infect Dis 1992;25:63; MMWR 1994;43(RR-14); Clin Infect Dis 1995;4:186)
Hepatitis A Single dose Havrix ≥ 2 wks	Vaccine (Havrix, SmithKline Beecham; VAQTA, Merck) is recommended for travel outside U.S., Canada, Western Europe, Japan, Australia, or New Zealand.

Continued

Category/vaccine	Comments
before travel or Twinrix (see HBV comment)	(NEJM 2004;350:476) Twinrix (hepatitis A and B): see below and hepatitis B
	Protective levels of antibody are usually achieved 2–4 wk after a single dose. A booster is recommended at 6–12 mo, but a single dose is considered adequate protection if given at least 2–4 wk before travel.
	Immunity after 2 doses lasts >20 yrs (Lancet 2003;362:1065. Boosters are not recommended.
	Immune globulin (0.02 mL/kg IM) is available from 800-843-7477 and is occasionally recommended in addition to HAV vaccine for travelers who need full protection before 4 weeks.
	Serology to determine susceptibility is not recommended.
Hepatitis B (1 mL IM × 3) or Twinrix (see comment)	HBV vaccine if travel to endemic areas, and there is risk of need for medical or dental care, travel >6 mo, sexual contact with local persons is likely, frequent returns, live with the local population or if contact with blood is likely. Major risk areas are Africa, Asia, Middle East, Southern & Western Pacific Islands, tropical S. America and the Caribbean (Med Letter Guidelines 2004;2:33). (All of these are high risk areas for HAV as well)
	Accelerated schedule is dosing at 0, 1, and 2 mo with a fourth dose at 12 mo (FDA approved for Energix-B)
	Immunity is lifelong but 3–6% of adults do not respond
	Twinrix is available for patients at risk for HAV and HBV. At least two doses must be given prior to travel. Accelerated schedule is 0, 1, 3 weeks with 4th dose at 12 mo or 0, 1 & 2 weeks and 4th doses at least 6 months after the first
	Risk is low.
Rabies Imovax (Aventist) or RabAlvert (Chiron) given at 0, 7 and 21–28 days	Consider human diploid cell rabies vaccine (HDCV), rabies vaccine absorbed (RVA), or purified chick embryo cell vaccine (PCEC) for travelers with occupational risk and those with extended travel to endemic area (Africa, India, Asia, parts of S. Amer)
Japanese encephalitis (JE-Vax, 1 mL SC × 3 in 2–4 wk) with last dose >10 days before travel	Vaccine recommended endemic areas with stays of >1 mo in rural rice-growing areas with extensive exposure to mosquitoes. Potential problem countries include Bangladesh, Cambodia, Indonesia, Laos, Malasia, Myanmar (Burma), Pakistan, China, Korea, Taiwan, Thailand, Singapore, eastern Russia, Vietnam, India, Nepal, Sri Lanka, and the Philippines (NEJM 1988;319:641)

Continued

Category/vaccine	Comments
	JE Vax is Formalin-inactivated, purified, mouse-brain–derived vaccine that causes urticaria, angioedema, or other serious reactions in 0.5% of recipients (MMWR 1993;42(RR-1):12) JE Vax is given in 3 doses over 2–4 weeks; last dose should be 10 days before departure due to unpredictable allergic effects Attack rate is low: <10 cases in U.S. travelers over 1985–95 (CID 2002;35:183)

Influenza
  Single dose
  ≥2 wks before
  travel
	Indicated for consideration in high risk persons traveling to Southern Hemisphere April–September
	
	Vaccination does not protect against Avian influenza; travelers to endemic areas should avoid live poultry markets, farms, and avoid eating poultry unless well cooked (MMWR 2004;53:97)

Measles (MMR 0.5 mL SC × 1)	Susceptible persons[b] should receive a single dose of MMR before travel

Meningococcal
  vaccine with
  serogroups A, C, Y,
  and W 135 (0.5 mL
  SC × 1)
	Recommended for travel to areas of epidemics, most frequently the "meningitis belt" in sub-Saharan Africa from Senegal & Guinea eastward to Ethiopia from Dec. to June (CID 2002;34:84)
	
	Saudi Arabia requires certificate of vaccination for pilgrims to Mecca or Medina
	
	Vaccine is single dose (Menomune-Aventist) and provides protection for ≥3 yr

Polio
  Single dose IVP
  ≥4 weeks before
  travel
	Travelers to developing Africa or the Indian subcontinent or areas of outbreaks should receive a primary series and inactivated polio vaccine (IVP) if not previously immunized
	
	If protection is needed within 4 wk, single dose eIPV is recommended.

[a]Diphtheria and tetanus toxoids adsorbed (for adult use). Primary series is 0.5 mL IM at 0, 4 wk and 6–12 mo; booster doses at 10-yr intervals are single doses of 0.5 mL IM. Adults who have not received at least three doses of Td should complete primary series. Persons with unknown histories should receive series.

[b]Persons are considered immune to measles if there is documentation of receipt of two doses of live measles vaccine after first birthday, prior physician diagnosis of measles, laboratory evidence of measles immunity, or birth before 1957.

[c]Persons are considered immune to mumps if they have a record of adequate vaccination, documented physician diagnosed disease, or laboratory evidence of immunity. Persons are considered immune to rubella if they have a record of vaccination after their first birthday or laboratory evidence of immunity. (A physician diagnosis of rubella is considered nonspecific.)

[d]Live virus vaccines: measles, rubella, yellow fever, oral polio vaccine.

D. Specific Vaccines

1. INFLUENZA VACCINE

Recommendations of Advisory Committee on Immunization (MMWR 2005;54:1–40).

Preparations: Inactivated egg-grown viruses that may be split (chemically treated to reduce febrile reactions in children) or whole. The 2005–6 trivalent vaccine contains A/California/7/2004 (H3N2), A/New Caledonia/20/99 (H1N1) and B/Shanghai/361/2002. For A/Calif/7/2004 a manufacturer may use A/New York/55/2004 and for B/Shanghai/361/2002 they may use B/Jiangsu/10/2003.

Flu mist: This is the first nasally administered vaccine in the U.S. It consists of live viruses including two strains of influenza A and one strain of influenza B. This was FDA approved in June 2003 for use in persons 5–49 years; a single dose is advocated for persons 9–49 years, persons >50, those with medical conditions that constitute indications for the vaccine, and persons with immunosuppression should use standard influenza vaccine since FluMist is a live virus vaccine and has not been tested in high risk populations. The cost is $46/dose.

Administration (older than 12 yr): Whole or split virus vaccine, 0.5 mL × 1 IM in the deltoid muscle, preferably mid-October to mid-November. Recommendations for the 2003–04 season are for preferential immunization of high risk persons in October to assure an adequate supply for this group. The needle should be ≥1 inch. Protection begins 2 wk post-vaccination and may last 6 mo, but antibody titers may fall below protective levels within 4 mo in elderly patients.

Effectiveness: At least 70–90% effective in preventing influenza in healthy persons (MMWR 1993;42(RR-5):1, Drugs 1997;54:841) when there is a good match between the vaccine antigens and the prevalent strain(s) of influenza. This has been achieved in 13 of the last 15 seasons. In elderly nursing home residents, the vaccine is 30–40% effective in preventing influenza and up to 80% effective in preventing influenza-related mortality (JAMA 1985;251:1136). Population-based studies show influenza vaccinations of persons >65 years are associated with a 20–30% reduction in hospitalization for heart disease and pneumonia and a 50% reduction in all-cause mortality (NEJM 2003;348:1322).

Target Group for Influenza Vaccine

Note: This list defines the two categories that should have the highest priority for initial vaccination in the event that supplies are limited.

Groups at increased risk for influenza-related complications

1. Persons > 50 yrs
2. Residents of nursing homes and other chronic care facilities housing persons of any age with chronic medical conditions
3. Persons with chronic disorders of the pulmonary or cardiovascular system, including those with asthma

4. Adults and children who required regular medical follow-up or hospitalization during the prior year due to chronic metabolic diseases (diabetes), renal dysfunction, hemoglobinopathies, or immunosuppression (including HIV infection)
5. **Persons with any condition that can compromise respiratory function or handling of secretions and are at risk for aspiration. These include disorders of cognitive function, spinal cord injury and other neuromuscular diseases.***
6. Children and teenagers who are receiving long-term aspirin therapy (risk of Reye's syndrome)
7. Women who will be in the second or third trimester of pregnancy during influenza season
8. Elderly and other high-risk persons embarking on international travel: Tropics—all year; Southern Hemisphere—April–September

Groups that can transmit influenza to high-risk patients

1. **All healthcare workers (New emphasis in 2005)** who have contact with high-risk patients
2. Providers of home care to high-risk persons
3. Household family members of high-risk persons

Contraindications

1. Severe allergy to eggs
2. Persons with acute febrile illness (delay until symptoms abate); persons with minor illnesses such as URIs may be vaccinated
3. Pregnancy: There has been no significant excess in the influenza-associated mortality among pregnant women since the 1957–58 pandemic (Am J Obstet Gynecol 1959;78:1172). Influenza vaccine is not routinely recommended, but pregnancy is not viewed as a contraindication in women with other high-risk conditions. A study of more than 2000 pregnant women who received influenza vaccine showed no adverse fetal effects (Int J Epidemiol 1973;2:229). Some experts prefer to vaccinate in the second trimester to avoid a coincidental association with spontaneous abortions unless the first trimester corresponds to the influenza season

Adverse Reactions for Influenza Vaccine

1. Soreness at the vaccination site for up to 2 days in about one-third
2. Fever, malaise, etc—infrequent and most common in those not previously exposed to influenza antigens, e.g., young children. Reactions begin 6–12 hr postvaccination and persist 1–2 days
3. Allergic reactions—rare and include hives, angioedema, asthma, anaphylaxis; usually allergy to egg protein
4. Guillain-Barré syndrome: 1976–77 influenza vaccine was associated with a statistically significant risk of Guillain-Barré syndrome. A review of the influenza vaccine for 1992–93 and 1993–94 showed the odds ratio for Guillain-Barré with vaccination was 1.8; this represents a risk of 1–2 cases/1 million persons vaccinated (MMWR 1998;47(RR–6); NEJM 1998;339:1797)

* New category in 2005

2. RABIES PREVENTION

Recommendation of Advisory Committee on Immunization Practice (MMWR 1999; 48:(RR–1))

Experience: From 1980 to 1997 there were a total of 36 cases of human rabies in the U.S.—12 from dogs outside the U.S. and 21 from bats. Rabies in wildlife (primarily racoons, skunks, and bats) account for >85% of animal rabies in the U.S. The major animal source in Asia, Africa, and Latin America is dogs. Rabies is now rare in domestic animals in the U.S., although >80% of exposures that qualify for post-exposure rabies prevention treatment are dog and cat contacts (JAMA 2000;284:1001). **Greatest risk is bats including bat exposure with no clear bite; these account for all five rabies cases acquired in the U.S. from 1998–2000 (MMWR 2000;49:1111). A review of 26 cases of bat variant rabies indicated that only two were associated with known bat bites (CID 2002;35:738). The revised recommendations are for rabies prophylaxis for a bat bite, but also for situations where there is a reasonable possibility that a bite has occurred (MMWR 2002;51:828).** Rabies was transmitted to four organ transplant recipients from a single donor with enigmatic encephalitis in 2004 (MMWR 2004;53:33). There has never been a confirmed case of human-human transmission (MMWR 2004;53:33). There are 6 reported rabies survivors; none are known to be neurologically intact (Lancet 2004;363:595).

Rabies biologics

1. <u>Vaccines:</u> Neutralizing antibodies are produced in 7–10 days and persist ≥2 yr

Vaccine	Name	Source
Human diploid cell vaccine (HDCV) IM Intradermal	Imovax Rabies Imovax Rabies ID	Pasteur Merieux Connaught 800-822-2463
Rabies vaccine absorbed (RVA) IM	Rabies Vaccine Adsorbed (RVA)	Bio Port Corp 517-327-1500
Purified chick embryo cell vaccine (PCEC) IM	Rab Avert Rabipur	Chiron Corp 800-244-7668

2. <u>Rabies immune globulin</u> (RIG): Provides rapid passive immunity with a half-life of 21 days

Rabies immune globulin product	Source
Imogam Rabies-HT	Pasteur-Merieux Connaught 800-822-2463
BayRab	Bayer Corp 800-288-8370

Cost: AWP cost for five doses of any of the three vaccines is $735–$760; for rabies immune globulin the cost is about $700 for a 70-kg patient.

RABIES POSTEXPOSURE PROPHYLAXIS—UNITED STATES

Note: In reality, the major risk for rabies is from a dog bite that takes place in the developing world or a bat exposure (with or without a bite) in the U.S. These recommendations do not account for the latter experience.

Animal type	Evaluation and disposition of animal	Postexposure prophylaxis recommendations
Dogs and cats	Healthy and available for 10 days' observation	Should not begin prophylaxis unless animal develops symptoms of rabies[a]
	Rabid or suspected rabid	Immediate vaccination
	Unknown (escaped)	Consult public health officials
Skunks, raccoons, bats, foxes, and most other carnivores	Regarded as rabid unless animal proven negative by laboratory test[b]	Consider immediate vaccination
Livestock, small rodents and lagomorphs (rabbits and hares), large rodents (woodchucks and beavers), and other mammals	Consider individually	Consult public health officials. Bites of squirrels, hamsters, guinea pigs, gerbils, chipmunks, rats, mice, other small rodents, rabbits, and hares almost never require antirabies treatment

[a]During the 10-day holding period, begin postexposure prophylaxis at the first sign of rabies in the dog, cat, or ferret that has bitten someone. If animal exhibits clinical signs of rabies, it should be euthanized immediately and tested.

[b]Animal should be euthanized and tested as soon as possible. Holding for observation is not recommended. Discontinue vaccine if immunofluorescence test results of animal are negative.

RABIES POSTEXPOSURE TREATMENT SCHEDULE
MMWR 1998;47:4

Vaccination status	Treatment[a]
Not previously vaccinated	Local wound cleaning: Postexposure treatment should begin with immediate thorough cleansing of all wounds with soap and water. If available, a virucidal agent such as a povidone-iodine solution should be used to irrigate the wounds (J Am Acad Dermatol 1995;33:1019)
	RIG: 20 IU/kg body weight. If anatomically feasible, full dose should be infiltrated around wound and the rest should be given IM at a site distant from vaccine administration. RIG and vaccine should not be administered in the same syringe. Because RIG may partially suppress active production of antibody, no more than recommended dose should be given
	Vaccine: HDCV, RVA—1.0 mL or PCEC IM (deltoid area),[b] one each on days 0, 3, 7, 14, and 28

Continued

Vaccination status	Treatment[a]
Previously vaccinated[c]	Local wound cleaning: All post-exposure treatment should begin with immediate thorough cleansing of all wounds with soap and water. If available, a virucidal agent such as a povidone-iodine solution should be used to irrigate the wounds. RIG: RIG should **not** be administered Vaccine: HDCV, RVA, or PCEC 1.0 mL IM (deltoid area); one each on days 0 and 3

[a]Regimens are applicable for all age groups, including children.
[b]Deltoid area is the only acceptable site of vaccination for adults and older children. For younger children, the outer aspect of the thigh may be used. Vaccine should never be administered in gluteal area.
[c]Any person with a history of pre-exposure vaccination with HDCV, RVA, or PCEC; prior post-exposure prophylaxis with HDCV, RVA, or PCEC; or previous vaccination with any other type of rabies vaccine and a documented history of antibody response in the prior vaccination.

3. TETANUS-DIPHTHERIA ± PERTUSSIS VACCINE
Recommendations of Advisory Committee on Immunization Practices (MMWR 1991;40(RR-10))

Vaccine: Inactivated toxoid vaccine tetanus and diphtheria toxoids adsorbed (Td) are preferred to tetanus toxoid because most adults who need tetanus toxoid are susceptible to diphtheria (Mayo Clin Proc 1999;74:381). The primary series is 0.5 mL IM doses at 0 time, 1–2 mo, and 6–12 mo. Doses should not be repeated if the schedule is delayed. Booster doses are recommended at 10-yr intervals. A new vaccine: Tetanus toxoid, reduced diphtheria toxoid and acellular pertussis vaccine, adsorbed (Boostrix) was FDA approved in 2005. It is recommended for single dose administration for adolescents age 10–18 yrs. There is speculation that this will be the vaccine for boosting at 10 year intervals in adults (in place of DT) (Ann Intern Med 2005;142:832).

Cost: Td adsorbed, 0.5 mL—$9.75.

Susceptibility: Antigenic response to TD is good but is reduced in elderly patients. Current estimates are that 27% of U.S. persons >70 yr are unprotected against diphtheria and tetanus (NEJM 1995;332:761). Pertussis accounts for 12–32% of cough illnesses that last over 6 days or over 1 month according to 6 published studies (Ann Intern Med 2005;142:832). It is estimated that there are >1 million cases of pertussis/yr. in the US. (CID 2004;39:20)

Adverse reactions: Pain and tenderness at injection site; systemic reactions are rare. The frequency of local reactions increases with increases in the number of doses given.

Contraindications: Anaphylactic reaction or neurologic reaction to prior Td dosing. Persons with a history of an Arthrus reaction or fever >39.4°C should not receive Td more than once every 10 yr. Persons who report reactions to a "tetanus shot" before 1938 probably received equine antitoxin and can receive the current vaccine tetanus prophylaxis.

TETANUS PROPHYLAXIS
MMWR 1991;40(RR-12):1–94

History of	Clean, minor wounds		Other[b]	
tetanus toxoid	Td[a]	TIG[a]	Td[a]	TIG[a]
Unknown or <3 doses	Yes	No	Yes	Yes
≥3 doses[c]	No unless >10 yr since last dose	No	No, unless >5 yr since last dose	No

[a]Td. tetanus toxoid; TIG. tetanus immune globulin.

[b]Wounds contaminated with dirt, stool, soil, saliva, etc; puncture wounds; avulsions; from missiles, crushing, burns and frostbite.

[c]If only three doses of toxoid, a fourth should be given.

---

4. PNEUMOCOCCAL VACCINE
Advisory Committee on Immunization Practices, CDC (MMWR 1997;46(RR-8)).

Vaccine: 23 valent polysaccharide vaccine for the *S. pneumoniae* contains antigens responsible for 87% of bacteremic pneumococcal disease in the U.S. The 23 types (Danish nomenclature) follow: 1, 2, 3, 4, 5, 6B, 7F, 8, 9N, 9V, 10A, 11A, 12F, 14, 15B, 17F, 18C, 19A, 19F, 20, 22F, 23F, and 33F. Six serotype (6B, 9V, 14, 19A, 19F, 23F) account for most antibiotic resistance and are included in the vaccine. Most adults show a 2× rise in type-specific antibody at 2–3 wk after vaccination.

Efficacy: Seven systematic reviews of Pneumovax between 1994 and 2002 show no decrease in mortality or in rates of pneumococcal pneumonia in high risk patients (elderly or immunosuppressed) who are the target of current vaccine policies (see below) (BMJ 2002;325:292). A more recent report shows efficacy in reducing invasive pneumococcal disease (primarily pneumococcal bacteremia), but not pneumonia or pneumococcal pneumonia (NEJM 2003;348:1747)

Preparation and cost: Pneumovax (Merck Human Health) — $16/ dose.

Recommendations for adults:
1. Immunocompetent adults at increased risk of pneumococcal disease or its complications because of chronic illness (e.g., cardiovascular disease, pulmonary disease, diabetes, alcoholism, cirrhosis, or cerebrospinal fluid leaks) or who are ≥65 yr old. Current recommendations are to review risks for pneumococcal disease at the 50th birthday because 30–40% have medical conditions that merit vaccine.

2. Immunocompromised adults at increased risk of pneumococcal disease or its complications (e.g., splenic dysfunction or anatomic asplenia, lymphoma, Hodgkin's disease, multiple myeloma, chronic renal failure, nephrosis organ transplant recipients, HIV infection, and other conditions associated with immunosuppression).

3. Persons in special environments or social settings with identified risk of pneumococcal disease (Native Americans, homeless, etc).

4. Patients with HIV infection should be given vaccine early during disease for adequate antibody response.

Note: 1) Vaccine should be given at least 2 wk before elective splenectomy; 2) vaccine should be given as long as possible before planned immunosuppressive treatment; 3) hospital discharge is a convenient time for vaccination because two-thirds of patients with serious pneumococcal infections have been hospitalized within the prior 5 yr; 4) may be given simultaneously with influenza vaccine (separate injection sites).

Adverse reactions:

1. Pain and erythema at injection site: 50%.

2. Fever, myalgia, severe local reaction: <1%.

3. Anaphylactoid reactions: 5/million; severe reactions: Estimated frequency of anaphylactoid reactions is 5/million. A meta-analysis of 7531 pneumococcal vaccine recipients in nine trials showed no patients had severe fever or anaphylactic reactions. There have been no cases of Guillain-Barré syndrome. Arthrus reactions are more common with revaccination at <4 yr.

4. Frequency of severe reactions is increased with revaccination <13 mo after primary vaccination; severe reactions are no more frequent when revaccination occurs >4 yr after primary vaccination.

Revaccination: This is recommended at 5 yr for adults who are immunosuppressed or have asplenia and those who were <65 yr when first vaccinated. Frequency of local reactions is 3.3× higher with revaccination (JAMA 1999;281:243).

Pneumococcal conjugate vaccine (Prevnar): 7 valent conjugate vaccine with antigens for serotypes 4, 6B, 9V, 14, 18C, 19F, and 23F. These account for 80% of invasive pneumococcal disease in children <6 yr in the U.S. Use is currently restricted to pediatrics.

---

5. VARICELLA VACCINE
Recommendations of Advisory Committee on Immunization Practice (MMWR 1996;45(RR-11); MMWR 1999;48(RR-6))

Morbidity in adults: Approximately 5–8% of adults are susceptible; about 75% of adults with a negative history for chickenpox have antibody indicating prior exposure (JAMA 1991;266:2724). Chickenpox is more severe in young adults; risks are greatest in pregnant and immuno-compromised hosts (Ann Intern Med 1980;93:414).

Zoster vaccine: The VA Cooperative Study #403 examined the efficacy and safety of a more patent varicella vaccine (0.5 mL of live attenuated Oka/Merck VZV vaccine in a controlled trial with 38,546 immunocompetent adults ≥60 yrs. (NEJM 2005;352:2271). Results showed a 51% reduction in the frequency of zoster and a reduction in symptoms in those who got zoster including postherpetic neuralgia.

Vaccine: VARIVAX—live attenuated virus vaccine (for prevention of varicella)

Note: Vaccine must be stored frozen at $< -15°C$ to maintain potency. Once reconstituted it must be used within 30 min

Dose: Adult—0.5 mL SC $\times$ 2 separated by 4–8 wk

Cost: $65.40/dose

Efficacy: Seroconversion rate in adults is 78% with one dose; 99% with two doses. Protection at 7–10 yr is 70–90% against infection and 95% against severe disease. Impact in rates of zoster is unknown. It is speculated that reactivation of the vaccine strain causes mild disease and boosted immunity (Nature Med 2000;6:451). There are reports of vaccine failure that are expected to occur more frequently as the period of time from vaccination increases (NEJM 2002;347:1909). A concern is the possible confusion with smallpox (NEJM 2002;347:1962)

Indications: Susceptible adults in rank order are in the following categories (Ann Intern Med 1996;124:35).

1. Health care workers
2. Susceptible household contacts of immunosuppressed persons
3. Persons living or working in areas where transmission of VZV is likely—teachers of young children, day care employees, staff members in institutional settings
4. Young adults in closed or semiclosed populations—military personnel, college students, inmates and staff of prisons and jails
5. Nonpregnant women of childbearing potential
6. International travelers
7. Adolescents or adults living in households with children

Cost effective analysis: Serologic testing in adults and vaccinating seronegatives would be cost effective only for those 20–29 yr. Assumptions were cost of vaccination—$78, cost of serology—$20, cost for outpatient treatment of chickenpox—$80 plus acyclovir at $124 (Am J Med 2000;108:723)

Contraindications:

1. Pregnancy or this possibility within 1 mo
2. Immunosuppressed patients
3. Miscellaneous: Active tuberculosis; persons who have received blood products within 6 mo (passive immunity precludes antibody response); persons with anaphylactic reactions to gelatin or neomycin

Adverse reactions:

Fever >100°F: 10%
Local reaction at injection site: 30% in 0–2 days
Varicella-like rash at injection site: In 6–20 days reported in 37/100,000 vaccine doses; 3% in clinical trials

120

Generalized varicella rash: 10% in 7–21 days; this usually consists of <10 lesions fasting ≥3 days and may be source of VZV transmission to susceptible contacts

Transmission: Transmission of the vaccine strain is a theoretical risk but is documented in only three cases out of 15 million vaccine doses distributed; all three were mild (MMWR 1999;48(RR-6)).

Post-exposure prophylaxis: Should be given within 3 days of exposure. Comparative cost and efficacy with other postexposure strategies follow:

Strategy	Time from exposure	Cost	Efficacy
Vaccine	3 days	$40	70–90%
Acyclovir 40–80 mg/kg	7–9 days	$120	80–85%
ZIG 625 units IM	4 days	$400	90%

6. HEPATITIS B VACCINE

MMWR 1987;36:353–366; MMWR 1987;37:342–351; MMWR 1991;40(RR-13); Guide for Adult Immunization, American College of Physicians 3rd Edition, 1994:74–83; NEJM 1997; 336:196; Mayo Clin Proc 1997;74:377; MMWR 1999;48:33; MMWR 2001;50(RR-1)

Vaccine preparations

1. Recombivax HB (Merck & Co): Recombinant vaccine produced by *Saccharomyces cerevisiae* (baker's yeast) and available since July 1986; 10 or 40 μg HBsAg/mL; usual adult dose is three 1-mL doses (10 μg) at 0, 1, and 6 mo; three 1-mL doses (40 μg) for dialysis patients
2. Engerix-B (Glaxo SmithKline): Recombinant vaccine available since 1989; 20 μg HBsAg/mL; usual adult dose regimen is three 1-mL doses (20 μg) at 0, 1, and 6 mo; alternative schedule is four 1-mL doses (20 μg) at 0, 1, 2, and 12 mo (for more rapid induction of immunity)
3. Twinrix (Glaxo SmithKline): bivalent vaccine with Havrix (HAV vaccine, 720 ELISA units/ml) + Engerix-B (20 μg HBsAg/ml); usual adult regimen is 3 1 mL doses at 0, 1, and 6 mo.

Cost: Recombivax HB @ $57/dose (10 μg); Engerix-B @ $55/dose (20 μg); Twinrix @ $92/dose for HAV and HBV)

Adverse reactions: Injection site reactions in up to 20%. Systemic reactions are uncommon; anaphylaxis is rare, but epinephrine should be available for immediate use. Fever is reported in 1–6% of HBV vaccine recipients. Hypersensitivity to yeast and to thimerosal are contraindications to HBV vaccine. HBV vaccine appears to play no role in the etiology or relapses of multiple sclerosis (NEJM 2001;344:319; NEJM 2001;344:327)

Pre-exposure vaccination:

1. Regimen. Three IM doses (deltoid) at 0 time, 1 mo, and 6 mo; 0, 2 and 4 mo; or 0, 1, and 4 mo. There must be ≥4 wk between dose #1 and #2, ≥8 wk between dose #2 and #3, and >4 mo between #1 and #3. If series is delayed, start where you left off. Usual adult dose is 1 mL (20 μg Engerix B or 10 μg Recombivax HB); hemodialysis

patients and possibly other immunocompromised patients should receive 2–4 × the usual adult dose (usually 40 μg doses of either recombinant vaccine preparation). HBV deposited into fat rather than muscle results in lower seroconversion rates, so needle length is important. Needles for all men and for women 60–90 kg should be 2.5 cm, for women >90 kg should be 3.8 cm, and for women <60 kg should be 1.6 cm (JAMA 1997;277:1709).

2. <u>Response rate</u>. >95% of young, healthy adults develop adequate antibody response (>10 mIU/mL). Non-response is greater with age over 40 yr, with certain HLA haplotypes, smoking history, obesity, HIV infection, hemodialysis, and accelerated schedule (JAMA 1993;270:2935); response rates are 50–70% in persons with HIV infection; 60–70% with renal failure; 70–80% in diabetics; and 60–70% with chronic liver disease. Age-related response rates show >95% seroconversion rates in 20-yr-olds, 86% in 40-yr-olds, and 47% in persons >60 yr (Am J Prev Med 1998;15:73). A meta-analysis of 24 studies with 11,037 vaccine recipients showed a continuous risk of non-response above 30 years. (CID 2002;35:1368). This review also showed that a booster dose substantially improved the response rate. If the schedule is interrupted it may be resumed with good results providing the second and third doses are separated by ≥2 mo.

3. <u>Post-vaccination serologic testing</u>. Recommended for some persons whose subsequent clinical management depends on this knowledge (e.g., health care workers, dialysis patients, infants born to HBsAg-positive mothers) and for vaccine recipients who have decreased response rates: Age >30 yr, renal failure, HIV infection, diabetes, and chronic liver failure. When done, test at 1–6 mo after last dose. Studies in Taiwan show serologic titer decrease of about 10% per year, but efficacy persists (JID 2003;187:134).

4. <u>Revaccination</u>. Revaccination based on measurements of serologic response is controversial. One point-of-view is that persons at risk, including health care workers, should have periodic antibody measurements with boosters if levels are below 10mIU/mL (Arch Intern Med 1999;159:1481). The contrary view from the ACIP is that antibody levels do not measure immunologic memory and that immunologic protection lasts more than 12 yr regardless of antibody levels (Clin Microbiol Rev 1999;12:351; Arch Intern Med 2000;160:3170). If done, revaccination of nonresponders will produce response in 15–25% with one additional dose and in 30–50% with three doses (Ann Intern Med 1982;97:362). 13–60% of responders lose detectable antibody within 9 yr. New ACIP recommendations include routine postvaccination serologic testing for healthcare workers, patients with HIV infection and hemodialysis patients. Response is defined as HBsAb levels of >10 mIU/mL (MMWR 2001;50:RR-1) Testing is done at ≥1 month after the 3rd dose.

5. <u>Prevaccination serologic testing</u>. Testing groups at highest risk is usually cost-effective if the prevalence of HBV markers is >20% (see table below). Routine testing usually consists of one antibody test: Either

anti-HBc or anti-HBs. Anti-HBc fails to detect persons immune from prior vaccination and anti-HBs (only) will falsely identify HBsAg as susceptible. Average wholesale price of three-dose vaccine regimen is $165–$213; usual cost of serologic testing for anti-HBs or anti-HBc is $12–$20.

Prevalence of Hepatitis B Serologic Markers

Population group	HBsAg (%)	Any marker (%)
Immigrants/refugees from areas of high HBV endemicity	13	70–85
Alaska/Pacific Islands natives	5–15	40–70
Clients in institutions for the developmentally disabled	10–20	35–80
Users of illicit parenteral drugs	7	60–80
Sexually active homosexual men	6	35–80
Household contacts of HBV carriers	3–6	30–60
Patients of hemodialysis units	3–10	20–80
Health-care workers—frequent blood contact	1–2	15–30
Prisoners (male)	1–8	10–80
Staff of institutions for developmentally disabled	1	10–25
Heterosexuals with multiple partners	0.5	5–20
Health-care workers—no or infrequent blood contact	0.3	3–10
General population (NHANES II)		
Blacks	0.9	14
Whites	0.2	3

6. <u>Side effects</u>. Pain at injection site (3–29%) and fever >37.7°C (1–6%). Note: These side effects are no more frequent than in placebo recipients in controlled studies. Experience in more than 4 million adults shows rare cases of Guillain-Barré syndrome with plasma-derived vaccine and no serious side effects with recombinant vaccines. Adverse reactions should be reported to 800-822-7967.
7. <u>Vaccine efficacy</u>. 80–95% for preventing HBV infection in gay men and virtually 100% if protective antibody response (≥10 mIU/mL) is achieved.

Candidates for pre-exposure vaccination:
<u>All infants and children by the age of 18 yr</u>
<u>Persons with occupational risk</u>
    Now defined by the Occupational Safety and Health Administration, these include health care workers and many public service workers. For persons in health care fields, vaccination should be completed during training before students encounter blood
<u>Persons with lifestyle risk</u>
    Heterosexual persons with multiple partners (more than one partner in the preceding 6 mo) or any sexually transmitted disease, homosexual and bisexual men, injecting drug users
<u>Special patient groups</u>
    Hemophiliac persons
    Hemodialysis patients

Environmental risk factors

Household and sexual contacts of HBV carriers, clients and staff of institutions for the developmentally disabled, prison inmates, immigrants and refugees from areas where HBV is highly endemic, international travelers to HBV endemic areas who are health care workers, who will reside there more than 6 mo, or who anticipate sexual contact with local persons

Pregnant women (MMWR 1991;40(RR-13)): Risk of HBV transmission from HBsAg-positive pregnant woman to infant is 10–85% depending on HBeAg status. Perinatal infection has a 90% risk of chronic HBV infection and 25% mortality due to liver disease—cirrhosis or hepatocellular carcinoma. Children who do not acquire HBV perinatally are at increased risk for person-to-person spread during the first 5 yr. Over 90% of these infections can be prevented using active and passive immunizations. Recommendations follow.

1. All pregnant women should be tested for HBsAg during an early prenatal visit
2. Infants born to HBsAg-positive mothers should receive HBIG (0.5 mL) IM × 1 (preferably within 12 hr of delivery) and HB vaccine (0.5 mL) IM × 3 (5 µg Recombivax or 10 µg Engerix-B) at 0 time (concurrent with HBIG) at 1–2 mo, and at 6 mo. Test infants for HBsAg and antiHBs at 12–15 mo
3. Infants of HBsAg-negative mothers and children <11 yr should receive routine vaccination with three doses of Recombivax (2.5 µg) or Engerix-B (10 µg)

Postexposure vaccination: (MMWR 1991;40(RR-13)):

Acute exposure to blood: Occupational exposure
Definition of exposure is percutaneous (needlestick, laceration, or bite) or permucosal (ocular or mucous membrane) exposure to blood. Recommendations depend on HBsAg status of source and vaccination/vaccine response of exposed person.
Note: HBIG, when indicated, should be given as soon as possible, and value beyond 7 days post-exposure is unclear.

RECOMMENDATIONS FOR POSTEXPOSURE PROPHYLAXIS FOR PERCUTANEOUS OR PERMUCOSAL EXPOSURE TO HEPATITIS B, UNITED STATES

| Exposed person | Treatment when source is | | |
	Hepatitis B surface antigen positive	Hepatitis B surface antigen negative	Source not tested or unknown
Unvaccinated	HBIG; × 1[a] and initiate HB vaccine**	Initiate HB vaccine[b]	Initiate HB vaccine[b]
Previously vaccinated known responder	Test exposed for anti-HBs 1. If adequate,[c] no treatment 2. If inadequate, HB vaccine booster dose	No treatment	No treatment

Continued

	Treatment when source is		
Exposed person	Hepatitis B surface antigen positive	Hepatitis B surface antigen negative	Source not tested or unknown
Known nonresponder	HBIG × 2 or HBIG × 1 plus 1 HB vaccine dose	No treatment	If known high-risk source, may treat as if source were HBsAg positive
Response unknown	Test exposed for anti-HBs 1. If inadequate,[c] HBIG × 1 + HB vaccine booster dose 2. If adequate, no treatment	No treatment	Test exposed for anti-HBs 1. If inadequate, HB vaccine booster dose 2. If adequate, no treatment

HBIG, hepatitis B immunoglobulin.

[a]HBIG dose 0.06 mL/kg IM.

[b]For HB vaccine dose, see p 121.

[c]Adequate antiHBs is 10 SRU by radioimmunoassay or positive by enzyme immunoassay (MMWR 1993;42:707).

[d]Antibody to hepatitis B surface antigen.

POST-EXPOSURE IMMUNOPROPHYLAXIS WITH OTHER TYPES OF EXPOSURES
(MMWR 40(RR-13):9, 1991)

Type of exposure	Immunoprophylaxis	Comments
Perinatal (HBsAg-positive mother)	HBIG + vaccination	HBIG + vaccine within 12 hr of birth
Sexual contact— acute HBV	HBIG (0.06 mL/kg) ± vaccination	HBIG efficacy 75%; all susceptible partners should receive HBIG and start vaccination within 14 days of last exposure; testing susceptibility with anti-HBc recommended if it does not delay prophylaxis >14 days. Vaccination is optimal if exposed person is not in a high-risk category and sex partner is HBsAg negative at 3 mo
Sexual contact— chronic carrier (HBsAg × 6 mo)	Vaccination[a]	
Household contact— acute HBV	None unless there is sexual contact or blood exposure (sharing toothbrushes, razors, etc)	With known exposure; HBIG plus vaccination
Household contact— chronic carrier (HBsAg × 6 mo)	Vaccination[a]	

[a]1 mL IM × 3 at 0, 1, and 6 mo.

7. SMALLPOX VACCINATION

Recommendations for Using Smallpox Vaccine in a Pre-Event Vaccination Program: Supplemental Recommendations of the Advisory Committee on Immunization Practices (ACIP) and the Healthcare Infection Control Practices Advisory Committee (HICPAC) [CDC MMWR 2003;52:RR-7]:

Vaccination Method: The bifurcated needle is inserted into the vaccine vial to obtain a small droplet of vaccine which is delivered with 2–3 punctures (primary vaccination) or 15 punctures (revaccination) with sufficient force to allow a trace of blood after 15–20 seconds.

Normal Response: Most of the local reaction and significant complications occur at 5–15 days after vaccination, which corresponds with the time of viral replication and the immune response. Adverse events are much less frequent with revaccination and are most common in older perons who have not been vaccinated for decades or those with cellular immune deficiencies. With primary vaccination, the maximal inflammation and induration occurs at 6–8 days with a pustule, ulcer, or scab. Revaccination in a highly immune person may cause a lesion similar to that seen with a positive Tine test, and full resolution may occur at day three with nothing evident at 6–8 days. This may reflect good immunity or poor technique; it is called "equivocal response" and requires revaccination.

Contact vaccinia: Vaccinia virus can be recovered from the vaccination site from the time of the papule (2–5 days after vaccination) until the scab separates (14–21 days after vaccination); maximal shedding is at 4–14 days after vaccination and might be of shorter duration with revaccination.

Nosocomial transmission of vaccina: This has rarely been described and the majority of cases involve direct person-to-person transmission; the 2003 experience with 24,000 healthcare workers who received smallpox vaccination and continued to provide patient care showed no nosocomial transmission.

Contraindications: The vaccine is contraindicated in potential recipients with the following conditions or household contacts with these conditions: (1) history of eczema or atopic dermatitis; (2) other acute, chronic, or exfoliative skin conditions including burns, impetigo, varicella-zoster, HSV, severe acne or psoriasis; (3) immunosuppression (HIV, leukemia, lymphoma, generalized malignancy, solid organ transplantation, cellular or humoral immunodeficiencies or therapy with alkylating agents, antimetabolites, radiation, or high dose steroids); (4) pregnancy; and (5) persons with coronary artery disease. The vaccine is contraindicated for potential recipients (but not household contacts) who are breast-feeding, are less than one year of age (not recommended for persons under 18 years), and those who are allergic to a vaccine component.

Pregnancy: The risk is small but fetal vaccinia is serious. During 1932–72, there were 20 affected pregnancies; 18 in vaccine recipients and 2 with contact vaccinia. Of the 20 pregnancies, 7 occurred during the first trimester and 13 occurred in the second trimester; only one of the 20 pregnancies was maintained to term and three survived. The vaccine is contraindicated in women who are pregnant or plan pregnancy within four weeks. A urine pregnancy test should be available on the day scheduled for vaccination. Inadvertent vaccination during pregnancy or pregnancy within four weeks should not be used as reason to terminate pregnancy.

HIV infection: There has been one reported case of disseminated vaccinia in a patient with AIDS. There were also 732 recruits vaccinated between 1981 and 1985 who subsequently had positive serology in 1985–88 without known consequences. This gives a frequency of serious adverse events in this population of 0.14%. The 2003 military experience included inadvertent vaccination of 10 HIV-infected recruits with CD4 counts $> 300/mm^3$; all had "takes" and none had complications. Vaccination is not recommended with HIV infection; mandatory HIV testing is not recommended, but the test should be available.

Major Adverse Events: (See Ann Intern Med 2003;138:488)

1. Encephalitis: Develops at 5–15 days after primary vaccination. The mortality rate is about 25%, residual sequelae are noted in 25%, the virus is rarely detected in brain or CSF, natural history is completed in two weeks, it is not progressive and is managed with supportive care only. This is more common in children under one year of age and accounts for the delay in vaccination to the second year of life per a policy in the mid 1960s.

2. Progressive vaccinia: In the 1960s, this was most common in persons with leukemia or agammaglobulinemia. At present, the greatest concerns are for people with HIV, organ transplants, cancer chemotherapy, and other iatrogenic immunosuppressive disorders. The complication is characterized by continued viral replication with continuous enlargement and metastasis. Treatment is with VIG and possibly cidofovir.

3. Eczema vaccinatum: The condition is characterized by widespread vaccinal lesions in patients with eczema or history of eczema. This complication in the 1960s was more common with contact vaccinia than a complication in vaccine recipients due to exclusion of these patients for immunization. Treatment is with VIG, which reduces the mortality rate from 10% to about 1% with supportive care similiar to that given to burn victims.

4. Accidental implantation: This occurs when patients touch the vaccination site and then touch another anatomical site. The greatest concern is ocular involvement; about 6% with vaccinia in the eye develop vaccinal keratitis. VIG is controversial because of animal studies that suggest an antigen-antibody cause.

5. Fetal vaccinia: This complication is exceedingly rare. Pregnant women exposed to smallpox should be vaccinated because smallpox is associated with a mortality rate in pregnant women of up to 90% and fetal wastage nearly 100%.

6. <u>Cardiac</u>: Myocarditis at 1–3 weeks postvaccination. Most common with primary vaccination in white men in 20's; all military recruits with this complication in 2003 recovered without sequelae. Ischemic cardiac events (14 cases) and dilated cardiomyopathy (4 cases) were noted in the 2003 experience with about 500,000 vaccinations but were probably unrelated.

Treatment of Adverse Events: Clinical trials with VIG or any other antiviral agent have not been done with humans. Cidofovir may be used because of its in vitro activity against vaccinia.

EXPERIENCE WITH SMALLPOX VACCINATION IN 2003

The following table summarizes the adverse events encountered with vaccination of 450,293 military recruits in 2003 (JAMA 2003;289:3278)

	Reactions n = 450,293	Rate/ million	Historic Rate/ million
Mild/temporary			
Generalized vaccinia	36	80	45–212
Erythema multiforme	1	—	—
Inadvertent self inoculation	48	107	606
Contact vaccinia	21	47	8–27
Moderate-serious			
Encephalitis	1	2.2	2.6–8.7
Progressive vaccinia	0	0	1.5
Eczema vaccination	0	0	38
Myocarditis	37	82	100*

*Based on Finnish military recruit study. Acta Med Scand 1983;213:65.

8. MENINGOCOCCAL VACCINE (see p 130)

Continued

E. Immune Globulins

RECOMMENDED TREATMENT

(Adapted from Guide for Adult Immunization, American College of Physicians, 3rd Edition, Philadelphia, 1994:86; and MMWR 1994;43(RR-1), pp 5, 177)

Infection	Indication	Preparation	Recommendation
Botulism	Treatment and prophylaxis of ingestion of botulism toxin	Equine Ab types A, B, and E	CDC: 404-639-3670
CMV	Treatment and prophylaxis of CMV in transplant recipients	CMV-IVIG	150 mg/kg IV <72 hr, 100 mg/kg at 2, 4, 6, 8 wk; 50 mg/kg 12 and 16 wk
		or IVIG*	2–6 g over 10–12 wk
Diphtheria	Early diphtheria	Diphtheria antitoxin	20,000–120,000 units IM or IV depending on location and severity of disease Connaught 800-822-2463
Hepatitis A	Family and sexual contacts Outbreaks: Institutional or day care Travelers to developing countries	Immune globulin*	0.02 mL/kg IM up to 2 mL Travel—0.02 mL/kg for travel <3 mo; 0.06 mL/kg for >3 mo
Hepatitis B	Percutaneous or mucosal exposure Sexual contacts with HBsAg carriers or acute HBV infection	HBIG*	0.06 mL/kg IM ×1, then vaccinate with HBV vaccine
Measles	Nonimmune contacts of acute cases <6 days previously	Immune globulin*	0.25 mL/kg IM up to 15 mL healthy host 0.50 mL/kg IM up to 15 mL immunocompromised host
Rabies	Exposure to rabid or potentially rabid animal	HRIG*	20 IU/kg IM Connaught 800-822-2463
Tetanus	Significant exposure unimmunized	TIG*	250 units IM (prophylaxis)
	Clinical tetanus	TIG*	3000–6000 units (therapy)
Vaccinia	Severe reaction to vaccinia vaccination	VIG*	CDC 404-639-3670
Varicella-zoster	Immunosuppressed or newborn contact	VZIG*	125 units/10 kg IM up to 625 units Available from state health departments

*Human antibodies.

F. RECOMMENDATIONS FOR USE OF VACCINES IN IMMUNOCOMPROMISED HOST

Recommendation of the Advisory Committee on Immunization Practices of the CDC (MMWR 2004;53:Q1; Clin Micro Rev 1998;11:1)

Vaccine	Routine (not immuno-compromised)[a]	HIV infection/AIDS	HIV[a] response with CD4 <200	Organ transplantation, chronic immuno-suppressive therapy, severely immuno-compromised[b]	Asplenia	Renal failure, alcoholism, alcoholic cirrhosis, and diabetes	Pregnancy
Td	Recommended	Recommended	Reduced	Recommended	Recommended	Recommended	Recommended
MMR(MR/M/R)[c]	Use if indicated	Contraindicated	Poor	Contraindicated	Use if indicated	Use if indicated	Contraindicated
Hepatitis B	Use if indicated	Recommended[d]	Reduced	Use if indicated	Use if indicated	Use if indicated[c]	Use if indicated
Pneumococcal	Recommended if ≥65 yr old	Recommended with CD4 >200	Poor	Recommended	Recommended	Recommended	Use if indicated
Meningococcal	Use if indicated	Use if indicated	No data	Use if indicated	Recommended	Use if indicated	Use if indicated
Influenza	Recommended if ≥65 yr old	Recommended	Poor	Recommended	Recommended	Recommended	Recommended
Varicella	Use if indicated	Contraindicated	No data	Contraindicated	Use if indicated	Use if indicated	Contraindicated

[a]Non-routine vaccines:

Contraindicated vaccines for organ transplant recipients, chronic medication induced immunosuppression (alkylating agents, radiation, chronic prednisone, anti-metabolites), severe immunosuppression (congenital immunodeficiency, AIDS, leukemia, lymphoma, aplastic anemia or generalized malignancy): BCG, OPV, smallpox, typhoid TY21a, and yellow fever.

Use if indicated in above population: eIPV, cholera, plague, typhoid, inactivated rabies, anthrax

Patients with renal failure, alcoholism; cirrhosis or asplenia may receive the following vaccines if indicated: BCG, OPV, smallpox, typhoid TY21a, yellow fever, cholera, plague, rabies, anthrax

[b]Severe immunosuppression can be the result of congenital immunodeficiency, HIV infection, leukemia, lymphoma, generalized malignancy, or therapy with alkylating agents, antimetabolites, radiation, or large doses of corticosteroids.

[c]See discussion of MMR.

[d]Patients with renal failure on dialysis or HIV infection should have their anti-HBs response tested after vaccination, and those found not to respond should be revaccinated with three doses.

PROPHYLACTIC ANTIBIOTICS IN SURGERY:
Based on the consensus statement of the Surgical Infection Project from the CDC, Centers for Medicare and Medicaid with experts in infection control, surgical infection & epidemiology (Clin Infect Dis 2004;38:1706)

Table 1: Principles of Surgical Infection Prevention

Issue	Consensus position
Antibiotic timing	Infusion of abx should begin within 60 minutes before initial surgical incision
Duration	Discontinue within 24 hours after end of surgery
Dosing	Initial dose based on body weight or body mass index. Second intra-operative dose if surgery exceeds 2 half lives of abx
Betalactam allergy	History should be adequate. The alternative is skin testing.

Table 2: Dose and timing of second dose (usually when surgery exceeds 2 half lives)

Agent	Standard dose	Maximum adult dose	Half life (hr) Nl renal	Renal failure
Aztreonam	1 gm	2 gm	1.5–2	6
Ciprofloxacin	400 mg	400 mg	3.5–5	5–9
Cefazolin	1–2 gm	>80 kg–2 gm	1.2–2.5	40–70
Cefuroxime	1.5 gm	50 mg/kg	1–2	15–22
Cefoxotin	1–2 gm	20–40 mg/kg	.5–1.1	6.5–23
Cefotetan	1–2 gm	20–40 mg/kg	2.8–4.6	13–25
Clindamycin	600–900 mg	3–6 mg/kg	2–5.1	3.5–5.0
Erythro base	1 gm	9–13 mg/kg	0.8–3	5–6
Gentamicin	1.5 mg/kg	1.7 mg/kg	2–3	50–70
Neomycin	1 gm	20 mg/kg	—	—
Metronidazole	0.5–1 gm	15 mg/kg	6–14	7–21
Vancomycin	1 gm	10–15 mg/kg	4–6	40–400

Table 3: Recommendations by surgical procedure

Adapted from Med Lett 2001;43:93; Clin Infect Dis 2001;33 Suppl 2:578; Arch Intern Med, 2003;163:972; Clin Infec Dis 2002;35:26; NEJM 1986;315:1129–1138; Rev Infect Dis Suppl 1991;10, 13:S779; Mayo Clin Proc 1992;67:288; Clin Proc 1992;67:288; CID 1992;15:S 313; Arch Surg 1993;128:79; and Antibiotic Guidelines, Johns Hopkins Hospital 2005

Type of surgery	Preferred regimen*	Alternative	Comment
CARDIOTHORACIC			
Cardiovascular, coronary bypass, valve surgery	Cefazolin 1–2 g IV pre-op ± q4h intraop*, or Cefuroxime 1.5 g IV pre-op ± q6h intraop	Vancomycin 1 g IV pre-op infused over 60 min** Clindamycin 600–900 mg IV	Likely pathogens: *S. epidermidis, S. aureus, Corynebacterium*, Gram-negative bacilli. Single doses are as effective as multiple doses provided high serum concentrations are maintained throughout the procedure (Eur J Clin Microbiol Infect Dis 1994;13:1033). Main benefit is reduced rates of wound infections Some recommend a second dose at time of removal from bypass
Pacemaker insertion, defibrillator implant	Cefazolin 1–2 g IV pre-op*	Vancomycin 1 g IV pre-op infused over 60 min**	Likely pathogens: As above Meta-analysis of 7 controlled studies showed prophylaxis reduced infections associated with pacemaker implantation (Circulation 1998;97:1796)
Peripheral vascular surgery, abdominal aorta, and legs or any procedure involving a prosthesis including coronary stents and grafts for hemodialysis	Cefazolin 1–2 g IV pre-op	Vancomycin 1 g pre-op infused over 60 min** ± gentamicin Clindamycin 600–900 mg IV	Likely pathogens: *S. aureus, S. epidermidis*, Gram-negative bacilli, clostridia. Prophylaxis recommended for procedures on abdominal aorta and procedures on leg that include groin incision or amputation for ischemia and any vascular procedure involving a prosthesis (Scand J Infect Dis 1998;30:547) Many use prophylaxis with any vascular prosthetic material

Continued

Type of surgery	Preferred regimen	Alternative	Comment
Carotid or brachial artery	None		
Thoracic surgery: Lobectomy, pneumonectomy	Cefazolin 1–2 g IV pre-op **or** Cefuroxime 1.5 g IV pre-op	Vancomycin 1 g IV pre-op infused over 60 min** or Clindamycin 600 mg IV pre-op	Efficacy of prophylaxis antibiotics is not established [RID 1991;13 (Suppl 10):S869]. Some studies show decreased rates of wound infection but no reduction in pneumonia or empyema
GASTROINTESTINAL			
Esophageal dilatation or sclerotherapy	Cefazolin 1–2 g IV pre-op	Cefoxitin 1–2 g IV pre-op Clindamycin 600 mg IV pre-op	Likely pathogens: Gram-negative bacilli, Gram-positive cocci, anaerobes Antibiotic prophylaxis common practice, but proof of efficacy is lacking
Gastric surgery (high risk only)	Cefazolin 1–2 g IV pre-op	Clindamycin 600 mg IV + gentamicin 1.7 mg/kg	Likely pathogens: Enteric Gram-negative bacilli, Gram-positive cocci. Prophylaxis advocated for high risk that is usually due to reduced gastric acidity or motility—obstruction, treatment with H_2-blocker or proton pump inhibitor, hemorrhage, gastric cancer, gastric bypass and morbid obesity. Prophylaxis is usually given for percutaneous gastrostomy but efficacy not established (Gastroenterol 2000;95:3133) Prophylactic antibiotics are not indicated for uncomplicated duodenal ulcer surgery (Ann Intern Med 1987;107:824)
Biliary tract (high risk only) ERCP: See comment	Cefazolin 1–2 g IV pre-op	Gentamicin 1.7 mg/kg pre-op × 1 or q8h × 3	Likely pathogens: Enteric Gram-negative bacilli, enterococci, clostridia. Traditionally advocated only for high risk—acute cholecystitis, obstructive jaundice, nonfunctioning gallbladder, common duct stones, or age >70 yr.

Continued

Type of surgery	Preferred regimen	Alternative	Comment
			Meta-analysis of 42 studies showed benefit to high-risk and low-risk patients (Br J Surg 1990;77:283).
			ERCP—one study showed benefit of 1–3 piperacillin doses in patients with cholestasis (CID 1995;20:1236)
			Laparoscopic cholecystectomy: Prophylactic antibiotics are not indicated (Arch Surg 1999; 65:226; Arch Surg 1999;134:611)
Colorectal	Neomycin 1 g po and erythromycin 1 g po at 1 PM, 2 PM, and 11 PM the day before surgery (19,18, and 11 hr pre-op) ± cefoxitin 2 g IV or cefotetan 2 g IV	Cefoxitin 1–2 g IV Cefotetan 1–2 gm IV Cefazolin 1–2 gm IV plus metronidazole 0.5 gm IV Betalactam allergy: Clindamycin 600–900 mg + gentamicin 1.5 mg/kg, aztreonam 1–2 gm, ciprofloxacin 400 mg or levofloxacin 750 mg Metronidazole 0.5–1 gm + gentamicin 1.5 mg/kg ciprofloxacin 400 mg or levofloxacin 750 mg	Likely pathogens: Enteric Gram-negative bacilli, anaerobes. Many U.S. surgeons use both an oral and a parenteral prep plus bowel cleansing (Dis Colon Rectum 1990;33:154). Although this is not recommended (Can J Surg 2002;45:173) Oral prep with metronidazole + neomycin or kanamycin is probably as effective as erythromycin + neomycin [RID 1991;13 (Suppl 10):815)
Penetrating trauma abdomen	Cefoxitin 1–2 g IV immediately, then q6h or cefotetan 1–2 g IV q12h or clindamycin 900 mg IV + gentamicin 1.7 mg/kg immediately, then q8h	Ticarcillin-clavulanate or piperacillin-tazobactam or combination of an aminoglycoside + metronidazole	Likely pathogens: Enteric Gram-negative bacilli, anaerobes. Patients with intestinal perforation should receive these agents for 2–5 days. Most studies use suboptimal doses of aminoglycosides [RID 1991; 13(Suppl 10):S847]. If laparotomy shows no bowel injury, one dose is adequate

Continued

Type of surgery	Preferred regimen	Alternative	Comment
Appendectomy	Cefoxitin 1–2 g IV pre-op or cefotetan 1–2 g IV	Metronidazole 1 g IV or clindamycin 600 mg IV ± gentamicin 1.7 mg/kg	Likely pathogens: Enteric Gram-negative bacilli, anaerobes. For perforated or gangrenous appendix continue regimen for 3–5 days. For nonperforated appendix 1–4 doses are adequate [RID 1991; 13(Suppl 10):S813]
Laparotomy, lysis of adhesions, splenectomy, etc without GI tract surgery	None		
GYNECOLOGY AND OBSTETRICS			
Vaginal and abdominal hysterectomy	Cefazolin 1–2 g IV pre-op or Cefotetan 1–2 g IV pre-op or Cefoxitin 1 g IV pre-op	Metronidazole 0.5–1 gm IV Clindamycin 600–900 mg + gentamicin 1.5 mg/kg, aztreonam 1–2 gm, ciprofloxacin 400 mg or levofloxacin 750 mg	Likely pathogens: Enteric Gram-negative bacilli anaerobes, group B streptococci, enterococcus. Efficacy of prophylaxis is established for vaginal and abdominal hysterectomy (Infect Dis Obstet Gynecol 2000;8:230) Single dose appears to be as effective as multiple doses.
Cesarean section	Cefazolin 1 g IV after clamping cord	Cefoxitin 2 g IV or cefotetan 2 g IV or clindamycin 900 mg IV or metronidazole 0.5 g IV after clamping cord	Likely pathogens as above. Greatest benefit is with high risk C-sections: procedures done after ROM or onset of labor and emergency procedures. In the US, give antibiotics after clamping cord
Abortion (first trimester, high risk only)	First trimester: Doxycycline 100 mg po before and 200 mg po 30 min after or aqueous penicillin G 2 mil units IV	Metronidazole 500 mg po × 3 doses in perioperative period	Likely pathogens as above. Efficacy shown for first and second trimester abortions (Drugs 1991;41:19) and high-risk patients—prior PID, gonorrhea, or multiple sex partners.

Continued

135

Type of surgery	Preferred regimen	Alternative	Comment
	Second trimester: Cefazolin 1 g IV		For patients with *N. gonorrhoeae* or *C. trachomatis*, treat STD with minimum delay in abortion (Am J Obstet Gynecol 1984;150:689)
			A meta-analysis showed benefit with prophylaxis for all therapeutic abortions (Obstet Gynecol 1996;87:884)
Dilation and curettage	Cefazolin 1 g IV pre-op (see comment)		Complicated procedures only
Cystocele or rectocele repair	None		
Tubal ligation	None		
HEAD AND NECK			
Tonsillectomy ± adenoidectomy	None		Controlled studies are limited
Rhinoplasty	None		
Major surgery with entry via oral cavity or pharynx	Clindamycin 600–900 mg IV ± gentamicin 1.7 mg/kg IV pre-op*	Cefazolin 1–2 g IV pre-op* Cefuroxime 1.5 g IV pre-op*	Likely pathogens: *S. aureus*, streptococci, oral anaerobes. Controlled study showed cefazolin dose of 2 g superior to 0.5 g (Ann Surg 1988;207:108). Meta-analysis showed single dose of clindamycin alone was most effective (Plast Reconstr Surg 1991;87:429). Another showed ampicillin-sulbactam (Unasyn) more effective than clindamycin (Arch Otolaryngol Head Neck Surg 1992;118:1159)
ORTHOPEDIC SURGERY			
Joint replacement	Cefazolin 1–2 g IV pre-op*	Vancomycin 1 g IV pre-op infused over 60 min**	Likely pathogens: *S. aureus, S. epidermidis.* Efficacy of prophylaxis is established (Lancet 1996; 347:1133; RID 1991;10:S42). Antibiotic-impregnated cement is controversial. Preblended cement with antibiotics is indicated for second stage of a 2 stage revision for total joint arthroplasty after removal of active infection

Continued

Type of surgery	Preferred regimen	Alternative	Comment
Open reduction of fracture/ internal fixation	Cefazolin 1–2 g IV 1 g q8h × 1–3 days (closed hip fracture) or 10 days (open hip fracture)	Vancomycin 1 g IV pre-op infused over 60 min** repeat q12h × 1–3 days (closed hip fractures) or 10 days (open hip fracture)	Likely pathogens: *S. aureus; S. epidermidis*. Efficacy established for compound or open fractures treated with screws, plates, or wires and surgical repair of closed fractures (Lancet 1996; 347:1133; Pharmacother 1991;11:157) Antibiotics are not indicated for arthroscopic surgery (Orthopedics 1997;20:133)
Compound fracture	Cefazolin 1–2 g IV q8h × 5–10 days or nafcillin 1–2 g q4h	Vancomycin 1 g IV q12h** or clindamycin 900 mg IV q8h	Start treatment immediately and continue 5–10 days
Amputation of leg	Cefazolin 1–2 g IV or cefoxitin 1–2 g or cefotetan 1–2 g IV pre-op*	Clindamycin 600 mg IV + gentamicin 1.7 mg/kg IV or Vancomycin 1 g IV pre-op infused over 60 min**	Likely pathogens: *S. aureus*, enteric Gram-negative bacilli, Clostridia Efficacy of prophylaxis is established (J Bone Joint Surg 1985;67:800)
NEUROSURGERY			
Cerebrospinal fluid shunt	Cefazolin 1–2 g IV pre-op ± second dose at 4 hr.	Clindamycin 600 mg IV pre-op ± second dose at 4 hr	Likely pathogens: *S. aureus, S. epidermidis*. Efficacy of antimicrobials supported with meta-analysis (CID 1993;17:98); agents used most were trimethoprim-sulfamethoxazole, cloxacillin, and cephalosporins for ≤48 hr. Some studies fail to show efficacy (Lancet 1994;344:1547)
Craniotomy	Cefazolin 1–2 g pre-op	Vancomycin 1 g IV over 60 min pre-op**	Likely pathogens: *S. aureus, S. epidermidis* Efficacy established (J Neurosurg 1990;13:383; Neurosurgery 1994;35:484), advocated even for low-risk procedures except where infection rates are <0.1% (Neurosurg 1989;24:401). Preferred drugs do not cross blood-brain barrier well presumably because most are soft tissue infections (Neurosurg Clin North Am 1992;3:355)

Continued

137

Type of surgery	Preferred regimen	Alternative	Comment
Spinal surgery	None		Rates of infection are too low for demonstrable benefit with lumbar discectomy; infection rates are higher and use of antibiotics more common with fusion, insertion of foreign material, or prolonged procedures, but benefit is not established (Spine 2000;25:2544)
OCULAR	Gentamicin, tobramycin, ciprofloxacin, ofloxacin or neomycin-gramicidin-polymyxin B as eye drops over 2–24 hr Cefazolin 100 mg subconjunctivally		Likely pathogens: *S. aureus, S. epidermidis,* streptococcus, enteric Gram-negative bacilli, *Pseudomonas* Most use eye drops but some give subconjunctival injection of cefazolin, cefuroxime, ceftazidime, vancomycin, or ciprofloxacin (Mayo Clin Proc 1997;72:149) Post-operative: 5% povidone-iodine ophthalmic soln may be more effective than topical antibiotics (Am J Ophthalmol 1995;119:701) There is no consensus on best antibiotics or route of administration (Cornea 1999;18:383) There is no evidence of efficacy with procedures that do not invade the globe
UROLOGY Prostatectomy Sterile urine (high risk only)	Ciprofloxacin 500 mg po or 400 mg IV or gatifloxacin 400 mg po or IV		Likely pathogens: Enteric Gram-negative bacilli and enterococcus Prophylaxis is not usually recommended if pre-op urine is sterile Cefazolin sometimes advocated for open prostatectomy (Urol Clin North Am 1990;17:595)
Infected urine	Continue agent active in vitro or give single pre-operative dose		Sterilization of urine before surgery is preferred

Continued

Type of surgery	Preferred regimen	Alternative	Comment
Radical retropubic prostatectomy or nephrectomy	Cefoxitin 1–2 g IV or cefotetan 1–2 g IV pre-op	Clindamycin 600 mg IV pre-op	
Prostatic biopsy	None		
Dilation of urethra	None		
MISCELLANEOUS			
Inguinal hernia repair	Cefazolin 1 g IV pre-op (see comment)		One study showed benefit of cefonicid, 1 g IV 30 min pre-op (NEJM 1990;322:153); sequel study showed diverse antibiotics (primarily cefazolin) in high-risk patients was beneficial (JID 1992;166:556) Prophylaxis is not generally recommended (Med Lett 2001;43:91)
Mastectomy	Cefazolin 1 g IV pre-op (see comment)		One study showed benefit of cefonicid for breast surgery (NEJM 1990;322:153); Greatest risks were radical mastectomy and axillary node dissection: Most authorities do not recommend prophylaxis (Med Lett 2001;43:91)
Traumatic wound	Cefazolin 1–2 g IV q8h		Likely pathogens: *S. aureus*, group A strep, clostridia

*Pre-op usually indicates administration with induction of anesthesia. Intra-op dose often given with prolonged procedures. Optimal duration is usually unclear, but most studies show a single dose is adequate. Use of more than a single pre-operative dose is arbitrary and usually discouraged. When repeat dosing: cefazolin q4h, cefoxitin q4h, cefotetan q8h, clindamycin q8h, vancomycin q12h. With cefazolin, obese patients should receive 2 g (Surgery 1989;106:750).

**Vancomycin preferred for hospitals with a high rate of wound infections caused by methicillin-resistant *S. aureus* or *S. epidermidis* and for patients with allergy to penicillins or cephalosporins. Hypotension is a complication with rapid infusion and may occur even if infused over 60 min. Treat with Benadryl and further slowing of infusion (J Thorac Cardiovasc Surg 1992;104:1423). Hospitals should reduce all unnecessary vancomycin use due to concern for possible promotion of vancomycin-resistant enterococci.

PREVENTION OF BACTERIAL ENDOCARDITIS
Recommendations of the American Heart Association, Infectious Diseases
Society of America, American Dental Association, American Academy of Pediatrics,
and American Society for Gastrointestinal Endoscopy (JAMA 1997;277:1794;
CID 1997;25:1448; Med Lett 2001;43:98)

CARDIAC CONDITIONS
Cardiac conditions considered at risk (not all inclusive)

a. High Risk

    Prosthetic cardiac valve, including bioprosthetic and homograph valves

    Prior endocarditis

    Complex cyanotic congenital heart disease

    Surgically constructed systemic pulmonary shunts

b. Moderate Risk

    Rheumatic and other acquired valvular dysfunction (even after valve surgery)

    Hypertrophic cardiomyopathy (IHSS)

    Mitral valve prolapse with valve regurgitation (patients with mitral valve prolapse associated with thickening and/or redundancy of the valve may be at increased risk, especially men age $\geq$45 yr)

Prophylaxis not recommended

    Isolated secundum atrial septal defect

    Surgical repair without residual >6 mo of secundum atrial defect, ventricular septal defect, or patent ductus or arteriosus (without residual beyond 6 mo)

    Prior coronary bypass surgery

    Mitral valve defect without regurgitation (see above)

    Physiologic or functional heart murmurs

    Prior rheumatic fever without valve disease

    Cardiac pacemakers and implanted defibrillators

    Prior Kawasaki's disease without valve dysfunction

PROCEDURES
Endocarditis prophylaxis recommended

    Dental procedures: Extractions; periodontal procedures—surgery, scaling, root planing, probing; dental implant, root canal, subgingival placement of antibiotic strips; initial placement of orthodontic bands; intraligamentary local anesthetic injections, and tooth cleaning if bleeding is anticipated

    Note: Three major studies have challenged the benefit of prophylactic antibiotics before dental procedures to prevent endocarditis (Arch Intern Med 1992;152: 1869; Lancet 1992;339:135; and Ann Intern Med 1998;129:761). Some authorities recommend prophylaxis only with extractions and gingival surgery and only when the risk is a prosthetic valve or previous endocarditis (Ann Intern Med 1998;129:829).

    Tonsillectomy and adenoidectomy

    Surgical procedures that involve intestinal or respiratory mucosa

    Bronchoscopy with a rigid bronchoscope

    Sclerotherapy for esophageal varices*

    Esophageal dilation*

Endoscopic retrograde cholangiography with biliary obstruction*
Surgical procedures that involve intestinal mucosa*
Gallbladder surgery*
Cystoscopy
Urethral dilation

Endocarditis prophylaxis not recommended**
  Dental procedures: Restorative dentistry, local anesthesia, intracanal
    endodontic treatment, placement of rubber dams, suture removal,
    placement of removable prosthodontic or orthopedic appliances,
    fluoride treatments, impressions, orthodontic appliance adjustment,
    shedding of primary teeth
  Endotracheal intubation
  Tympanostomy tube insertion
  Bronchoscopy with flexible bronchoscopy with or without biopsy**
  Transesophageal echocardiography
  Endoscopy of GI tract with or without biopsy**
  Cardiac catheterization including balloon angiopathy
  Transesophageal echocardiography**
  Implanted cardiac pacemakers, defibrillators, and coronary stents
  Incision and drainage of prepped sites
  Circumcision
  Vaginal hysterectomy**
  Vaginal delivery**
  Cesarean section
  Genitourinary surgery in uninfected tissue: urethral catheterization,
    uterine dilation and curettage, therapeutic abortion, sterilization
    procedures, or insertion or removal of intrauterine device

*Prophylaxis is recommended for high risk patients and is considered optional for medium-risk patients.
**Prophylaxis is optional for high-risk patients.

RECOMMENDED REGIMENS
Based on recommendations of the American Heart Association
(JAMA 1997;227:1794; Med Letter 2005;47:57)

Dental, oral and upper respiratory procedures

Standard
  Amoxicillin: 2.0 g po 1 hr before procedure
  Alternatives: Penicillin V, 2 g po 1 hr pre-procedure; then 1 g 6 hr after first dose

Amoxicillin or penicillin allergy
  Clindamycin 600 mg po 1 hr pre-procedure or
  Cephalexin or cefadroxil, 2 g po 1 hr pre-procedure or
  Azithromycin or clarithromycin, 500 mg po 1 hr pre-procedure

Cannot take oral medications
  Ampicillin 2.0 g IM or IV 30 min pre-procedure

Amoxicillin or penicillin allergy and unable to take oral medicines
  Clindamycin 600 mg IV within 30 min pre-procedure or
  Cefazolin 1 g IM or IV within 30 min pre-procedure

Genitourinary or gastrointestinal procedures

High risk*: Ampicillin, 2 g IM or IV plus gentamicin 1.5 mg/kg IM or IV ≤ 30 min of start-ing procedure; 6 hr later ampicillin 1 g IV or amoxicillin 1 g po

High risk plus penicillin allergy: Vancomycin 1 g IV over 1–2 hr plus gentamicin 1.5 mg/kg IV or IM (≤120 mg) complete infusion within 30 min of starting procedure

Moderate risk: Amoxicillin, 2 g po 1 hr pre-procedure or ampicillin 2.0 g IM or IV within 30 min of starting procedure

Moderate risk plus penicillin allergy: Vancomycin 1 g IV over 1–2 hr; complete infusion within 30 min of starting the procedure

*High risk: Prosthetic valve, history of endocarditis or surgically constructed systemic shunts or conduits or complex cyanotic congenital heart disease.

MISCELLANEOUS ISSUES (CID 1997;25:1454)

Target organisms: Upper respiratory tract procedures—*S. viridans*; GI and GU procedures—*E. faecalis*

Patients already receiving an antibiotic: Pick from a different class. Thus, if receiving a beta-lactam, use clindamycin, clarithromycin, or axithromycin

Anticoagulated patients: Avoid IM injections of antibiotics

Procedures involving infected tissue: Treat cause of infection

Cardiac surgery candidates: Antibiotic prophylaxis advocated, usually a first generation cephalosporin or vancomycin

Cardiac transplant recipients: Experience is very limited, but most treat as the moderate-risk category

Endocarditis experience: Most cases of strep viridans endocarditis have not followed dental procedures; most procedure related endocarditis occurs within 2 wk of the procedure

Effectiveness of prophylaxis: Efficacy of prophylaxis has never been shown (CID 1999;29:1). Nevertheless, most infectious disease-trained physi-cians follow these guidelines, mainly because of the liability risk rather than the supporting science (CID 2002;34:1621).

PROPHYLAXIS FOR DENTAL, GASTROINTESTINAL, OR GENITOURINARY PROCEDURES IN PATIENTS WITH PROSTHETIC JOINTS

1. Analysis by Gillespie showed no evidence of benefit (Infect Dis Clin North Am 1990;4:465).

2. Review in CID 1995;20:1420: Patients with prosthetic joints do not require prophylaxis for dental, gastrointestinal, or genitourinary procedures; possible exceptions are long procedures, surgery in infected area (e.g., periodontal disease), and other procedures with a high risk of bacteremia (Med Lett 1995;37:79; J Bone Joint Surg 1996;78-A:1755).

3. Updated statement of American Academy of Orthopedic Surgeons and American Dental Association (J Am Dent Assoc 1997;128:1004): Prophylaxis is not indicated for dental patients with pins, plates, and screws, and it is not routinely indicated for most dental patients with total joint replacements. However, it is advisable to consider prophylaxis in a small number of patients who may be at potential increased risk of hematogenous total joint infection.

PREVENTION OF DISEASES ASSOCIATED WITH TRAVEL

A. INTERNATIONAL TRAVEL DIRECTORY: CDC TRAVEL HOTLINE AND FAX INFORMATION SERVICE

Travel advise	877-394-8747	24 hr/d voice mail
Traveler's Health FAX service	888-232-3299	24 hr/d automated FAX service (patients and providers)
Travel information	www.cdc.gov/ travel/diseases	Select "Traveler's Health"
Malaria—Prevention and management	770-488-7100	
Travel—Emergency consultation	770-488-7100	24 hr/d service
CDC Parasitic Diseases Drug Service	404-639-3670	Drugs for special use

B. TRAVELER'S DIARRHEA *(Adapted from Med Letter Guidelines 2004;2:33; NEJM 1993;328:1821; CID 1993;16:616; Infect Dis Clin North Am 1998;12:301)*

1. **Risk**
   High-risk areas (incidence 20–50%): Developing countries of Latin America, Africa, Middle East, and Asia
   Intermediate risk: Southern Europe and some Caribbean islands
   Low risk: Canada, Northern Europe, Australia, New Zealand, United States

2. **Agents** (JID 2002;185:497)

E. coli (enterotoxigenic—most common, enteroinvasive, enteroadherent)	Rotavirus (Mexico)
	Norovirus (cruise ships)
Shigella	Giardia (North America and Russia)
Campylobacter jejuni	
Aeromonas (especially Thailand)	Cryptosporidium (Russia)
Plesiomonas shigelloides	E. histolytica (Rare)
Salmonella sp	
Non-cholera Vibrios (coastal Asia)	

3. **Prevention**
   Safe foods: Food served fresh and steaming hot; dry food (e.g., bread); hyperosmolar food (e.g., jellies, acidic fruits); fruit that is self-peeled; alcoholic beverages; carbonated beverages; water that is filtered and iodinized
   Avoid: Salads, cold foods, sauces, cream-filled desserts, raw vegetables, unpeeled fruit, cooked food that is not served steaming hot, raw seafood, raw meat, soft cheeses, tapwater, ice

4. **Antimicrobial prophylaxis** *(CID 2000;31:1079):* Generally not recommended except some immuno-suppressed patients—give once daily ciprofloxacin 500 mg, levofloxacin 500 mg, ofloxacin 300 mg or norfloxacin 400 mg

5. **Treatment of traveler's diarrhea** *(CID 2000;31:1079)[a] and CDC (www.cdc.gov/ travel accessed 7/30/05)*

Clinical feature	Treatment options
Mild or moderate diarrhea: ≤ 3 loose stools/8 hrs with no fever or blood	No treatment or loperamide 4 mg, then 2 with each loose stool up to 16 mg/d
Severe: ≥ 3 loose stools/8 hrs, or diarrhea associated with fever or bloody stools	Loperamide + fluoroquinolone[b] 1. Norfloxacin 400 mg po bid × 3 d 2. Ciprofloxacin 500 mg po bid × 3 d 3. Levofloxacin 500 mg qd × 3 d 4. Azithromycin 1000 mg × 1 or 500 mg qd × 3d (CID 2003;37:1165) Pregnancy: Loperamide + azithromycin 1000 mg × 1 or 500 mg qd × 3 d

[a] The 3-day course of treatment appears superior to single dose treatment for salmonellosis (AAC 1989;33:1101; JID 1992;165:1557) and for shigellosis due to *S. dysenteriae* type 1 (Ann Intern Med 1992;117:727). A study of shigellosis in Thailand failed to show loperamide is contraindicated when given with a quinolone (Ann Intern Med 1985;102:582).

6. **Oral rehydration:** Potable fruit juice, caffeine-free soft drinks, salted crackers. Severe symptoms: WHO Oral Rehydration Salts. Ingredients/L water: NaCl 3.5 g (3/4 tsp), trisodium citrate 2.9 g (could use 1 tsp baking soda) and glucose 20 g, KCl 1.5 g (1 cup orange juice or bananas). Packets of oral rehydration salts are available from Cera Products, Jessup, MD (888-237-2598) and Jianas Bros, Kansas City, MO (816-421-2880)
7. **Antibiotic resistance:** Rate of resistance by *Shigella, Salmonella,* and *E. coli* is 50–90% for tetracycline and 35–76% for TMP-SMX (Infect Dis Clin North Am 6:333, 1992). Quinolone resistance is 20–60% for *C. jejuni* (Emerg Infect Dis 2001;7:24)

C. MALARIA PROPHYLAXIS *(CDC Health Information for International Travel 2004, U.S. Department of Health and Human Services, Med Letter Guidelines 2004;2:33; MMWR 2005;54:25)*

CDC Malaria Hotline: Recommendations for prevention and case management—770-488-7788 (8 AM–4:30 PM EST) Emergency hotline for treatment guidance after hours—770-488-7100; www.cdc.gov/

Risk areas: Most areas of Central and South America, Hispaniola, sub-Saharan Africa, the Indian subcontinent, Southeast Asia, the Middle East, and Oceania. During 2003 there were 1,278 reported cases of malaria in the U.S. including 53% *P. falciparum*, 23% *P. vivax*, 3.6% *P. malariae*, and 2.6% *P. ovale* and 18% undetermined (MMWR 2005;54:25). Areas of acquisition included Africa (73%), Asia (11%), Central America and Caribbean (8%). Of the 1278 cases at least 17% were U.S. citizens who claimed they received malaria prophylaxis. There were 7 deaths attributed to malaria for a mortality rate of 0.5%.

Drug resistance of *P. falciparum* to chloroquine (CRPF) is probable or confirmed in all countries with *P. falciparum* except Central America west of the Panama Canal Zone, Haiti, the Dominican Republic, Northern Argentina, Mexico, most of China, and most of the Middle East. Resistance to both Fansidar and chloroquine is widespread in Thailand, Myanmar (formerly Burma), Cambodia, and the Amazon basin of South America and has been reported in sub-Saharan Africa. Resistance to mefloquine has been reported primarily in Thailand borders with Myanmar and Cambodia. There is no documented resistance to tetracycline.

Advice to travelers *(Med Letter Guideline 2004;2:33)*
   1. Personal protection:
      a. Transmission is most common between dusk and dawn.
      b. Precautions include remaining in well-screened areas and using mosquito nets, clothing that covers most of the body, insect repellent containing DEET on exposed areas, and pyrethroid containing insect spray for environs and clothing. Long acting DEET is now available as Ultrathon; provides protection for 6–12 hrs. Permethrin may also be sprayed on clothing; bednets, tents, sleeping bags, etc. On clothes, it persists several weeks even with laundering. On nets and tents etc. it lasts 6 months.

Drugs to Prevent Malaria in Areas of Chloroquine-resistant
P. falciparum (adapted from *Med Letter Guidelines 2004;2:33*)

Drug	Regimen & cost (AWP) for 14 day stay
Mefloquine[a]	250 mg q wk beginning 1–2 wk before travel, during travel and 4 wk after leaving $70
Doxycycline[b]	100 mg daily beginning 1–2 days before travel, during travel, and 4 wk after leaving $35
Atovaquone/proguanil[c] (Malarone)	250/100 mg (1 tab) daily beginning 1–2 days before travel, during travel, and 1 wk after returning $108
Chloroquine sensitive[e] Chloroquine	500 mg (300 mg base) 1–2 wk before travel, during travel and 4 wk after travel $27

[a]Mefloquine: Serious psychiatric side effects reported. Contraindications include major psychiatric illness, seizures or cardiac conduction disorders. The drug should be stopped if the patient has anxiety depression, confusion or restlessness.

Contraindications include pregnancy and travelers with history of epilepsy or psychiatric disorders. This drug is safe during the second and third trimesters of pregnancy (JID 1994;169:595); experience in first trimester is limited. Mefloquine resistance is reported in Thai-Cambodian and Thai-Myanmar border and western Cambodia.

[b]Doxyclycline: Efficacy is similar to mefloquine (Ann Intern Med 1997;126:963). Patients must be warned of photosensitivity and GI intolerance.

[c]Malarone is the best tolerated (BMJ 2003;327:1078)

[d]Use of chloroquine in areas with chloroquine-resistant *P. falciparum* should be accompanied by Fansidar to promptly treat febrile illness. Chloroquine and proguanil may be used in pregnancy.

[e]Haiti, Dominican Republic, Central America west of the Panama Canal, and Middle East.

COUNTRIES WITH A RISK OF MALARIA* *(Reprinted from Med Guidelines 2004;2:33)*

AFRICA

Angola	Guinea	Sudan
Benin	Guinea-Bissau	Swaziland
Botswana	Kenya	Tanzania
Burkina Faso	Liberia	Togo
Burundi	Madagascar	Uganda
Cameroon	Malawi	Zambia
Central African Republic	Mali	**Zimbabwe
Chad	Mauritania	
Comoros	**Mauritius	
Congo	Mayotte (French territorial collectivity)	
Côte d'Ivoire	Mozambique	
Democratic Republic of the Congo (formerly Zaire)	Namibia	
Djibouti	Niger	
Equitorial Guinea	Nigeria	
**Eritrea	Rwanda	
**Ethiopia	São Tomé and Principe	
Gabon	Senegal	
Gambia	Sierra Leone	
Ghana	Somalia	
	**South Africa	

AMERICAS

**Argentina	**Mexico	
**Belize	Nicaragua	
**Bolivia	**Panama	
Brazil	**Paraguay	
**Colombia	**Peru	
**Costa Rica	**Suriname	
**Dominican Republic	**Venezuela	
**Ecuador		
**El Salvador		
French Guiana		
**Guatemala		
Guyana		
Haiti		
**Honduras		

ASIA

Afghanistan	**Korea	
Armenia	**Kyrgyzstan	
**Azerbaijan	**Laos	
Bangladesh	**Malaysia	
**Bhutan	**Myanmar	
Cambodia	**Nepal	
**China, People's Republic	Pakistan	
East Timor	**Philippines	
**Georgia	**Saudi Arabia	
India	Sri Lanka	
**Indonesia	**Syria	
**Iran	Tajikistan	
**Iraq	**Thailand	
	**Turkey	
	**Turkmenistan	
	**Uzbekistan	
	**Viet Nam	
	**Yemen	

OCEANIA

Papua New Guinea
Solomon Islands
Vanuatu

*Only includes countries for which prophylaxis is recommended. For more information: The Medical Letter's Advice for Travelers CD-ROM or CDC at 1-888-232-3228.
**No malaria in urban areas.

146

D. VACCINES *(See pp 99–104 for complete listing)*

Indication: Susceptibility (anti-HBcAg negative) and travel to area where HBV endemicity is high or moderate plus: visits frequent, long stays, medical or dental care, or unprotected sex with residents

Prevalence of HAV and HBV (Med Letter 2001;43:67)

	HAV prevalence	HBV prevalence
U.S., Canada, Australia, Japan, northern and western Europe	Low	Low
Caribbean	Moderate	Moderate; high in Haiti and Dominican Republic
Central America	High	
South America	High	High in Amazon River basin
Eastern and southern Europe and Russia	Moderate	Moderate
Middle East	High	Moderate
Africa	High	Moderate–high
Asia (except Japan)	High	Moderate–high

TREATMENT OF FUNGAL INFECTIONS
(Adapted from Medical Letters Treatment Guide Antifungal Drugs 2005; 3:7)

FUNGUS-PREFERRED TREATMENT	ALTERNATIVES
Aspergillus—treat 6–12 mo • Amphotericin B* 1.0–1.5 mg/kg/d × 10 wks • Voriconazole 6 mg/kg IV q 12 h × 1 d; then 4 mg/kg q12 h, then 200 mg po bid × 10 wks	• Itraconazole 200 mg IV bid × 2 days, then 200 mg IV qd × 12 days or 200 mg po tid × 3 d; then 200 mg po bid • Caspofungin 70 mg IV × 1d then 50 mg IV qd × 10 wks
Blastomycosis—treat 6-12 mo Itraconazole 200 mg po bid × 6–12 wks Ampho B* 0.5–1 mg/kg/d IV × 6–12 wks	• Fluconazole 400–800 mg po/d

Candidiasis**
  1. Thrush or esophageal—treat 1–3 wks
    • Fluconazole 200 mg IV or po,
      then 100 mg/d × 1–3 wks
    • Ampho B* 0.3–0.5 mg/kg/d × 1–3 wks
    • Caspofungin 50 mg/d IV × 1–3 wks
  2. Vulvovaginal—treat 1–7 days
    • Topical therapy × 1–7 d
    • Systemic: Fluconazole 150 mg po × 1
  3. Urinary—treat 7–14 d
    • Fluconazole 200 mg IV or po qd × 7–14 d
      Ampho B* 0.3–0.5 mg/kg/d IV × 7–10 d
  4. Fungemia—treat until afebrile 2 wks & BC negative
    • Fluconazole 400–800 mg/d IV then po
    • Caspofungin 70 mg IV × 1, then 50 mg IV qd
    • Ampho B 0.5–1 mg/kg/d
	• Itraconazole 200 mg po qd × 1–3 wks
	• Voriconazole 200 mg po bid × 1–3 wks
	
	• Itraconazole 200 mg po bid × 1 day
	• Ketoconazole 200 mg po bid × 5 d
	
	• Flucytosine 25 mg/kg/d po × 7–14 d

Coccidioidomycosis—treat >1 yr • Itraconazole 200 mg bid po • Fluconazole 400–800 mg qd • Amphoteracin B* 0.5–0.7 mg/kg/d	

Cryptococcus Acute treatment - 2 wks. then
8 additional wks
• <u>Acute:</u> Ampho B* 0.5–1 mg/kg/d IV
  ± flucytosine 100 mg/kg/d po
• Phase 2: Fluconazole 400 mg
  po/d × 8 wks
• Maintenance: Fluconazole 200 mg
  po/d
	• Itraconazole 200 mg bid po; bid po;
	
	• Ampho B 0.5–1 mg/kg IV/wk

Fusariosis • Ampho B* 1.–1.5 mg/kg/d IV • Vorticonazole 6 mg/kg IV q 12 h × 1 day, then 4 mg/kg q 12 h	
Histoplasmosis: Treat 6–8 months • Itraconazole 200 mg po bind × 6–18 mo • Ampho B* 0.5–1.0 mg/kg/d IV × 10–12 wks Maintenance: Itraconazole 200 mg/d po 200 mg po × 1 wk/mo	• Fluconazole 400–800 mg po/d • Ampho B 0.5–1 mg/kg/wk

Continued

FUNGUS—PREFERRED TREATMENT	ALTERNATIVES
Mucomycosis—Treat 6–10 mo Ampho B* 1–1.5 mg/kg/d IV × 6–10 wks	• Posaconazole 200 mg qid po

Onychomycosis
• Terbinafine 250 mg po/d × 12 wks
• Itraconazole 200 mg/d po × 3 mo
  then 200 mg/d po × 1 wk/mo
	• Fluconazole 150–300
	  mg po/wk × 6–12 mo.

Paracocoidoidomycosis
• Itraconazole 100–200 mg po/d
  × 6–12 mo
	• Ketoconazole 200–400
	  mg po once/d × 6–12 mo.

Pseudallescheriasis
• Voriconazole: 6 mg/kg q
  12 h × 1 day, then 4 mg/kg
  q 12 h; then 200 mg po bid
	• Itraconazole 200 mg
	  IV bid × 2 d, then
	  IV qd or po tid
	  × 3 d, then po bid

Sporotrichosis
Cutaneous: Itraconazole 200 mg/d
  po × 3–6 mo
Extracutaneous: Ampho B
  0.5–0.7 mg/kg/d IV ×
  6–12 wks <u>or</u>
  Itraconazole 200 mg po
  bid × 12 mo
	• SSKI 1–5 ml po tid

Tinea pedis
  Terbinafine cream applied
  bid × 1–2 wks <u>or</u>
  Topical azole (miconazole,
  clotrimazole, econazole)
  applied daily × 4 wks
	• Fluconazole 150 mg q wk

*Amphoteracin B doses
  Abelcet: 5 mg/kg/d
  AmBisome: 3–5 mg/kg/d; doses up to 15 mg/kg
    have been used. For cryptococcal meningitis use
    6 mg/kg/d	

***C. albicans* is usually sensitive to fluconazole; *C. krusei* is usually resistant; *C. glabrata* may require high doses. *C. lusitaniae* may be resistant to *Amphoteracin*

COMPARISON OF ANTIFUNGAL AGENTS

Antifungal agents	Amphotericin (Fungizone)	Flucytosine (Ancobon)	Ketoconazole (Nizoral)	Fluconazole (Diflucan)	Itraconazole (Sporanox)	Voriconazole	Caspofungin (Cancidas)
Oral bioavailability	Nil	>80%	75%	>80%	>70%	95%	Nil
Effect of gastric achlorhydria	—	—	Reduced absorption	—	Reduced absorption	—	—
Serum half-life	15 days	3–6 hr	6–10 hr	24–30 hr	30–45 hr	3 hr	9–11 hr
Half-life—anuria	15 days	70 hr	6–10 hr	100 hr	30–45 hr (contraindicated)	18 hr	9–11 hr
Urine level (active agent)	3%	80%	<2–4%	80%	<1%	<2%	1%
CSF levels (% serum)	3%	75%	<10%	70–90%	<1%	>50%	?
Usual dose/d	25–50 mg IV/day	100 mg/kg/d	200–400 mg po/day	100–200 mg IV or po/day	200–400 mg IV or po/day	200 mg po bid 6 mg/kg IV q 12 h × 2 then 4 mg/kg IV q12h	70 mg IV, then 50 mg/d IV
Main side effect	Renal failure Infusion reactions chills, fever	Neutropenia Colitis	GI intolerance Hepatitis	GI intolerance Alopecia	GI intolerance Hepatitis Hypokalemia Cardiomyopathy	Visual change-reversible	Hepatotoxicity (rare)
Main uses	All systemic fungal infections	Cryptococcal meningitis	Candida Histo, Blasto Cocci Paracocci	Candida; Cryptococcus	Aspergillosis Blastomycosis Histoplasmosis Candida	Aspergillosis Candida Fusaria Zygomyces	Candida Aspergillosis
Cost (average wholesale)/d (2005)	$23/50 mg Ampho $480–1320/3 g lipid preps.	$100/7 g po	$4/200 mg po	$28/400 mg po $162/400 mg IV	$40/400 mg po $203/200 mg IV	$32/200 mg po $315/day IV	$373/50 mg IV

COMPARISON OF AMPHOTERICIN PREPARATIONS
LIPID FORMULATIONS OF AMPHOTERICIN B: IDSA GUIDELINES
(CID 2000;30:653; CID 2003;37:415)

Potential advantages compared with conventional amphotericin B: Increased daily dose (up to 10-fold); high tissue concentration, especially in RE system (lungs, spleen, liver), reduced infusion related reactions (especially AmBisome), substantial decrease in nephrotoxicity

Disadvantages compared with conventional amphotericin B: the lipid-based formulations are **much** more expensive: Amphotericin B: $20/d; AmBisome: $800–$1500/d; Abelcet: $640/d; Amphotec: $480–640/d (average wholesale price, 2005)

Indications (See IDSA Guidelines, CID 2000;30:653)
1. Patients receiving amphotericin B who develop renal dysfunction (creatinine > 2.5 mg/mL), severe infusion related adverse events or disease progression despite >500 mg total dose of amphotericin
2. Patients who require amphotericin therapy with baseline creatinine >2.5 mg/mL
3. Some immunocompromised patients with life-threatening mold disease (aspergillosis or zygomycosis)

Update: Some argue it is time to embrace the lipid preparations as the new standard since experience shows that these preparations are as active or more active than amphotericin B desoxycholate, they are superior for some and are clearly less toxic (CID 2003;37:415)

COMPARISON OF LIPID-BASED AMPHOTERICIN PREPARATIONS
(CID 2003;37:415)

Preparation	Amphotec (ABCD)	Abelset (ABLC)	AmBisome (LAmB)
FDA approval	Invasive aspergillosis plus contraindication or failure with Ampho B	Invasive fungal infections plus contraindications or failure with Ampho B	Empiric RX in neutropenic patients Cryptococcal meningitis with AIDS Candida, Crypto, and Aspergillis infection plus failure or contraindication with Ampho B
Dose—FDA approved	3–4 mg/kg/day	5 mg/kg/day	3 mg/kg/d—empiric therapy 3–5 mg/kg systemic fungal disease 4 mg/kg cryptococcal meningitis
Efficacy*			
Aspergillus	34%	46%	61%
Candidiasis	59%	75%	80%
Cryptococcosis	45%	67%	100%
Tissue penetration**			
Liver	2×	2×	0.5–1×
Kidney	0.1×	0.2×	0.2×
Lung	—	2×	0.2×
Brain	0.1	0.1	1.2×
C_{max}	3.1 µg/mL	1.7 µg/mL	83 µg/mL
Usual AWP (/day)	$400–500	$800–850	$950–1300

* Efficacy based on non-comparative clinical trials

**Tissue concentrations relative to amphotericin B

SPECTRUM OF ACTIVITY OF ANTIFUNGAL AGENTS
(Based on in vitro sensitivity tests and animal models)

	Aspergillus	Blastomyces	Candida albicans	Candida krusei	Chromomycosis agents	Cryptococcus	Coccidioides	Histoplasma	Paracoccidioides	Phycomyces (mucormycosis)	Pseudoallescheria boydii	Sporothrix	Zygomyces
Amphotericin B	+*	+*	+*	+*	–	+*	+*	+*	+	+*	–	+	*
Flucytosine	+	–	+	+	+*	+	–	+	+	–	–	+	–
Ketoconazole	–	+	+	–	+	+	+	+	+	–	–	+	–
Fluconazole	+	+*	+*	–	–	+*	+*	+*	+*	–	–	+*	+
Itraconazole	+	+*	+	–	+	+	+*	+*	+*	–	–	+*	+
Voriconazole	+	+	+	+	+	+	+	+	?	+	*	+	+
Caspofungin	+	–	+	+	–	–	–	–	–	–	–	–	–

* Preferred agent(s) for most clinical infections.

TREATMENT OF DERMATOPHYTIC FUNGAL INFECTIONS

Condition	Agents	Location	Treatment
Tinea corporis (ringworm)	T. rubrum T. mentagrophytes M. canis E. floccosum	Circular, erythema well demarcated with scaly, vesicular, or pustular border Non-hairy skin Pruritic	Topical agents: Miconazole, clotrimazole, econazole, naftifine, ciclopirox, or terbinafine bid or ketoconazole, oxiconazole, sulconazole qd for ≥4 wk. If no response then griseofulvin × 2–4 wk (see below)
Tinea cruris (Jock itch)	E. floccosum T. rubrum T. mentagrophytes	Erythema and scaly groin and upper thighs Pruritic	Topical agents as above. Loose fitting clothes Absorbent powder. Unresponsive cases: Griseofulvin × 2–4 wk
Tinea pedis (athlete's foot)	T. rubrum T. mentagrophytes E. floccosum	Foot, especially fissures between toes; scaly, vesicles, pustules ± nail involvement	Topical agents as above. Keep feet dry and cool Unresponsive cases: griseofulvin 4–8 wk
Tinea unguium (nail involvement)	T. rubrum T. mentagrophytes Candida T. soudanense	Nails, usually distal and lateral nail thickening with adjacent skin involved	Oral griseofulvin or ketoconazole 6–24 mo (until new nail) or itraconazole 200 mg bid × 1 wk × 2 (fingernails) separated by 3 wk; 200 mg/d × 12 wk or 200 mg bid × 1 wk/mo × 3–4 mo (toenails) (Med Lett 1996;38:5); terbinafine (Lamisil) 250 mg/d × 6 wk (fingernails) or 12 wk (toenails) (Med Lett 38:76, 1996) or butenafine (Mentax) (1%) topical qd × 4 wk (Med Lett 39:63, 1997)
Tinea capitis (ringworm—scalp)	T. tonsurans T. mentagrophytes T. verrucosum M. canis	Scaling and erythematous area of scalp with broken hairs and localized alopecia	Griseofulvin × 4–8 wk + 2.5% selenium sulfide shampoo 2×/wk. Alternative to griseofulvin is ketoconazole
Tinea versicolor	Malassezia furfur	Scaling oval macular and patchy lesions on upper trunk and arms; dark or light, fail to tan	Topical 2.5% selenium sulfide applied as thin layer over entire body × 1–2 hr or overnight for 1–2 wk, then monthly × 3; wash off. Alternatives: Topical clotrimazole, econazole, ketoconazole, naftifine, haloprogin, or oral ketoconazole

I. TUBERCULOSIS

Guidelines of CDC, American Thoracic Society, and Infectious Diseases Society of America (Am J Respir Crit Care Med 2003;167:603; MMWR 2003;52:RR-11; NEJM 2001;345:189; BMJ 2002;325:1282; Med Letter Treatment Guideline 2004;2:83)

A. Treatment

1. Four drug treatments preferred for initial empiric treatment: Isoniazid (INH), rifampin (Rif), pyrazinamide (PZA), and ethambutol (EMB).
2. Directly observed therapy (DOT) is preferred for all patients (AMJ Resp Crit Care Med 2004;170:561). Priorities for DOT: Pulmonary TB with positive smear, treatment failure, relapse, drug resistance, HIV co-infection, current or prior drug abuse, psychiatric illness, memory impairment, or prior non-adherence.
3. Susceptibility tests should be performed on the initial isolate and on any isolate obtained at 3 mo post-treatment (failure to convert).
4. Future therapy: Fluoroquinolones are the most promising new agents (BMJ 2002;325:1282).
5. Monitoring: Some recommend routine baseline LFTs and periodic monitoring due to hepatotoxicity of INH, PZA, and rifampin. Increases in ALT in up to 20%, but major liver disease in <1% (BMJ 2002;325:1282)
6. Relapse: Probability of relapse is <5%; most occur within 6 months and involve drug sensitive strains.
7. Resistant strains: Give 4 active drugs, usually 3 oral and one parenteral aminoglycoside.

REGIMEN OPTIONS FOR INITIAL TREATMENT OF TB AMONG ADULTS WITH DRUG SENSITIVE STRAINS

Phase 1 (8 weeks)	Phase 2* (4–7 months): Regimen, doses, minimal duration
8 weeks: INH/RIF/PZA/EMB 7 d/wk, 56 doses, 8 wks 5 d/wk, 40 doses, 8 wks	INH/RIF 7 d/wk, 126 doses or 5 d/wk, 90 doses, 18 wks INH/RIF 2×/wk, 36 doses, 18 wks INH/RPT, 1×/wk, 18 doses, 18 wks**
2 wk/6 week: INH/RIF/PZA/EMB 7 d/wk, 14 doses, 2 wks, then 2×/week, 12 doses, 6 wks	INH/RIF 2×/wk, 36 doses, 18 wks INH/RPT 1×/wk, 18 doses, 18 wks**
8 weeks: INH/RIF/PZA/EMB 3×/wk, 24 doses, 8 wks	INH/RIF 3×/wk, 54 doses, 18 wks
8 weeks: INH/RIF/EMB*** 7 d/wk, 56 doses or 5 d/wk, 40 doses, 8 wks	INH/RIF 7 d/wk, 217 doses or 5 d/wk, 155 doses, 31 wks INH/RIF 2×/wk, 62 doses, 31 wks

INH = Isoniazide, RIF = Rifampin, RPT = rifapentine, PZA = Pyrazinamide, EMB = Ethambutol

* Patients with cavitation at baseline and positive cultures at 2 months should receive 31 week continuation phase for total of 9 months.

**Not recommended for HIV infected patients.

***For patients with a contraindication to PZA (severe liver disease or gout)

RECOMMENDED FIRST LINE DRUGS

(Am Rev Respir Crit Care 2003;167:603; Medical Letter 2004;2:83)

Agent	Forms	Daily dose	Twice/thrice weekly dose	Cost/mo daily regimen	Adverse reactions	Comment
Isoniazid (INH)	Tabs: 50 mg, 100 mg, 300 mg Syrup: 50 mg/5 mL Vials: 1 g (IM)	5 mg/kg po or IM Max—300 mg, po or IV	15 mg/kg Max—900 mg	$1.50	Elevated ALT 10–20% clinical hepatitis* 0.6%, peripheral neuropathy 0.2%	Liver injury increased with RIF and/or PZA, EtOH, age Peripheral neuropathy is prevented with pyridoxine (50 mg/d) suggested for diabetes, HIV, uremia, alcoholism, malnutrition, pregnancy, or seizure disorder
Rifampin (RIF)	Caps: 150 mg, 300 mg Vials: 600 mg (IV)	10 mg/kg Max—600 mg po or IV	10 mg/kg Max—600 mg	$123	Orange discoloration of secretions and urine, purpura (rare) Hepatitis*, cholestatic Pruritis ± rash 6% Flu sx with 2×/wk	Multiple drug interactions: accelerates clearance of methadone, warfarin, corticosteroids, estrogens, ketoconazole, cyclosporine, phenytoin, oral hypoglycemics, protease inhibitors
Rifapentine	Tabs: 150 mg	—	10 mg/kg/wk Max—600 mg/wk	$48	Hepatotoxicity	Once weekly with INH for phase 2 which should be 7 mo.

		wt (kg)	Daily	2×/wk	3×/wk			
Pyrazinamide (PZA)	Tabs: 500 mg	40–55 56–75 76–90	1.0 g 1.5 g 2.0 g	2.0 g 3.0 g 4.0 g	1.5 g 2.5 g 3.0 g	$127	Hepatitis*—frequent with RIF + PZA Nongouty polyarthralgias Hyperuricemia (gout rare)	Severe liver injury in 6% given PZA + RIF Hyperuricemia is usually inconsequential
Ethambutol (EMB)	Tabs: 100 mg, 400 mg	40–55 56–75 76–90	0.8 g 1.2 g 1.6 g	2.0 g 2.8 g 4.0 g	1.2 g 2.0 g 2.4 g	$168	Optic neuritis, dose-related	Decreased acuity or red-green discrimination; dose-related

* All patients receiving INH, rifampin, and/or pyrazinamide should be instructed to report immediately any symptoms of hepatitis: anorexia, nausea, vomiting, jaundice, malaise, fever >3 days, or abdominal tenderness. Risk of hepatitis is greater with age >35 yr and daily alcohol use.

Agent	Forms	Daily dose* (maximum)	Adverse reactions	Monitoring/comments
Streptomycin	Vials	15 mg/kg/d* max-1 g/d Age >50 yrs 10 mg/kg/d 750 mg/d	Auditory, vestibular, and renal toxicity	Audiometry and vestibular tests at baseline and periodically; renal function tests
Capreomycin (Capastat)	Vials: 1 g	15 mg/kg IM max-1 g/d	Auditory, vestibular, and renal toxicity	Audiometry and vestibular tests at baseline and periodically; renal function; high frequency hearing loss in 3–10%
Kanamycin (Kantrex)	Vials: 75 and 500 mg, 1 g	15 mg/kg IV or IM max-1 g/d	Auditory, vestibular, (rare), and renal toxicity	Audiometry and vestibular tests at baseline and periodically;
Amikacin (Amikin)	Vials: 0.1, 0.5 and 1 g	15 mg/kg IV or IM max-1 g/d	Auditory, vestibular, and renal toxicity	Audiometry and vestibular tests at baseline and periodically; renal function
Ethionamide (Trecator)	Tabs: 250 mg	15–20 mg/kg in 2 doses max 500 mg bid po	GI intolerance, hepatotoxicity, photosensitivity, arthralgias, impotence, metallic taste	Hepatic enzymes monthly and D/C if transaminase ≥5 × upper limits normal. GI intolerance—may need to gradually increase dose and/or give hs and 30 min after antiemetic
Gatifloxacin (Tequin)	Caps: 400 mg	400 mg/d po, IV	GI intolerance	No monitoring for ADR
Moxifloxacin (Avelox)	Caps: 400 mg	400 mg/d po, IV	GI intolerance	No monitoring for ADR
Levofloxacin (Levoquin)	Caps: 500 and 750 mg	500 mg qd or bid po, IV	GI intolerance	No monitoring for ADR
PAS (Paser)	Tabs: 500 mg, 1 g	4–6 g po bid;	GI intolerance, hepatotoxicity, sodium load, hypersensitivity	Delayed release granules should be given with acidic food or drink
Cycloserine (Seromycin)	Caps: 250 mg	500–750 mg po bid; 10–15 mg/kg/d Max-500 mg bid	Psychosis, rash, convulsions	Assess mental status; some give pyridoxine (50 mg/250 mg cycloserine) to decrease psychiatric effects, seizures, and neuropathy

* Give IM or IV 5–7 days/wk × 2–4 months, then 2–3×/wk after culture conversion

B. Diagnostic Tests

1. AFB smear: Sensitivity of AFB stain with expectorated sputum, induced sputum and bronchoscopy aspirates are similar at 40–60% in culture positive cases (Am J Respir Crit Care Med 2000;162:2238). Specificity depends on the prevalence of TB and MOTT, but may be as low as 50% (J Clin Micro 1998;36:1046)

2. **Nucleic acid amplification** (NAA assays) (Am J Respir Crit Care Med 2001;164: 2020): Commercially available as MTB (Gen Probe) and Amplicor (Roche) at $50–100/assay. Sensitivity of NAA assays is 80–84% including virtually all smear-positive cases and about half of smear-negative/culture-positive cases. CDC recommendations (MMWR 2000;49:593):
   - AFB smear and NAA on the first sputum collected. If the smear is positive and the NAA is positive, TB is diagnosed with near 100% certainty.
   - If the smear is positive and the NAA is negative, the sputum should be tested for inhibitors by spiking the sample with lysed *M. tuberculosis* and repeat the assay. If inhibitors are not present, the patient is assumed to have MOTT.
   - If the smear is negative and the NAA is positive, additional sputum samples are recommended. If positive, the patient is presumed to have TB.
   - If both the smear and the NAA are negative, additional specimens should be tested by NAA and, if negative, TB is assumed to be excluded.
3. **AFB culture:** Frequency of false positive results in a review of 14 studies with >100 patients show a mean of 3.1% of positives were false positives (CID 2000;31:1390). The presumed mechanism is laboratory cross-contamination. The major clue is a single positive culture, especially if not supported by clinical observations.
4. **Broth-based cultures:** When combined with DNA probes, broth-based cultures are capable of detecting *M. tuberculosis* within two weeks with smear-positive cases and within three weeks with smear-negative cases (Am J Clin Path 2000;113:770; Diag Microbiol Infect Dis 2000;37:31)

C. Monitoring Drug Therapy
1. Monitoring for adverse drug reactions (ADRs)
   a. Most frequent reactions with standard 4 drug therapy are rash ± fever, hepatitis, and GI intolerance. The main cause of hepatotoxicity appears to be PZA (Am J Resp Crit Care Med 2003;167:1472). Ethambutol is a rare cause of toxicity except for occasional cases of dose-related vision changes.
   b. Recommendations
   - INH: Baseline and monthly LFTs if pre-existing liver disease, or development of abnormal LFTs that do not require discontinuing INH Monthly inquiries about symptoms that suggest hepatitis
   - RIF: No monitoring for ADRs
   - PZA: LFTs as for INH; uric acid is usually elevated, but usually is not consequential and monitoring is not recommended
   - EMB: Baseline visual acuity and Ishihara test of color discrimination. Inquire about vision changes at each monthly visit and warn to contact clinic immediately if vision changes. Monthly tests of acuity and color discrimination with doses >15–20 mg/kg for >2 months or with renal failure
2. Duration of therapy with drug-sensitive strains

Initial 8 week course: Identical for all patients

Continuation phase:
   - Cavitation or positive culture at 2 months

Cavitation	Positive culture at 8 wks	Duration continuation phase
+	−	4 mo.
−	+	4 mo.
+	+	7 mo.

   - No cavitation, negative culture at 2 months, negative HIV and no extrapulmonary TB: RIF/INH or RPT/INH × 4 mo.

- HIV or extrapulmonary TB: INH/RIF (only)
- Rationale: Risk for relapse with cavitation and/or positive sputum at 2 months using standard initial 4 drug initial phase and INH/RIF 2×/week × 16 weeks USPH study 22 (Lancet 2002;360:528).

Cavity	Sputum positive at 2 mo	Sputum negative at 2 mo
Yes	21% (n = 48)	5% (n = 150)
No	6% (n = 17)	2% (n = 181)

3. Treatment interruptions

Initial phase
Duration of interruption <14 days:
 Continue therapy, if not completed in 3 months—restart
Duration ≥14 days: Restart

Continuation phase:
≥80 doses: No additional therapy
<80% doses
 Duration of interruption <3 months:
  Continue, if not completed in 6 months—restart
 Duration of interruption ≥3 months:
  Restart 4 drug initial phase

4. **Evaluation of response:** Symptoms usually improve within 4 wk, and 85% of patients treated with INH-rifampin containing regimen convert sputum culturees to negative by the end of 2 mo. Sputum smear and culture should be performed at least monthly until conversion is documented. Weekly sputum smears with quantitation are encouraged. Patients with positive sputum cultures after 2 mo of treatment need reevaluation, drug susceptibility test, and directly observed treatment. If resistance noted, give at least two active drugs under DOT. Patients with negative cultures ≤2 mo should have one additional smear and culture at completion of treatment. Some recommend x-ray at 2–3 mo and at completion of treatment.

5. **Relapse:** Most relapses occur within 6 months and involve drug sensitive strains. Major risks are: (1) extent and severity of the lung disease as indicated by cavitation and bilateral infiltrates, and (2) positive cultures at two months (Lancet 2002;360:528).

D. Special Considerations With Treatment

1. **HIV Infection:** Concurrent treatment of TB and HIV is confounded by large pill burden (≥7 drugs), multiple drug toxicities (especially hepatitis, GI intolerance, rash and fever) drug interactions with rifampin that precludes use of all PIs and NNRTIs except efavirenz, high rates of the immune reconstitution syndrome and elevated frequency of MDRTB. TB is always treated immediately. Principles of treatment of co-infected patients:

 Identical for general population except:
 - CD4 <100/mm^3: Continuation phase of TB treatment should be daily or 3×/week
 - Once weekly rifapentine regimen should not be used.
 - Positive cultures at 2 months: Strongly consider 7 month continuation phase (total 9 mo.)
 - In absence of prior HIV therapy and CD4 <200/mm^3: Delay antiretroviral drugs for 4–8 weeks. Baseline CD4 200–350/mm^3: delay HAART until TB therapy completed
 - RIF may be used with EFV; consider AZT/3TC/ABC/TDF or PI with rifabutin.

- Rifabutin combined with other PIs and NNRTI requires a dose adjustment of both. See: www.cdc.gov/nchstp/tb/ or www.medscape.com/updates/quickguide
- When starting NNRTI or PI in patient receiving RIF, substitute rifabutin 2 weeks prior to NNRTI or PI to give a 2 week washout period for RIF
- Immune reconstitution syndrome: Frequency in various series is 11–45% with average of 18%. Risks are low baseline CD4 (especially if <50/min^3), a good CD4 response, extrapulmonary TB and early antiretroviral therapy. Clinical features include high fever; increased adenopathy, CNS lesions, pulmonary infiltrates and/or pleural effusions. Treatment is symptomatic; if severe, give prednisone 1 mg/kg and reduce dose at 1–2 weeks.

2. Extrapulmonary TB*

Standard 4 drug initial phase followed by INH/RIF for 4–7 months except for CNS. TB which is treated 9–12 months.

Site	Duration	Steroids
Lymph nodes	6 months	No
Bone or joint	6–9 months	No
Pleural disease	6 months	No
Pericarditis	6 months	Recommended*
CNS TB	9–12 months	Recommended*
Disseminated	9–12 months	No
GU TB	6 months	No
Peritoneal	6 months	No

*(N Engl J Med 2004; 351:1741)

3. Culture negative suspected active TB

Low probability: No initial treatment
Culture negative at 2 mo and x-ray unchanged
- RIF ± INH × 4 mo.
- INH × 9 mo
- RIF/PZA × 2 mo

High probability
INH/RIF/EMB/PZA × 2 mo
- Culture negative at 2 mo. and x-ray improved: INH/RIF × 2 mo
- Culture negative and x-ray unchanged: D/C therapy

4. Pregnancy and breast feeding

Regimen: INH/RIF/EMB × 9 mo or standard treatment wit INH/RIF/EMB/PZA × 2 mo, then INH/RIF × 4 mo. The issue is the safety of PZA, which has no evidence of adverse effects in pregnancy, but inadequete experience to assure safety.

Streptomycin: Only anti-TB drug with documented harm to human fetuses.

5. Renal insufficiency

Drug	Dose with CrCl <30 cc/min
INH	Standard
RIF	Standard
RZA	25–35 mg/kg 3×/wk
EMB	15–25 mg/kg 3×/wk
Moxifloxacin	Standard (400 mg/d)
Gatifloxacin	200 mg qd

Continued

Drug	Dose with CrCl <30 cc/min
Levofloxacin	750–1000 mg 3×/week
Cycloserine	250 mg qd or 500 mg 3×/wk
Ethionamide	Standard
PAS	Standard
Aminoglycosides	12–15 mg/kg 2–3×/wk

6. **Hepatic disease**

Regimen excluding INH: RIF/PZA/EMB × 6 months
Regimen excluding PZA: INH/RIF/EMB × 2 months, then INH/RIF × 7 months
Regimen for severe liver disease:
- RIF/fluoroquinolone/cycloserine/aminoglycoside × 18 months or
- Streptomycin/EMB, fluoroquinolone/another second line drug × 18–24 months

7. **Drug-resistant TB**

Drug Resistance	Regimen
INH	RIF/PZA/EMB ± fluoroquinolone × 6 mo
INH/RIF	Fluoroquinolone/PZA/EMB/aminoglycoside ± alternative agent ± 18–24 mo
RIF	INH/PZA/EMB ± fluoroquinolone 9–12 mo
MDRTB	Suggested initial therapy for suspected MDRTB INH/RIF/EMB/PZA/aminoglycoside/fluoroquinalone (levofloxacin, gatifloxacin or moxifloxacin)/either ethionamide or PAS (Lancet 2004;363:474; Clin Infect Dis 2003;36 suppl 1:584). Consider surgical resection (Am J Resp Crit Care 2004;169:1103)

II. PREVENTIVE TREATMENT FOR TUBERCULOSIS INFECTION IN THE U.S.

ATS/CDC Statement Committee on Latent Tuberculosis Infection [MMWR 2000;49(RR-6); Am J Resp Crit Care Med 2000;161:S221; MMWR 2003;52:735)

A. Testing (NEJM 2002;347:1860)

1. **Testing methods:** The traditional method is the PPD skin test which has been used for more than 100 years. A new test has been approved by the FDA which mesures the release of interferon-gamma in blood following stimulation by PPD (JAMA 2001;286:1740). At present, the usual test is the traditional PPD skin test with the following characteristics:
   - Standard test: 5 tuberculin units given intracutaneously and read at 48–72 hours, although reading up to one week is considered accurate (ARRD 1986;134:1043).
   - BCG: In one study, only 8% of those given BCG vaccine at birth had a positive PPD skin test at 15 years (ARRD 1992;145:621). BCG is given in countries that have the highest incidence of tuberculosis making it difficult to discount a positive PPD. The current recommendation is to ignore BCG vaccination when interpreting PPD skin tests.
   - Sensitivity: 10–20% of persons with tuberculosis have negative skin tests (NEJM 1971;285:1506; Chest 1980;77:32).
   - Anergy testing: Most authorities no longer recommend it.
   - Boosting: The concern is that a negative test may boost the size of the reaction with a second test. The recommendation is that persons who

undergo annual PPD skin tests such as health care workers should undergo two-step testing on initial evaluation with the second PPD given one week after a negative test.

2. Indications for PPD

Risk	Example
Recent TB exposure	Recent close (>12 hours) contact with active case
	Health care workers with TB cases
Risk of TB infection	Prior residence in countries with high TB rates
	Homeless
	Residents of long-term care facilities
Risk of activation of latent infection	HIV infection
	Recent TB infection: children <4 years, PPD conversion (>10 mm induration) in ≤2 years, injection drug use, silicosis, renal failure, diabetes, immunosuppressive therapy, hematologic cancers, prior gastrectomy or jejunoileal bypass
	Malnourished or recent weight loss >10% ideal weight

B. Candidates for treatment of latent tuberculosis

Induration caterogy of PPD

≥5 mm   HIV infection
           Recent contacts of active TB
           Fibrotic changes on x-ray consistent with TB
           Immunosuppressed: Organ transplants and others with immuno-suppression including chronic prednisone (equivalent to 15 mg/d for ≥1 mo)

≥10 mm   Recent immigrants (<5 yr) from high prevalence area
           Injection drug users
           Residents and employees of prisons, jails, nursing homes, long term care facilities for elderly, hospitals, homeless shelters
           Mycobacteria lab personnel
           Patients with silicosis, diabetes, renal failure, leukemia, lymphoma, ca head or neck, weight loss >10%, gastrectomy and jejuroleal by-pass

≥15 mm   Persons with no risk factors (Note that targeted PPD skin testing should be done only in people with defined risks. It is often unclear why these people are tested and treatment is optional)

C. Prophylaxis regimens (MMWR 2003;52:735)

1. Recommended regimens
   INH 300 mg/d × 9 mo
   INH 300 mg/d × 6 mo (not for HIV co-infection or patients with fibrotic lesions on chest x-ray)
   INH 900 mg 2 ×/wk (DOT) × 9 mo
   INH 900 mg 2 ×/wk (DOT) × 6 mo (not for HIV co-infection or patients with fibrotic lesions on chest x-ray)
   Rifampin 600 mg/d × 4 mo (contacts of patients with INH resistant, rifampin susceptible strains)

<u>Note</u>: The 2 month course of RIF + PZA is no longer recommended due to high rates of hepatotoxicity (MMWR 2003;52:735)

<u>INH regimen</u>
- Efficacy: Studies of more than 70,000 participants show efficacy of about 60% in reducing active tuberculosis (Bibl Tuberc 1970;26:28). Most studies were done with one year of therapy; a study of INH for six months showed 65% efficacy (Bull WHO 1982;60:555).
- Hepatitis: Increases in serum transaminase levels occur in 10–20%, but symptomatic hepatitis is uncommon with about one case per 1,000 (JAMA 1992;281:1014). The risk increases with alcohol consumptoin and with increasing age, but age is no longer considered in the recommendations for treatment.
- Peripheral neuropathy: Allegedly occurs in up to 2% (Am Rev Tuberc 1954;70:504) and may be prevented with pyridoxine (Tubercle 1980; 61:191).
- Current recommendations: INH for 6–9 months in the usual dose of 300 mg/day, monthly clinical monitoring, baseline transaminase levels only in persons with risk factors for hepatitis, abstinence from alcohol during the INH course and suspension of treatment if transaminase levels exceed the upper limit of normal by five-fold. The alternative regimen is 900 mg twice weekly by directly observed therapy.

<u>Rifampin regimen</u>
- Efficacy: Thought to be equivalent to INH (ARRD 1992;145:36).
- Adverse reactions: Uncommon.
- Drug interactions: Common and often important.
- Current recommendations: 600 mg/day for four months with clinical monitoring at monthly intervals, baseline transaminase measurements only for persons at risk for hepatitis, and concern for drug interactions such as protease inhibitors, warfarin, contraceptive pills, and methadone.

D. Monitoring
<u>Laboratory monitoring: INH</u>
- No lab tests at baseline unless the following:
  HIV infection, pregnancy, or <3 mo postpartum, history of liver disease (HCV, HBV, alcoholic hepatitis, cirrhosis), persons who use EtOH daily
- Baseline lab tests: AST, ALT, and bilirubin
- Active hepatitis and end-stage liver disease are relative contraindications to INH and PZA
- Follow-up lab tests: symptoms of hepatotoxicity—D/C INH if AST/ALT ≥ 3× ULN + symptoms or AST/ALT >5 × ULN without symptoms

<u>Clinical monitoring</u>: Monitor for symptoms of hepatotoxicity at baseline and every mo for INH regimen.

III. ATYPICAL MYCOBACTERIA TREATMENT *(Recommendations of American Thoracic Society: Am Rev Respir Dis 1997;156:S1)* and *M. Iseman (personal communication 2003)*

Agent	Condition	Treatment and comment
M. kansasii	Pulmonary and extrapulmonary	RIF + EMB + INH ± AK 15–18 mo (AK for extensive disease)
		RIF + EMB × 9 mo
		RIF + EMB + clarithromycin or azithromycin × 9 mo
		RIF + EMB + AK × 9 mo
		Contraindication or resistance to RIF: EMB + CIP + clarithromycin

Continued

Agent	Condition	Treatment and comment

M. avium	Pulmonary and extrapulmonary	Clarithromycin or azithromycin + EMB + RIF ± AK × 18–24 mo
		Clarithromycin + EMB + CFZ ± AK × 18–24 mo
		RIF + EMB + CFZ ± AK ± ciprofloxacin × 18–24 mo
		  Use for macrolide resistance or intolerance
		Clarithromycin + EMB ± CFZ × 18–24 mo
		  Use for elderly patients with less extensive disease
		Note: Can substitute azithromycin for clarithromycin if intolerant of clarithromycin or to avoid interaction between clarithromycin and RIF
		Note: Twice weekly therapy is probably as effective as daily therapy—advantages include reduced cost and toxicity

M. fortuitum	Cutaneous and bone	<u>In vitro tests</u> required <u>Standard</u>: Amikacin (10–15 mg/kg/d) + cefoxitin (12 g/d) or imipenem ≥ 2 wk, then oral regimen based on vitro activity—usually clarithromycin (500 mg bid), doxycycline (100 mg bid), sulfamethoxazole (1 g tid) ± ciprofloxacin (500 mg bid) × ≥4 mo (cutaneous) or ≥6 mo (bone)* <u>Surgery</u>: Usually indicated for extensive disease and with foreign bodies
	Pulmonary	<u>Most lung disease</u> caused by rapid growers i.e. *M. abscessus* <u>*M. fortuitum*</u>: Two oral agents based on in vitro activity × 6–12 mo
M. abscessus	Cutaneous	<u>Standard</u>: Amikacin + cefoxitin or imipenem as above, then oral agent if any are active in vitro—usually clarithromycin ± clofazimine × ≥4 mo (cutaneous) or ≥6 mo (bone)* <u>Surgery</u>: As above
	Pulmonary	<u>Standard</u>: Amikacin + cefoxitin (as above) × 2–4 wk, then periodic parenteral treatment or clarithromycin for suppressive therapy* <u>Surgery</u>: May be curative for local disease (Am Rev Respir Dis 1993;148:1271)*
M. chelonae	Cutaneous	<u>Standard</u>: Tobramycin + cefoxitin (12 g/d) or imipenem × ≥ 2 wk, then oral agents based on in vitro activity especially clarithromycin (500 mg bid) monotherapy × 6 mo* (Am Intern Med 1993;119:482)
M. marinum	Cutaneous	<u>Standard</u>: Multiple regimens—clarithromycin (500 mg bid); doxycycline (100 mg bid); TMP-SMX (DS bid); rifampin (600 mg bid) + ethambutol (15 mg/kg/d)—all ≥3 mo* <u>Surgery</u>: Infections in closed space of hand and refractory infections
M. scrofulaceum	Lymphadenitis	Surgical excision; very resistant to drugs—INH, rifampin, streptomycin + cycloserine (rare in U.S.)
M. ulcerans	Buruli ulcer	Rifampin + amikacin (7.5 mg/kg IV bid) or ethambutol + TMP-SMX (1 DS tid) × 4–6 wk; surgical excision
M. haemophilum	Skin, soft tissue, osteomyelitis	Sensitive to ciprofloxacin, cycloserine, kanamycin, rifabutin; experience with treatment limited (Ann Intern Med 1994;120:118)
M. bovis	Pulmonary	As with *M. tuberculosis* but resistant to pyrazinamide

Continued

Agent	Condition	Treatment and comment
M. szulgae	Pulmonary, extrapulmonary	Same as M. kansasii (Thorax 1987;42:838)
M. malmoense	Pulmonary, disseminated	Clarithromycin + ethambutol + rifabutin ± strepto-mycin × 18–24 mo (Tubercle 1985;66:197; CID 1994;18:596)
M. xenopi	Pulmonary	Rifampin or rifabutin + clarithromycin ± streptomycin; surgery for relapses (Am Rev Respir Dis 1981;123:104; Tubercle 1988;69:47)
M. simiae	Pulmonary	Clarithromycin, ethambutol, rifabutin + streptomycin (need in vitro susceptibility tests)
M. smegmatis	Soft tissue, bone, etc	Ethambutol, amikacin, ciprofloxacin, sulfonamides, clofazimine, imipenem, doxycycline
M. gordonae	Pulmonary, disseminated	Combinations of rifampin, ethambutol, streptomycin ± INH, clofazimine, clarithromycin (AAC 1992;36:1987; Dermatology 1993;187:301)
M. genavense	Disseminated	Clarithromycin + other agents—INH, ethambutol, rifampin,ciprofloxacin, pyrazinamide (AIDS 1993;7:1357)

* Efficacy is established.

A. Doses

Amikacin: 12–15 mg/kg/day IV or IM or 15–22 mg/kg tiw
Azithromycin: 250–500 mg/day or 500 mg tiw
Cefoxitin: 2 g IV q8–12h
Ciprofloxacin: 500–750 mg bid, 750 mg qd or 750 mg tiw
Clarithromycin: 500–750 mg/d, 500 mg bid or 750 mg tiw
Doxycycline: 100 mg bid
Ethambutol: 25 mg/kg/d × 2 mo, then 15 mg/kg or 25–30 mg/kg tiw
Imipenem: 1 g IV q12h
Isonazid: 300–600 mg/d or 600 mg tiw
Levofloxacin: 500–750 mg/day or 750 mg tiw
Linezolid: 600 mg IV or po bid
Rifabutin: 150–300 mg/d or 300 mg tiw
Rifampin: 600 mg qd or 600 mg tiw

Streptomycin regimens

Wt/age	Initial 6–12 wks	Maintenance
>50 kg <50 yr	1 g 5×/wk	1 g 3×/wk
<50 kg <70 yr	500 mg 5×/wk	750 mg 2×/wk
>70 yr	750 mg 2×/wk	750 mg 2×/wk

B. Classification of atypical mycobacteria *(adapted from Am Rev Respir Crit Care Dis 1997;156:59)*

Clinical	Mycobacteria	Geography	Morphology	Other mycobacteria
Pulmonary	M. avium	Worldwide	Nonpigmented Slow growth	M. simiae, M. szulgai, M. fortuitum, M.
	M. kansasii	U.S., Europe coal mining	Pigmented	celatum, M. asaiticum, M. shimodii,
	M. abscessus	Mostly U.S.	Nonpigmented Rapid growth	M. haemophilum, M. smegmatis
	M. xenopi	Europe Canada	Pigmented Slow growth	
Lymphadenitis	M. avium	Worldwide	Nonpigmented	M. fortuitum, M.
	M. scrofulaceum	Worldwide	Pigmented	chelonae, M. ab-
	M. malmoense	U.K. Scand	Slow growth	scessus, M. kansasii, M. haemophilum
Skin	M. marium	Worldwide	Growth at 28–30°C	M. aviam, M. kansasii, M. nonchromo-
	M. fortuitum	Worldwide	Nonpigmented Rapid growth	genicum, M. smeg- matis,
	M. chelmae	Worldwide	Nonpigmented Rapid growth	M. hoemophilum
	M. abscessus	Worldwide	Nonpigmented Rapid growth	
	M. ulcerans	Australia SE Asia, Africa	Pigmented Slow growth	
Disseminated	M. avium	Worlwide	AIDS patients— 80% pigmented	M. xenopi, M. abscessus,
	M. kansasii	U.S.	Photochromogen	M. malmoense
	M. chelonae	U.S.	Nonpigmented	M. simiae,
	M. haemophilum	U.S. Australia	Nonpigmented Needs hemin, low temperature, and CO_2	M. genovense, M. marium, M. fortuitum, M. canspicum

Runyon classification

Group	Prior Runyon group	Agents	Growth rate (days)	Comments/sites of disease
Photochromogens (slow growing)	I	M. kansasii	10–21	Rare contaminant. Lung disease
		M. marium	7–14	Optimal growth at 32°C. Rare contaminant. Skin and soft tissue
		M. simiae	7–14	Rare human pathogen. Lung
		M. asiaticum	7–14	Rarely pathogenic
Scotochromogens (slow growing)	II	M. scrofula- ceum	10–28	Nearly disappeared from U.S. Lymphadenitis
		M. szulgae	12–28	Infrequent human pathogen. Lung
		M. gordonae	10–28	Rarely pathogenic. Environmental contaminant
		M. flavescens	7–10	Rarely pathogenic. Environmental contaminant

Continued

165

Group	Prior Runyon group	Agents	Growth rate (days)	Comments/sites of disease
Nonphotochromogens (slow growing)	III	*M. avium*	10–21	*M. avium* and *M. intracellulare* sometimes referred to as *M. avium* complex (MAC)
		M. intracellulare	10–21	
		M. ulcerans	28–60	Buruli ulcer (Australia and Africa)
		M. xenopi	14–28	Optimal growth at 42°C. Environmental contaminant. Lung
		M. malmoense	18–84	Infrequent human pathogen. Lung. Optimal growth at 20–32°C. Skin and soft tissue in immunosuppressed
		M. haemophilum		
		M. terrae complex	10–21	Rarely pathogenic. Environmental contaminant
		M. gastri	10–21	Rarely pathogenic. Environmental contaminant
		M. flavescens		Rarely pathogenic
		M. triviale	10–21	Environmental contaminant
Rapid growers	IV	*M. fortuitum*	3–7	Environmental contaminant. Ulcers
		M. chelonae	3–7	Environmental contaminant. Ulcers
		M. smegmatis	3–7	Rarely pathogenic
		M. phlei	3–7	Rarely pathogenic

DRUGS FOR TREATMENT OF PARASITIC INFECTIONS

*(Reproduced with permission from Medical Letter Handbook of
Antimicrobial Therapy 16th Edition 2002;120–143)*

Infection	Drug	Adult dosage
***Acanthamoeba* keratitis**		
Drug of choice:	See footnote 1	
AMEBIASIS (*Entamoeba histolytica*)		
asymptomatic		
Drug of choice:	Iodoquinol	650 mg tid × 20 d
or	Paromomycin	25–35 mg/kg/d in 3 doses × 7 d
Alternative:	Diloxanide furoate[2]	500 mg tid × 10 d
mild to moderate intestinal disease[3]		
Drug of choice:[4]	Metronidazole	500–750 mg tid × 7–10 d
or	Tinidazole[5]	2 g/d divided tid × 3 d
severe intestinal and extraintestinal disease[3]		
Drug of choice:	Metronidazole	750 mg tid × 7–10 d
or	Tinidazole[5]	800 mg tid × 5 d
AMEBIC MENINGOENCEPHALITIS, PRIMARY		
Naegleria		
Drug of choice:	Amphotericin B[6,7]	1 mg/kg/d IV, uncertain duration
Acanthamoeba		
Drug of choice:	See footnote 8	
Balamuthia mandrillaris		
Drug of choice:	See footnote 9	
Sappinia diploidea		
Drug of choice:	See footnote 10	
ANCYLOSTOMA caninum (Eosinophilic enterocolitis)		
Drug of choice:	Albendazole[7]	400 mg once
or	Mebendazole	100 mg bid × 3 d
or	Pyrantel pamoate[7]	11 mg/kg (max. 1 g) × 3 d
or	Endoscopic removal	
Ancylostoma duodenale, see HOOKWORM		
ANGIOSTRONGYLIASIS		
Angiostrongylus cantonensis		
Drug of choice:	See footnote 11	
Angiostrongylus costaricensis		
Drug of choice:	See footnote 12	
ANISAKIASIS(*Anisakis*)		
Treatment of choice:	Surgical or endoscopic removal	
ASCARIASIS (*Ascaris lumbricoides,* roundworm)		
Drug of choice:	Albendazole[7]	400 mg once
or	Mebendazole	100 mg bid × 3 d or 500 mg once
or	Pyrantel pamoate[7]	11 mg/kg once (max. 1 g)

Continued

Infection		Drug	Adult dosage
BABESIOSIS (*Babesia microti*)			
Drugs of choice:[13]		Clindamycin[7]	1.2 g bid IV or 600 mg tid po × 7–10 d
		plus quinine	650 mg tid po × 7 d
	or	Atovaquone[7]	750 mg bid × 7–10 d
		plus azithromycin[7]	600 mg po daily × 7–10 d

Balamuthia mandrillaris, see AMEBIC MENINGOENCEPHALITIS, PRIMARY

BALANTIDIASIS (*Balantidium coli*)			
Drug of choice:		Tetracycline[7,14]	500 mg qid × 10 d
Alternatives:		Metronidazole[7]	750 mg tid × 5 d
		Iodoquinol[7]	650 mg tid × 20 d

BAYLISASCARIASIS (*Baylisascaris procyonis*)		
Drug of choice:	See footnote 15	

BLASTOCYSTIS hominis infection		
Drug of choice:	See footnote 16	

CAPILLARIASIS (*Capillaria philippinensis*)		
Drug of choice:	Mebendazole[7]	200 mg bid × 20 d
Alternative:	Albendazole[7]	400 mg daily × 10 d

Chagas' disease, see TRYPANOSOMIASIS

Clonorchis sinensis, see FLUKE infection

CRYPTOSPORIDIOSIS (*Cryptosporidium*)		
Drug of choice:	See footnote 17	

CUTANEOUS LARVA MIGRANS (creeping eruption, dog and cat hookworm)			
Drug of choice:[18]		Albendazole[7]	400 mg daily × 3 d
	or	Ivermectin[7]	200 µg/kg daily × 1–2 d
	or	Thiabendazole	Topically

CYCLOSPORA infection		
Drug of choice:[19]	Trimethoprim- sulfamethoxazole[7]	TMP 160 mg, SMX 800 mg bid × 7–10 d

CYSTICERCOSIS, see TAPEWORM infection

DIENTAMOEBA fragilis infection			
Drug of choice:		Iodoquinol	650 mg tid × 20 d
	or	Paromomycin[7]	25–35 mg/kg/d in 3 doses × 7 d
	or	Tetracycline[7,14]	500 mg qid × 10 d
	or	Metronidazole	500–750 mg tid × 10 d

Diphyllobothrium latum, see TAPEWORM infection

DRACUNCULUS medinensis (guinea worm) infection		
Drug of choice:	Metronidazole[7,20]	250 mg tid × 10 d

Echinococcus, see TAPEWORM infection

Entamoeba histolytica, see AMEBIASIS

Continued

Infection	Drug	Adult dosage
ENTAMOEBA polecki infection		
Drug of choice:	Metronidazole[7]	750 mg tid × 10 d
ENTEROBIUS vermicularis (pinworm) infection		
Drug of choice:[21]	Pyrantel pamoate	11 mg/kg base once (max. 1 g); repeat in 2 weeks
or	Mebendazole	100 mg once; repeat in 2 weeks
or	Albendazole[7]	400 mg once; repeat in 2 weeks

Fasciola hepatica, see FLUKE infection

FILARIASIS[22]

Wuchereria bancrofti, Brugia malayi, Brugia timori

Drug of choice:[23,24]	Diethylcarbamazine[25]	Day 1: 50 mg, p.c.
		Day 2: 50 mg tid
		Day 3: 100 mg tid
		Days 4 through 14:
		6 mg/kg/d in 3 doses

Loa loa

Drug of choice:[24,26]	Diethylcarbamazine[25]	Day 1: 50 mg p.c.
		Day 2: 50 mg tid
		Day 3: 100 mg tid
		Days 4 through 21:
		9 mg/kg/d in 3 doses

Mansonella ozzardi
Drug of choice:[24] — See footnote 27

Mansonella perstans

Drug of choice:[24]	Mebendazole[7]	100 mg bid × 30 d
or	Albendazole[7]	400 mg bid × 10 d

Mansonella streptocerca

Drug of choice:[24,28]	Diethylcarbamazine*	6 mg/kg/d × 14 d
or	Ivermectin[7]	150 μg/kg once

Tropical Pulmonary Eosinophilia (TPE)

Drug of choice:	Diethylcarbamazine*	6 mg/kg/d in 3 doses × 21 d

Onchocerca volvulus (River blindness)

Drug of choice:	Ivermectin[29]	150 μg/kg once, repeated every 6 to 12 months until asymptomatic

FLUKE, hermaphroditic, infection

Clonorchis sinensis (Chinese liver fluke)

Drug of choice:	Praziquantel	75 mg/kg/d in 3 doses × 1 d
or	Albendazole[7]	10 mg/kg × 7 d

Fasciola hepatica (sheep liver fluke)

Drug of choice:[30]	Triclabendazole*	10 mg/kg once
Alternative:	Bithionol*	30–50 mg/kg × 10–15 doses

Fasciolopsis buski, Heterophyes heterophyes, Metagonimus yokogawai

Drug of choice:	Praziquantel[7]	75 mg/kg/d in 3 doses × 1 d

Metorchis conjunctus (North American liver fluke)[31]

Drug of choice:	Praziquantel[7]	75 mg/kg/d in 3 doses × 1 d

Continued

Infection	Drug	Adult dosage
Nanophyetus salmincola		
Drug of choice:	Praziquantel[7]	60 mg/kg/d in 3 doses × 1 d
Opisthorchis viverrini (Southeast Asian liver fluke)		
Drug of choice:	Praziquantel	75 mg/kg/d in 3 doses × 1 d
Paragonimus westermani (lung fluke)		
Drug of choice:	Praziquantel[7]	75 mg/kg/d in 3 doses × 2 d
Alternative:[32]	Bithionol*	30–50 mg/kg on alternate days × 10–15 doses
GIARDIASIS (*Giardia lamblia*)		
Drug of choice:	Metronidazole[7]	250 mg tid × 5 d
Alternatives:[33]	Quinacrine[2]	100 mg tid × 5 d (max. 300 mg/d)
	Tinidazole[5]	2 g once
	Furazolidone	100 mg qid × 7–10 d
	Paromomycin[7,34]	25–35 mg/kg/d in 3 doses × 7 d
GNATHOSTOMIASIS (*Gnathostoma spinigerum*)		
Treatment of choice:[35] Albendazole[7]		400 mg bid × 21 d
or	Ivermectin[7]	200 μg/kg/d × 2 d
or	Surgical removal	
GONGYLONEMIASIS (*Gongylonema sp.*)		
Treatment of choice:	Surgical removal	
or	Albendazole[7,36]	10 mg/kg/d × 3 d
HOOKWORM infection (*Ancylostoma duodenale, Necator americanus*)		
Drug of choice:	Albendazole[7]	400 mg once
or	Mebendazole	100 mg bid × 3 d or 500 mg once
or	Pyrantel pamoate[7]	11 mg/kg (max. 1 g) × 3 d
Hydatid cyst, see TAPEWORM infection		
Hymenolepis nana, see TAPEWORM infection		
ISOSPORIASIS (*Isospora belli*)		
Drug of choice:[37]	Trimethoprim-sulfamethoxazole[7]	160 mg TMP, 800 mg SMX bid × 10 d
LEISHMANIASIS[38]		
Drug of choice:[39]	Sodium stibogluconate*	20 mg Sb/kg/d IV or IM × 20–28 d[40]
or	Meglumine antimonate*	20 mg Sb/kg/d IV or IM × 20–27 d[40]
or	Amphotericin B[7]	0.5 to 1 mg/kg IV daily or every 2 d for up to 8 wks
or	Liposomal Amphotericin B[41]	3 mg/kg/d (days 1–5) and 3 mg/kg/d days 14, 21[42]
Alternatives:	Pentamidine	2–4 mg/kg daily or every 2 d IV or IM for up to 15 doses[43]
or	Paromomycin[44]*	Topically bid × 10–20 d

Continued

Infection		Drug	Adult dosage
LICE infestation (*Pediculus humanus, P. capitis, Phthirus pubis*)[45]			
Drug of choice:		1% Permethrin[46]	Topically
	or	0.5% Malathion[47]	Topically
Alternative:		Pyrethrins with piperonyl butoxide[46]	Topically
	or	Ivermectin[7,48]	200 μg/kg once

Loa loa, see FILARIASIS

MALARIA, Treatment of (*Plasmodium falciparum, P. ovale, P. vivax,* and *P. malariae*)
  Chloroquine-resistant *P. falciparum*[49]
    ORAL

Drugs of choice:		Quinine sulfate plus	650 mg q8h × 3–7 d[50]
		doxycycline[7,14]	100 mg bid × 7 d
		or plus	
		tetracycline[7,14]	250 mg qid × 7 d
		or plus	
		pyrimethamine-sulfadoxine[51]	3 tablets at once on last day of quinine
		or plus	
		clindamycin[7,52]	900 mg tid × 5 d
	or	Atovaquone/proguanil[53]	2 adult tablets bid × 3 d
Alternatives:[54]		Mefloquine[55,56]	750 mg followed by 500 mg 12 hrs later
		Halofantrine[57]*	500 mg q6h × 3 doses; repeat in 1 week[58]
		Artesunate[59]* plus	4 mg/kg/d × 3 d
		mefloquine[55,56]	750 mg followed by 500 mg 12 hrs later

  Chloroquine-resistant *P. vivax*[60]

Drug of choice:		Quinine sulfate plus	650 mg q8h × 3–7 d[50]
		doxycycline[7,14]	100 mg bid × 7 d
	or	Mefloquine[55,56]	750 mg followed by 500 mg 12 hrs later
Alternatives:		Halofantrine[57,61]*	500 mg q6h × 3 doses
		Chloroquine	25 mg base/kg in 3 doses over 48 hrs
		plus	
		primaquine[62]	2.5 mg base/kg in 3 doses over 48 hrs

  All *Plasmodium* except Chloroquine-resistant
    ORAL

Drug of choice:	Chloroquine phosphate[63]	1 g (600 mg base), then 500 mg (300 mg base) 6 hrs later, then 500 mg (300 mg base) at 24 and 48 hrs

Continued

Infection		Drug	Adult dosage*
MALARIA, Treatment of (*continued*)			
All *Plasmodium*			
PARENTERAL			
Drug of choice:[64]		Quinidine gluconate[65]	10 mg/kg loading dose (max. 600 mg) in normal saline slowly over 1 to 2 hrs, followed by continuous infusion of 0.02 mg/kg/min until oral therapy can be started
	or	Quinine dihydrochloride[65]	20 mg/kg loading dose IV in 5% dextrose over 4 hrs, followed by 10 mg/kg over 2–4 hrs q8h (max. 1800 mg/d) until oral therapy can be started
Alternative:		Artemether[66]*	3.2 mg/kg IM, then 1.6 mg/kg daily × 5–7 d
Prevention of relapses: *P. vivax* and *P. ovale* only			
Drug of choice:		Primaquine phosphate[62,67]	26.3 mg (15 mg base)/d × 14 d or 79 mg (45 mg base)/wk × 8 wks
MALARIA, Prevention of[68]			
Chloroquine-sensitive areas[49]			
Drug of choice:		Chloroquine phosphate[69,70]	500 mg (300 mg base), once/week[71]
Chloroquine-resistant areas[49]			
Drug of choice:		Mefloquine[56,70,72]	250 mg once/week[71]
	or	Doxycycline[7,70]	100 mg daily[73]
	or	Atovaquone/ Proguanil[53,70]	250 mg/100 mg (1 adult tablet) daily[74]
Alternatives:		Primaquine[7,62,75]	30 mg base daily
		Chloroquine phosphate	500 mg (300 mg base) once/week[71]
		plus proguanil[76]	200 mg once/day
Presumptive treatment			
		Atovaquone/proguanil[53]	2 adult tablets bid × 3 d[74]
	or	Pyrimethamnine-sulfadoxine[51]	Carry a single dose (3 tablets) for self treatment of febrile illness when medical care is not immediately available

MICROSPORIDIOSIS

    Ocular (*Encephalitozoon hellem, Encephalitozoon cuniculi, Vittaforma corneae [Nosema corneum]*)

Drug of choice:[65]		Albendazole[7]	400 mg bid
		plus fumagillin[77]*	

    Intestinal (*Enterocytozoon bieneusi, Encephalitozoon [Septata] intestinalis*)
    E. bieneusi[78]

Continued

Infection	Drug	Adult dosage
Drug of choice: *E. intestinalis*	Fumagillin*	60 mg/d po × 14 d
Drug of choice:	Albendazole[7]	400 mg bid × 21 d

Disseminated (*E. hellem, E. cuniculi, E. intestinalis, Pleistophora* sp., *Trachipleistophora* sp.)

Drug of choice:[79]	Albendazole[7]	400 mg bid

Mites, see SCABIES

MONILIFORMIS moniliformis infection

Drug of choice:	Pyrantel pamoate[7]	11 mg/kg once, repeat twice, 2 wks apart

Naegleria species, see AMEBIC MENINGOENCEPHALITIS, PRIMARY

Necator americanus, see HOOKWORM infection

OESOPHAGOSTOMUM bifurcum

Drug of choice:	See footnote 80	

Onchocerca volvulus, see FILARIASIS

Opisthorchis viverrini, see FLUKE infection

Paragonimus westermani, see FLUKE infection

Pediculus capitis, humanus, Phthirus pubis, see LICE

Pinworm, see ENTEROBIUS

PNEUMOCYSTIS carinii pneumonia (PCP)[81]

Drug of choice:	Trimethoprim-
	  sulfamethoxazole
		TMP 15 mg/kg/d, SMX
		  75 mg/kg/d, oral or IV in
		  3 or 4 doses × 14–21 d

Alternatives:	Primaquine[7,62]
	  plus clindamycin[7]
		30 mg base po daily × 21 days
		600 mg IV q6h × 21 days, or
		  300–450 mg po q6h × 21 days

or	Trimethoprim[7]
	  plus dapsone[7]
	Pentamidine
		5 mg/kg po tid × 21 days
		100 mg po daily × 21 days
		3–4 mg/kg IV daily ×
		  14–21 days

or	Atovaquone	750 mg bid po × 21 d

    Primary and secondary prophylaxis[82]

Drug of choice:	Trimethoprim-
	  sulfamethoxazole
		1 tab (single or double strength)
		  daily

Alternatives:[83]	Dapsone[7]	50 mg bid, or 100 mg daily
or	Dapsone[7] plus pyrimethamine[84]	50 mg daily or 200 mg each week 50 mg or 75 mg each week
or	Pentamidine aerosol	300 mg inhaled monthly via *Respirgard II* nebulizer
or	Atovaquone[7]	1500 mg daily

Roundworm, see ASCARIASIS

Sappinia Diploidea, see AMEBIC MENINGOENCEPHALITIS, PRIMARY

Continued

Infection	Drug	Adult dosage*
SCABIES (*Sarcoptes scabiei*)		
Drug of choice:	5% Permethrin	Topically
Alternatives:	Ivermectin[7,85]	200 µg/kg po once
	10% Crotamiton	Topically once/daily × 2
SCHISTOSOMIASIS (*Bilharziasis*)		
S. haematobium		
Drug of choice:	Praziquantel	40 mg/kg/d in 2 doses × 1 d
S. japonicum		
Drug of choice:	Praziquantel	60 mg/kg/d in 3 doses × 1 d
S. mansoni		
Drug of choice:	Praziquantel	40 mg/kg/d in 2 doses × 1 d
Alternative:	Oxamniquine[86]	15 mg/kg once[87]
S. mekongi		
Drug of choice:	Praziquantel	60 mg/kg/d in 3 doses × 1 d
Sleeping sickness, see TRYPANOSOMIASIS		
STRONGYLOIDIASIS (*Strongyloides stercoralis*)		
Drug of choice:[88]	Ivermectin	200 µg/kg/d × 1–2 d
Alternative:	Thiabendazole	50 mg/kg/d in 2 doses (max. 3 g/d) × 2 d[89]

TAPEWORM infection
—Adult (intestinal stage)

***Diphyllobothrium latum* (fish), *Taenia saginata* (beef), *Taenia solium* (pork), *Dipylidium caninum* (dog)**		
Drug of choice:	Praziquantel[7]	5–10 mg/kg once
Alternative:	Niclosamide	2 g once
***Hymenolepis nana* (dwarf tapeworm)**		
Drug of choice:	Praziquantel[7]	25 mg/kg once

—Larval (tissue stage)

***Echinococcus granulosus* (hydatid cyst)**		
Drug of choice:[90]	Albendazole	400 mg bid × 1–6 months
Echinococcus multilocularis		
Treatment of choice:	See footnote 91	
***Cysticercus cellulosae* (cysticercosis)**		
Treatment of choice:	See footnote 92	
Alternative:	Albendazole	400 mg bid × 8–30 d, can be repeated as necessary
or	Praziquantel[5]	50–100 mg/kg/d in 3 doses × 30 d

Toxocariasis, see VISCERAL LARVA MIGRANS		
TOXOPLASMOSIS (*Toxoplasma gondii*)[93]		
Drugs of choice:[94]	Pyrimethamine[95,96]	25–100 mg/d × 3–4 wks
	plus sulfadiazine	1–1.5 g qid × 3–4 wks
Alternative:[97]	Spiramycin*	3–4 g/d × 3–4 wks

Continued

Infection	Drug	Adult dosage
TRICHINOSIS (*Trichinella spiralis*)		
Drugs of choice:	Steroids for severe symptoms	200–400 mg tid × 3 d, then
	plus mebendazole[7]	400–500 mg tid × 10 d
Alternative:	Albendazole[7]	400 mg bid × 8–14 d
TRICHOMONIASIS (*Trichomonas vaginalis*)		
Drug of choice:[98]	Metronidazole	2 g once or 500 mg bid × 7 d
or	Tinidazole[5]	2 g once or 500 mg bid
***TRICHOSTRONGYLUS* infection**		
Drug of choice:	Pyrantel pamoate[7]	11 mg/kg base once (max. 1 g)
Alternative:	Mebendazole[7]	100 mg bid × 3 d
or	Albendazole[7]	400 mg once
TRICHURIASIS (*Trichuris trichiura*, whipworm)		
Drug of choice:	Mebendazole	100 mg bid × 3d or 500 mg once
Alternative:	Albendazole[7]	400 mg once[86]
TRYPANOSOMIASIS		
T. cruzi (American trypanosomiasis, Chagas' disease)		
Drug of choice:	Benznidazole*	5–7 mg/kg/d in 2 divided doses × 30–90 d
	Nifurtimox*	8–10 mg/kg/d in 3–4 doses × 90–120 d
T. brucei gambiense (West African trypanosomiasis, sleeping sickness) **hemolymphatic stage**		
Drug of choice:	Pentamidine isethionate[7]	4 mg/kg/d IM × 10 d
Alternative:	Suramin*	100–200 mg (test dose) IV, then 1 g IV on days 1, 3, 7, 14, and 21
or	Eflornithine*	
T. b. rhodesiense (East African trypanosomiasis, sleeping sickness) **hemolymphatic stage**		
Drug of choice:	Suramin*	100–200 mg (test dose) IV, then 1 g IV on days 1, 3, 7, 14, and 21
late disease with CNS involvement (*T. b. gambiense* or *T. b. rhodesiense*)		
Drug of choice:	Melarsoprol	2–3.6 mg/kg/d IV × 3 d; after 1 wk 3.6 mg/kg per day IV × 3 d; repeat again after 10–21 days
or	Eflornithine	
VISCERAL LARVA MIGRANS (Toxocariasis)		
Drug of choice:	Albendazole[7]	400 mg bid × 5 d
	Mebendazole[5]	100–200 mg bid × 5 d
Whipworm, see TRICHURIASIS		
Wuchereria bancrofti, see FILARIASIS		

*Availability problems.

1. For treatment of keratitis caused by *Acanthamoeba,* concurrent topical use of 0.1% propamidine isethionate (Brolene) plus neomycin-polymyxin B-gramicidin ophthalmic solution has been successful (SL Hargrave et al, Ophthalmology 1999;106:952). In addtion, 0.02% topical polyhexamethylene biguanide (PHMB) and/or chlorhexadine has been used successfully in a large number of patients (G Tabin et al, Cornea 2001;20:757; YS Wysenbeek et al, Cornea 2000;19:464). PHMB is available from Leiters Park Avenue Pharmacy, San Jose, CA (800-292-6773).

2. The drug is not available commercially, but as a service can be compounded by Medical Center Pharmacy, New Haven, CT (203-688-6816) or Panorama Compounding Pharmacy 6744 Balboa Blvd, Van Nuys, CA 91406 (800-247-9767).

3. Treatment should be followed by a course of iodoquinol or paromomcycin in the dosage used to treat asymptomatic amebiasis.

4. Nitazoxanide (an investigational drug in the U.S. manufactured by Romark Laboratories, Tampa, Florida, 813-282-8544, www.romarklabs.com) 500 mg bid × 3 d is also effective for treatment of amebiasis (JF Rossignol et al, J Infect Dis 2001;184:381).

5. A nitro-imidazole similar to metronidazole, but not marketed in the U.S., tinidazole appears to be at least as effective as metronidazole and better tolerated. Omidazole, a similar drug, is also used outside the U.S.

6. A *Naegleria* infection was treated successfully with intravenous and intrathecal use of both amphotericin B and miconazole, plus rifampin (J Seidel et al, N Engl J Med 1982;306:346). Other reports of successful therapy are questionable.

7. An approved drug, but considered investigational for this condition by the U.S. Food and Drug Administration.

8. Strains of *Acanthamoeba* isolated from fatal granulomatous amebic encephalitis are usually susceptible *in vitro* to pentamidine, ketoconazole (Nizoral), flucytosine (Ancobon), and (less so) to amphotericin B. Chronic *Acanthamoeba* meningitis has been successfully treated in 2 children with a combination of oral trimethoprim/sulfamethoxazole, rifampin, and ketoconazole (T Singhal et al, Pediatr Infect Dis J 2001;20:623), and in an AIDS patient with fluconazole and sulfadiazine combined with surgical resection of the CNS lesion (M Seijo Martinez et al, J Clin Microbiol 2000;38:3892). Disseminated cutaneous infection in an immunocompromised patient has been treated successfully with IV pentamidine isethionate, topical chlorhexidine and 2% ketoconazole cream, followed by oral itraconazole (Sporanox) (CA Slater et al, N Engl J Med 1994;331:85).

9. A free-living leptomyxid ameba that causes subacute to chronic granulomatous CNS disease. *In vitro* pentamidine isethionate 10 µg/mL is amebastatic (CF Denney et al, Clin Infect Dis 1997;25:1354). One patient, according to Medical Letter consultants, was successfully treated with clarithromycin (Biaxin) 500 mg tid, fluconazole (Diflucan) 400 mg once daily, sulfadiazine 1.5 g q6h, and flucytosine (Ancobon) 1.5 g q6h.

10. A recently described free-living ameba not previously known to be pathogenic to humans. It was successfully treated with azithromycin, IV pentamidine, itraconazole, and flucytosine (BB Gelman et al, JAMA 2001;285:2450).

11. Most patients have a self-limited course and recover completely. Analgesics, corticosteroids, and careful removal of CSF at frequent intervals can relieve symptoms (FD Pien and BC Pien, Int J Infect Dis 1999;3:161; V Lo Re and SJ Gluckman, Clin Infect Dis 2001;33:e112). In a recent report, mebendazole and a glucocorticosteroid appeared to shorten the course of infection (H-C Tsai et al, Am J Med 2001;111:109). No drug is proven to be effective and some patients have worsened when given thiabendazole, albendazole, mebendazole, or ivermectin.

12. Mebendazole has been used in experimental animals.

13. Exchange transfusion has been used in severely ill patients and those with high (>10%) parasitemia (JC Hatcher et al, Clin Infect Dis 2001;32:1117). Combination therapy with atovaquone and azithromycin is as effective as clindamycin/quinine and may be better tolerated (PJ Krause et al, N Engl J Med 2000;343:1454). Concurrent use of pentamidine and trimethoprim-sulfamethoxazole has been reported to cure an infection with *B. divergens,* the most common *Babesia* species in Europe (D Raoult et al, Ann Intern Med 1987;107:944)

14. Use of tetracyclines is contraindicated in pregnancy and in children younger than 8 years old.
15. No drugs have been demonstrated to be effective. Albendazole 25 mg/kg/d × 10 d started up to 3 d after possible infection might prevent clinical disease and is recommended for children with known exposure (ingestion of racoon stool or contaminated soil) (MMWR Morb Mortal Wkly Rep 2002;50:1153). Mebendazole, thiabendazole, levamisole (Ergamisol) and ivermectin could also be tried. Steroid therapy may be helpful, especially in eye and CNS infections. Ocular baylisascariasis has been treated successfully using laser photocoagulation therapy to destroy the intraretinal larvae.
16. Clinical significance of these organisms is controversial, but metronidazole 750 mg tid × 10 d or iodoquinol 650 mg tid × 20 d has been reported to be effective (DJ Stenzel and PFL Borenam, Clin Microbiol Rev 1996;9:563). Metronidazole resistance may be common (K Haresh et al, Trop Med Int Health 1999;4:274). Trimethoprim-sulfamethoxazole is an alternative regimen (UZ Ok et al, Am J Gastroenterol 1999;94:3245).
17. Three days of treatment with nitazoxanide (see footnote 4) may be useful for treating cryptosporidial diarrhea in immunocompetent patients. The recommended dose in adults is 500 mg bid, in children 4–11 years old, 200 mg bid, and in children 1–3 years old, 100 mg bid (JA Rossignol et al, J Infect Dis 2001;184:103). A small randomized, double-blind trial in symptomatic HIV-infected patients found paromomycin similar to placebo (RG Hewitt et al, Clin Infect Dis 2000;3:1084).
18. G Albanese et al, Int J Dermatol 2001;40:67.
19. HIV-infected patients may need higher dosage and long-term maintenance. In cases of cotrimoxazole intolerance, ciprofloxacin 500 mg bid × 7 d has been effective (R-I Verdier et al, Ann Intern Med 2000;132:885).
20. Not curative, but decreases inflammation and facilitates removing the worm. Mebendazole 400–800 mg/d for 6 days has been reported to kill the worm directly.
21. Since all family members are usually effected, treatment of the entire household is recommended.
22. Endosymbiotic *Wolbachia* bacteria may have a role in filarial development and host response, and may represent a new target for therapy (HF Cross et al, Lancet 2001;358:1873). Doxycycline 100 mg daily 6 weeks has eradicated *Wolbachia* and led to sterility of adult worms in onchocerciasis (A Hoerauf et al, Lancet 2000;355:1241).
23. Most symptoms caused by the adult worm. Single-dose combination of albendazole (400 mg) with either ivermectin (200 μg/kg) or diethylcarbamazine (6 mg/kg) is effective for reduction or suppression of *W. bancrofti* microfilaremia (MM Ismail et al, Trans R Soc Trop Med Hyg 2001;95:332; TB Nutman, Curr Opin Infect Dis 2001;14:539).
24. Antihistamines or corticosteroids may be required to decrease allergic reactions due to disintegration of microfilariae in treatment of filarial infections, especially those caused by *Loa loa*.
25. For patients with no microfilariae in the blood, full doses can be given from day one.
26. In heavy infections with *Loa loa*, rapid killing of microfilariae can provoke an encephalopathy. Apheresis has been reported to be effective in lowering microfilarial counts in patients heavily infected with *Loa loa* (EA Ottesen, Infect Dis Clin North Am 1993;7:619). Albendazole or ivermectin have also been used to reduce microfilaremia; albendazole is preferred because of its slower onset of action (AD Klion et al, J infect Dis 1993;168:202; M Kombila et al, Am J Trop Med Hyg 1998;58:458). Albendazole may be useful for treatment of loiasis when diethylcarbamazine is ineffective or cannot be used but repeated courses may be necessary (AD Klion et al, Clin Infect Dis 1999;29:680). Diethylcarbamazine, 300 mg once weekly, has been recommended for prevention of loiasis (TB Nutman et al. N Engl J Med 1988;319:752).
27. Diethylcarbamazine has no effect. Ivermectin, 200 μg/kg once, has been effective.
28. Diethylcarbamazine is potentially curative due to activity against both adult worms and microfilariae. Ivermectin is only active against microfilariae.
29. Annual treatment with ivermectin 150 μg/kg can prevent blindness due to ocular onchoceriasis (D Mabey et al, Ophthalmology 1996;103:1001).
30. Unlike infections with other flukes, *Fasciola hepatica* infections may not respond to praziquantel. Triclabendazole, a veterinary fasciolide, may be safe and effective but data are limited (CS

Graham et al, Clin Infect Dis 2001;33:1). It is available from Victoria Pharmacy, Zurich, Switzerland, 41-1-211-24-32. It should be given with food for better absorption.

31. JD MacLean et al, Lancet 1996;347:154.

32. Triclabendazole may be effective in a dosage of 5 mg/kg once daily for 3 days or 10 mg/kg twice in one day (M Calvopiña et al, Trans R Soc Trop Med Hyg 1998;92:566). See footnote 30.

33. In one study, nitazoxanide (see footnote 4) was as effective as metronidazole and has been used successfully in high doses to treat a case of *Giardia* resistant to metronidazole and albendazole (JJ Ortiz et al, Aliment Pharmacol Ther 2001;15:1409; P Abboud et al, Clin Infect Dis 2001;32:1792). Albendazole 400 mg daily × 5 d may be effective (A Hall and Q Nahar, Trans R Soc Trop Med Hyg 1993;87:84; AK Dutta et al, Indian J Pediatr 1994;61:689). Bacitracin zinc or bacitracin 120,000 units bid for 10 days may also be effective (BJ Andrews et al, Am J Trop Med Hyg 1995;52:318). Combination treatment with standard doses of metronidazole and quinacrine given for 3 weeks has been effective for a small number of giardiasis in pregnancy.

34. Not absorbed; may be useful for treatment of giardiasis in pregnancy.

35. F Chappuis et al, Clin Infect Dis 2001;33:e17; P Nontasut et al, Southeast Asian J Trop Med Public Health 2000;31:374.

36. One patient has been successfully treated with albendazole (ML Eberhard and C Busillo, Am J Trop Med Hyg 1999;61:51).

37. Immunosuppressed patiens: TMP/SMX qid × 10 d followed by bid × 3 weeks. In sulfonamide-sensitive patients, pyrimethamine 50–75 mg daily in divided doses has been effective. HIV-infected patients may need long-term maintenance. Ciprofloxacin 500 mg bid × 7 d has also been effective (R-I Verdier et al, Ann Intern Med 2000;132:885).

38. Treatment dosage and duration vary based on the disease symptoms, host immune status, species, and the area of the world where infection was acquired. Cutaneous infection is due to *L. mexicana, L. tropica, L. major, L. braziliensis*; mucocutaneous is mostly due to *L. braziliensis*, and visceral is due to *L. donovani* (Kala-azar), *L. infantum, L. chagasi*. Dosage range listed includes many, but not all possibilities.

39. For treatment of kala-azar, oral miltefosine 100 mg daily for 4 weeks was 97% effective after 6 months in one study. Gastrointestinal adverse effects are common and the drug is contraindicated in pregnancy (TK Jha et al, N Engl J Med 1999;341:1795). In an uncontrolled trial, oral miltefosine was effective for the treament of American cutaneous leishmaniasis at a dosage of about 2.25 mg/kg/day for 3–4 wks. "Motion sickness" was the most frequent adverse effect (J Soto et al, Clin Infect Dis 2001;33:e57).

40. May be repeated or continued. A longer duration may be needed for some forms of visceral leishmaniasis (BL Herwaldt, Lancet 1999;354:1191).

41. Three preparations of lipid-encapsulated amphotericin B have been used for treatment of visceral leishmaniasis. Largely based on clinical trials in patients infected with *L. infantum,* the FDA approved liposomal amphotericin B (AmBisome) for treatment of visceral leishmaniasis (A Meyerhoff, Clin Infect Dis 1999;28:42; JD Berman, Clin Infect Dis 1999;28:49). Amphotericin B lipid complex (Abelcet) and amphotericin B cholesteryl sulfate (Amphotec) have also been used with good results. Limited data in a few patients suggest that liposomal amphotericin B may also be effective for mucocutaneous disease (VS Amato et al, J Antimicrob Chemother 2000;46:341; RNR Sampaio and PD Marsden, Trans R Soc Trop Med Hyg 1997;91:77). Some studies indicate that *L. donovani* resistant to pentavalent antimonial agents may respond to lipid-encapsulated amphotericin B (S Sundar et al, Ann Trop Med Parasitol 1998;92:755).

42. The dose for immunocompromised patients with HIV is 4 mg/kg/d (days 1–5) and 4 mg/kg/d on days 10, 17, 24, 31, 38. The relapse rate is high, suggesting that maintenance therapy may be indicated.

43. For *L. donovani*: 4 mg/kg once day × 15 doses; for cutaneous disease: 2 mg/kg once/day × 7 or 3 mg/kg once/day × 4 doses.

44. Topical paromomycin can only be used in geographic regions where cutaneous leishmaniasis species have low potential for mucosal spread. A formulation of 15% paromomycin and 12% methylbenzethonium chloride (Leshcutan) in soft white paraffin for topical use, has been reported to be effective in some patients against cutaneous leishmaniasis due to *L. major* (O Ozgoztasi and I Baydar, Int J Dermatol 1997;36:61; BA Arana et al, Am J Trop Med Hyg 2001;65:466).

45. For infestation of eyelashes with crab lice, use petrolatum. For pubic lice, treat with 5% permethrin or ivermectin as for scabies (see p 297).

46. A second application is recommended one week later to kill hatching progeny. Some lice are resistant to pyrethrins and permethrin (RJ Pollack, Arch Pediatr Adolesc Med 1999;153:969)

47. RJ Roberts et al, Lancet 2000;356:540.

48. Ivermectin is effective against adult lice but has no effect on nits (TA Bell, Pediatr Infect Dis J 1998;17:923).

49. Chloroquine-resistant *P. falciparum* occur in all malarious areas except Central America west of the Panama Canal Zone, Mexico, Haiti, the Dominican Republic, and most of the Middle East (chloroquine resistance has been reported in Yemen, Oman, Saudi Arabia, and Iran).

50. In Southeast Asia, relative resistance to quinine has increased, and the treatment should be continued for 7 days.

51. Fansidar tablets contain 25 mg pyrimethamine and 500 mg sulfadoxine. Resistance to pyrimethamine-sulfadoxine has been reported from Southeast Asia, the Amazon basin, sub-Saharan Africa, Bangladesh, and Oceania.

52. For use in pregnancy.

53. Atovaquone plus proguanil is available as a fixed-dose combination tablet: adult tablets (250 mg atovaquone/100 mg proguanil, Malarone) and pediatric tablets (62.5 mg atovaquone/25 mg proguanil, Malarone Pediatric). To enhance absorption, it should be taken within 45 minutes after eating (S Looareesuwan et al, Am J Trop Med Hyg 1999;60:533). Although approved for once daily dosing, to decrease nausea and vomiting the dose for treatment is usually divided in two.

54. For treatment of multiple drug-resistant *P. falciparum* in Southeast Asia, especially Thailand, where resistance to mefloquine and halofantrine is frequent, a 7-day course of quinine and tetracycline is recommended (G Watt et al, Am J Trop Med Hyg 1992;47:108). Artesunate plus mefloquine (C Luxemburger et al, Trans R Soc Trop Med Hyg 1994;88:213), artemether plus mefloquine (J Karbwang et al, Trans R Soc Trop Med Hyg 1995;89:296), mefloquine plus doxycycline or atovaquone/proguanil may also be used to treat multiple-drug-resistant *P. falciparum.*

55. At this dosage, adverse effects including nausea, vomiting, diarrhea, dizziness, disturbed sense of balance, toxic psychosis, and seizures can occur. Mefloquine is teratogenic in animals and should not be used for treatment of malaria in pregnancy. It should not be given together with quinine, quinidine, or halofantrine, and caution is required in using quinine, quinidine, or halofantrine to treat patients with malaria who have taken mefloquine for prophylaxis. The pediatric dosage has not been approved by the FDA. Resistance to mefloquine has been reported in some areas, such as the Thailand-Myanmar and -Cambodia borders and in the Amazon basin, where 25 mg/kg should be used.

56. In the U.S., a 250-mg tablet of mefloquine contains 228 mg mefloquine base. Outside the U.S., each 275-mg tablet contains 250 mg base.

57. May be effective in multiple drug-resistant *P. falciparum* malaria, but treatment failures and resistance have been reported, and the drug has caused lengthening of the PR and QTc intervals and fatal cardiac arrhythmias. It should not be used for patients with cardiac conduction defects or with other drugs that may affect the QT interval, such as quinine, quinidine and mefloquine. Cardiac monitoring is recommended. Variability in absorption is a problem; halofantrine should not be taken one hour before to two hours after meals because food increases its absorption. It should not be used in pregnancy.

58. A single 250-mg dose can be used for repeat treatment in mild to moderate infections (JE Touze et al, Lancet 1997;349:255).

59. K Na-Bangchang, Trop Med Int Health 1999;4:602.

60. *P. vivax* with decreased susceptibility to chloroquine is a significant problem in Papua-New Guinea and Indonesia. There are also a few reports of resistance from Myanmar, India, Thailand, the Solomon Islands, Vanuatu, Guyana, Brazil, Colombia, and Peru.

61. JK Baird et al, J Infect Dis 1995;171:1678.

62. Primaquine phosphate can cause hemolytic anemia, especially in patients whose red cells are deficient in glucose-6-phosphate dehydrogenase. This deficiency is most common in African, Asian, and Mediterranean peoples. Patients should be screened for G-6-PD deficiency before treatment. Primaquine should not be used during pregnancy.

179

63. If chloroquine phosphate is not available, hydroxychloroquine sulfate is as effective; 400 mg of hydroxychloroquine sulfate is equivalent to 500 mg chloroquine phosphate.

64. Exchange transfusion has been helpful for some patients with high-density (>10%) parasitemia, altered mental status, pulmonary edema, or renal complications (KD Miller et al, N Engl J Med 1989;321:65).

65. Continuous ECG, blood pressure, and glucose monitoring are recommended, especially in pregnant women and young children. For problems with quinidine availability, call the manufacturer (Eli Lilly, 800-821-0538) or the CDC Malaria Hotline (770-488-7788). Quinidine may have greater antimalarial activity than quinine. The loading dose should be decreased or omitted in those patients who have received quinine or mefloquine. If more than 48 hours of parenteral treatment is required, the quinine or quinidine dose should be reduced by ⅓ to ½.

66. Artemether-Quinine Meta-Analysis Study Group, Trans R Soc Trop Med Hyg 2001;95:637. Not available in the U.S.

67. Relapses have been reported with this regimen, and should be treated with a second 14-day course of 30 mg base/day. In Southeast Asia and Somalia the higher dose (30 mg base/day) should be used initially

68. No drug regimen guarantees protection against malaria. If fever develops within a year (particularly within the first two months) after travel to malarious areas, travelers should be advised to seek medical attention. Insect repellents, insecticide-impregnated bed nets and proper clothing are important adjuncts for malaria prophylaxis.

69. In pregnancy, chloroquine prophylaxis has been used extensively and safely.

70. In addition, for prevention of attack after departure from areas where P. vivax and P. ovale are endemic, which includes almost all areas where malaria is found (except Haiti), some experts prescribe primaquine phosphate 26.3 mg (15 mg base)/d or, for children, 0.3 mg base/kg/d during the last two weeks of prophylaxis. Others prefer to avoid the toxicity of primaquine and rely on surveillance to detect cases when they occur, particularly when exposure was limited or doubtful. See also footnotes 62 and 67.

71. Beginning one to two weeks before travel and continuing weekly for the duration of stay and for four weeks after leaving.

72. The pediatric dosage has not been approved by the FDA, and the drug has not been approved for use during pregnancy. However, it has been reported to be safe for prophylactic use during the second or third trimester of pregnancy and possibly during early pregnancy as well (CDC Health Information for International Travel, 2001–2002, page 113; BL Smoak et al, J Infect Dis 1997;176:831). Mefloquine is not recommended for patients with cardiac conduction abnormalities. Patients with a history of seizures or psychiatric disorders should avoid mefloquine (Medical Letter 1990;32:13). Resistance to mefloquine has been reported in some areas, such as Thailand; in these areas, doxycycline should be used for prophylaxis. In children less than eight years old, proguanil plus sulfisoxazole has been used (KN Suh and JS Keystone, Infect Dis Clin Pract 1996;5:541).

73. Beginning 1–2 days before travel and continuing for the duration of stay and for 4 week after leaving. Use of tetracyclines is contraindicated in pregnancy and in children less than eight years old. Doxycycline can cause gastrointestinal disturbances, vaginal moniliasis, and photosensitivity reactions.

74. GE Shanks et al, Clin Infect Dis 1998;27:494; B Lell et al, Lancet 1998;351:709. Beginning 1 to 2 days before travel and continuing for the duration of stay and for 1 week after leaving. In one study of malaria prophylaxis, atovaquone/proguanil was better tolerated than mefloquine in nonimmune travelers (D Overbosch et al, Clin Infect Dis 2001;33:1015).

75. Several studies have shown that daily primaquine beginning one day before departure and continued until 7 days after leaving the malaria area provides effective prophylaxis against chloroquine-resistant P. falciparum (JK Baird et al, Clin Infect Dis 2001;33:1990). Some studies have shown less efficacy against P. vivax. Nausea and abdominal pain can be diminished by taking with food.

76. Proguanil (Paludrine—Wyeth Ayerst, Canada; AstraZeneca, United Kingdom), which is not available in the U.S. but is widely available in Canada and Europe, and is recommended mainly for use in Africa south of the Sahara. Prophylaxis is recommended during exposure and for four

weeks afterwards. Proguanil has been used in pregnancy without evidence of toxicity (PA Phillips-Howard and D Wood, Drug Saf 1996;14:131).

77. Ocular lesions due to *E. hellem* in HIV-infected patients have responded to fumagillin eyedrops prepared from Fumidil-B, a commercial product (Mid-Continent Agrimarketing Inc., Olathe, Kansas, 800-547-1392) used to control a microsporidial disease of honey bees (MC Diesenhouse, Am J Ophthalmol 1993;115:293). For lesions from *V. corneae*, topical therapy is generally not effective and keratoplasty may be required (RM Davis et al, Ophthamology 1990;97:953).

78. Oral fumagillin (see footnote 77, Sanofi Recherche, Gentilly, France) has been effective in treating *E. bieneusi* (J-M Molina et al, AIDS 2000;14:1341), but has been associated with thrombocytopenia. Highly active antiretroviral therapy (HAART) may lead to microbiologic and clinical response in HIV-infected patients with microsporidial diarrhea (NA Foudraine et al, AIDS 1998;12:35; A Carr et al, Lancet 1998;351:256). Octreotide (Sandostatin) has provided symptomatic relief in some patients with large volume diarrhea.

79. J-M Molina et al, J Infect Dis 1995;171:245. There is no established treatment for *Pleistophora*.

80. Albendazole or pyrantel pamoate may be effective (HP Krepel et al, Trans R Soc Trop Med Hyg 1993;87:87).

81. In severe disease with room air $PO_2 \le 70$ mm Hg or Aa gradient ≥ 35 mm Hg, prednisone should also be used (S Gagnon et al, N Engl J Med 1990;323:1444; E Caumes et al, Clin Infect Dis 1994;18:319).

82. Primary/secondary prophylaxis in patients with HIV can be discontinued after CD4 count increases to >200 10^6/L for more than 3 months (HIV/AIDS Treatment Information Service, U.S. Department of Health and Human Services 2001; www.hivatis.org).

83. An alternative trimethoprim/sulfamethoxazole regimen is one DS tab 3×/week. Weekly therapy with sulfadoxine 500 mg/pyrimethamine 25 mg/leucovorin 25 mg was effective PCP prophylaxis in liver transplant patients (J Torre-Cisneros et al, Clin Infect Dis 1999;29:771).

84. Plus leucovorin 25 mg with each dose of pyrimethamine.

85. Effective for crusted scabies in immunocompromised patients (M Larralde et al, Pediatr Dermatol 1999;16:69; A Patel et al, Australas J Dermatol 1999;40:37; O Chosidow, Lancet 2000;355:819).

86. Oxamniquine has been effective in some areas in which praziquantel is less effective (FF Stelma et al, J Infect Dis 1997;176:304). Oxamniquine is contraindicated in pregnancy.

87. In East Africa, the dose should be increased to 30 mg/kg, and in Egypt and South Africa to 30 mg/kg/d × 2 d. Some experts recommend 40–60 mg/kg over 2–3 days in all of Africa (KC Shekhar, Drugs 1991;42:379).

88. In immunocompromised patients or disseminated disease, it may be necessary to prolong or repeat therapy or use other agents. A veterinary parenteral formulation of ivermectin was used in one patient (PL Chiodini et al, Lancet 2000;355:43).

89. This dose is likely to be toxic and may have to be decreased.

90. Patients may benefit from or require surgical resection of cysts. Praziquantel is useful preoperatively or in case of spill during surgery. Percutaneous drainage with ultrasound guidance plus albendazole therapy has been effective for management of hepatic hydatid cyst disease (MS Khuroo et al, N Engl J Med 1997;337:881; O Akhan and M Ozman, Eur J Radiol 1999;32:76).

91. Surgical excision or the PAIR (Puncture, Aspirate, Inject, Re-aspirate) technique is the only reliable means of cure. Reports have suggested that in non-resectable cases, use of albendazole or mebendazole can stabilize and sometimes cure infection (W Hao et al, Trans R Soc Trop Med Hyg 1994;88:340; WHO Group, Bull WHO 1996;74:231).

92. Initial therapy or parenchymal disease with seizures should focus on symptomatic treatment with anticonvulsant drugs. Treatment of parenchymal disease with albendazole and praziquantel is controversial and randomized trials have not been conclusive. Obstructive hydrocephalus is treated with surgical removal of the obstructing cyst or CSF diversion. Prednisone 40 mg daily may be given in conjunction with surgery. Arachnoiditis, vasculitis or cerebral edema is treated with prednisone 60 mg daily or dexamethasone 4–16 mg/d combined with albendazole or praziquantel (AC White, Jr, Annu Rev Med 2000;51:187). Patients with subarachnoid cysts or

giant cysts in the fissures should receive albendazole for at least 30 days (JV Proano et al, N Engl J Med 2001;345:879). Any cysticercocidal drug may cause irreparable damage when used to treat ocular or spinal cysts, even when corticosteroids are used. An ophthalmic exam should always be done before treatment to rule out intraocular cysts.

93. In ocular toxoplasmosis with macular involvement, corticosteroids are recommended for an anti-inflammatory effect on the eyes.

94. To treat CNS toxoplasmosis in HIV-infected patients, some clinicians have used pyrimethamine 50 to 100 mg daily (after a loading dose of 200 mg) with a sulfadiazine and, when sulfonamide sensitivity developed, have given clindamycin 1.8 to 2.4 g/d in divided doses instead of the sulfonamide (JS Remington et al, Lancet 1991;338:1142; BJ Luft et al, N Engl J Med 1993;329:995). Atovaquone plus pyrimethamine appears to be an effective alternative in sulfa-intolerant patients (JA Kovacs et al, Lancet 1992;340:637). Treatment is followed by chronic suppression with lower dosage regimens of the same drugs. For primary prophylaxis in HIV patients with <100 CD4 cells, either trimethoprim-sulfamethoxazole, pyrimethamine plus dapsone or atovaquone with or without pyrimethamine can be used. Primary/secondary prophylaxis may be discontinued when the CD4 count increases to >200 × 10^6/L for more than 3 months (HIV/AIDS Treatment Information Service US Department of Health and Human Services 2001; (www.hivatis.org). See also footnote 95.

95. Plus leucovorin 10 to 25 mg with each dose of pyrimethamine.

96. Congenitally infected newborns should be treated with pyrimethamine every two or three days and a sulfonamide daily for about one year (JS Remington and G Desmonts in JS Remington and JO Klein, eds, *Infectious Disease of the Fetus and Newborn Infant*, 5th ed, Philadelphia: Saunders, 1995, p 290).

97. For prophylactic use during pregnancy. If it is determined that transmission has occurred *in utero*, therapy with pyrimethamine and sulfadiazine should be started. Pyrimethamine is a potential teratogen and should be used only after the first trimester.

98. Sexual partners should be treated simultaneously. Metronidazole-resistant strains have been reported and should be treated with metronidazole 2–4 g/d × 7 –14 d. Desensitization has been recommended for patients allergic to metronidazole (MD Pearlman et al, Am J Obstet Gynecol 1996;174:934). High dose tinidazole has also been used for the treatment of metronidazole-resistant trichomoniasis (JD Sobel et al, Clin Infect Dis 2001;33:1341).

MANUFACTURERS OF SOME ANTIPARASITIC DRUGS

ALBENDAZOLE—*Albenza* (GlaxoSmithKline)

§**ARTEMETHER**—*Artenam* (Arenco, Belgium)

§**ARTESUNATE**—(Guilin No. 1 Factory, People's Republic of China)

ATOVAQUONE—*Mepron* (GlaxoSmithKline)

ATOVAQUONE/PROGUANIL—*Malarone* (GlaxoSmithKline)

BACITRACIN—many manufacturers

§**BACITRACIN-ZINC**—(Apothekernes Laboratorium A.S., Oslo, Norway)

§**BENZNIDAZOLE**—*Rochagan* (Roche, Brazil)

†**BITHIONOL**—*Bitin* (Tanabe, Japan)

CHLOROQUINE HCl and CHLOROQUINE PHOSPHATE—*Aralen* (Sanofi), others

CROTAMITON—*Eurax* (Westwood-Squibb)

DAPSONE—(Jacobus)

†**DIETHYLCARBAMAZINE CITRATE USP**—(University of Iowa School of Pharmacy)

§**DILOXANIDE FUROATE**—*Furamide* (Boots, United Kingdom)

§**EFLORNITHINE** (Difluoromethylornithine, DFMO)—*Ornidyl* (Aventis)

FURAZOLIDONE—*Furoxone* (Roberts)

§**HALOFANTRINE**—*Halfan* (GlaxoSmithKline)

IODOQUINOL—*Yodoxin* (Glenwood), others
IVERMECTIN—*Stromectol* (Merck)
MALATHION—*Ovide* (Medicus)
MEBENDAZOLE—*Vermox* (McNeil)
MEFLOQUINE—*Lariam* (Roche)
§**MEGLUMINE ANTIMONATE**—*Glucantime* (Aventis, France)
†**MELARSOPROL**—*Mel-B* (Specia)
METRONIDAZOLE—*Flagyl* (Searle), others
§**MILTEFOSINE**—(Zentaris)
†**NIFURTIMOX**—*Lampit* (Bayer, Germany)
*__**NITAZOXANIDE**—*Cryptaz* (Romark)
§**ORNIDAZOLE**—*Tiberal* (Roche, France)
OXAMNIQUINE—*Vansil* (Pfizer)
PAROMOMYCIN—*Humatin* (Monarch); *Leshcutan* (Teva Pharmaceutical Industries, Ltd., Israel; (topical formulation not available in U.S.)
PENTAMIDINE ISETHIONATE—*Pentam 300, NebuPent* (Fujisawa)
PERMETHRIN—*Nix* (GlaxoSmithKline), *Elimite* (Allergan)
PRAZIQUANTEL—*Biltricide* (Bayer)
PRIMAQUINE PHOSPHATE USP
§**PROGUANIL**—*Paludrine* (Wyeth Ayerst, Canada; AstraZeneca, United Kingdom); in combination with atovaquone as *Malarone* (GlaxoSmithKline)
§**PROPAMIDINE ISETHIONATE**—*Brolene* (Aventis, Canada)
PYRANTEL PAMOATE—*Antiminth* (Pfizer)
PYRETHRINS and PIPERONYL BUTOXIDE—*RID* (Pfizer), others
PYRIMETHAMINE USP—Daraprim (GlaxoSmithKline)
§**QUININE DIHYDROCHLORIDE**
QUININE SULFATE—many manufacturers
†**SODIUM STIBOGLUCONATE**—*Pentostam* (GlaxoSmithKline, United Kingdom)
*__**SPIRAMYCIN**—*Rovamycine* (Aventis)
†**SURAMIN SODIUM**—(Bayer, Germany)
THIABENDAZOLE—Mintezol (Merck)
§**TINIDAZOLE**—Fasigyn (Pfizer)
*__**TRICLABENDAZOLE**—*Egaten* (Novartis, Switzerland)
TRIMETREXATE—*Neutrexin* (US Bioscience)

---

*Available in the U.S. only from the manufacturer.
§Not available in the U.S.
†Available under an Investigational New Drug (IND) protocol from the CDC Drug Service, Centers for Disease Control and Prevention, Atlanta, Georgia 30333; 404-639-3670 (evenings, weekends, or holidays: 404-639-2888).

TREATMENT OF VIRAL INFECTIONS

A. HERPESVIRUS GROUP *(Med Lett 2002;44:9; NEJM 1999;340:1255; Lancet 2001;357:1513; Med Lett 2002;44:95)*

Virus	Regimen*	Comment
HERPES SIMPLEX		
Genital—primary	<u>Acyclovir</u>: 400 mg po tid × 7–10 days, ($32) <u>Severe</u>: 5 mg/kg IV q8h × 5–7 days <u>Valacyclovir</u>: 1 g po bid 7–10 days ($124) <u>Famciclovir</u>: 250 mg po tid × 7–10 days ($89)	Shortens duration of pain, reduces viral shedding and reduces duration of systemic symptoms (Med Lett 1995;37:117). Avoid sex until no visible lesions; effect of treatment on transmission is unknown Valacyclovir and acyclovir are equally effective (AAC 1995;35:181)
Genital—recurrent	<u>Acyclovir</u>: 800 mg tid × 2 d ($16) or 400 mg tid × 3–5 ($30) <u>Valacyclovir</u>: 500 mg po qd × 3 days ($29) <u>Famciclovir</u>: 125 mg po bid × 3–5 days ($29)	Slight benefit, but only if started early (MMWR 1993;RR-14:23) preferably within 24 hr (Arch Intern Med 1996;156:1729) Higher doses may be required in HIV-infected patients
Genital—prophylaxis	<u>Acyclovir</u>: 400 mg po bid ($109/mo) <u>Valacyclovir</u>: 500–1000 mg qd ($145/mo) <u>Famciclovir</u>: 250 mg po bid ($255/mo) <u>Immunocompromised</u>: acyclovir 200–400 mg po 3–5×/d ($218)	Indicated with ≥6 recurrences/yr. Good efficacy and good safety profile with acyclovir prophylaxis up to 7 yr (JAMA 1991;265:747; Arch Dermatol 1993;129:582; JID 1994;169:1338). Decreases HSV shedding between relapses (Ann Intern Med 1996;124:8) Daily dose should be titrated to lowest dose that prevents recurrences Cost data are for a 30 day supply Prophylaxis may reduce risk of HIV transmission
Perirectal	<u>Acyclovir</u>: 800 mg po tid × 7–10 days ($126)	
Labialis—prophylaxis	<u>Acyclovir</u>: 400 mg po bid or 200 mg 5 ×/d ($25/wk)	Effective for sun-induced episodes (Ann Intern Med 1993;118:268)
Labialis—treatment	<u>Acyclovir po</u>: 400 mg po 5×/d × 5 days ($45) <u>Famciclovir po</u>: 500 mg po bid × 7 days ($119) <u>Valacyclovir po</u>: 2 g po q12h × 1 day ($35) <u>Acyclovir 5% ointment</u>: 5×/d × 4 d ($33) <u>Penciclovir 1% cream</u>—topical q2h while awake × 4 days ($23)	Results are best with patient-initiated therapy Med Lett preference between creams is docosanol, which compared with penciclovir is less expensive, applied less frequently (5×/d vs q2h), and over-the-counter. Med Lett preference among all treatments is valacyclovir based on efficacy and convenience (2002;44:95)

Continued

Virus	Regimen	Comment
	Docosanol 10% cream, topical 5×/d ($16)	
Encephalitis	Acyclovir: IV-10–15 mg/kg q8h × 14–21 days ($3,540)	High rates of long-term morbidity in survivors (NEJM 1986;314:144)
Mucocuteaneous in immuno-competent host	Acyclovir: 5 mg/kg IV q8h × 5 days	Alternatives: Acyclovir 400 mg po 5×/d × 10 days Valacyclovir 1 g po tid × 10 days Famciclovir 500 mg po bid × 7 days
Mucocutaneous progressive/ compromised host	Acyclovir 5 mg/kg q8h IV × 7–14 d ($900) Acyclovir 400 mg po 5×/d × 7–10 d ($63) Famciclovir 500 mg po bid × 7–10 d ($119) Valganciclovir 0.5–1 gm po bid × 7–10 d ($68)	AIDS patients often require preventative therapy with acyclovir 200–400 mg po 3–5×/d indefinitely
Burn wound	Acyclovir: IV—5 mg/kg q8h × 7 days; po—200 mg 5×/d × 7–14 days	
Prophylaxis—high-risk patients	Acyclovir: IV—5 mg/kg q8h; po—200–400 mg 3–5×/d	Organ and bone marrow transplant recipients; treat seropositive patients for 1–3 mo post-transplant (NEJM 1989;320:1381)
Keratitis	Trifluridine: Topical (1%) 1 drop q2h up to 9 drops day × 10 days ($95)	Ophthalmologist should supervise treatment. Alternative is vidarabine 3% ointment, 1/2 inch ribbon 5×/d.
Acyclovir-resistant	Foscarnet: IV—40 mg/kg q8h × 14–21 days ($1500) Topical trifluridine for accessible lesions using 1% ophthalmic solution tid (Lancet 1992;340:1040)	Thymidine kinase deficient strains are most common cause of resistance and are almost always from immunosuppressed patients unresponsive to acyclovir (NEJM 1991;325:551; NEJM 1989;320:293; J Infect Dis 1990;161:1078). Most acyclovir-resistant strains are also resistant to famciclovir, penciclovir, and ganciclovir, but respond to foscarnet (CID 1998;27:1525) Foscarnet-resistant HSV may become acyclovir susceptible (JID 1994;109:193); most acyclovir-resistant HSV are resistant to penciclovir (Famciclovir) and ganciclovir

VARICELLA-ZOSTER (see Ann Intern Med 130:922, 1999)

Virus	Regimen	Comment
Chickenpox, adult immunocompetent	Valacyclovir: 1 g po tid × 7 d ($185)	Must treat within 24 hr of exantham; efficacy established (Ann Intern Med 1992;117:358)
Chickenpox, or zoster adult immunosuppressed	Acyclovir: 10 mg/kg IV q8h × 7 days ($1600)	Treat as quickly as possible
Pneumonia	Acyclovir: IV 10 mg/kg q8h × 7 days ($1600)	Efficacy not clearly established but appears best if treatment is initiated within 36 hr of admissions (RID 1990;12:788)

Continued

Virus	Regimen	Comment
Dermatomal or disseminated zoster; immunosuppressed	Acyclovir: IV 10 mg/kg q8h × 7 days ($1600)	Indications to treat are greater for severe disease, early disease, or zoster in immuno-suppressed host (NEJM 1983;308:1448; AmJ Med 1988;85 Suppl 2A:84; Infect Dis Clin Pract 1993;2:100) Treatment can be started as long as new lesions are forming Foscarnet for acyclovir-resistant strains, 60 mg/kg IV 2–3 ×/day for 7–14 days (NEJM 1993;308:1448)
Normal host	Valacyclovir: 1 g po tid × 7 days ($185) Acyclovir: 800 mg po 5×/d × 7–10 days ($121) Famciclovir: 500 mg po tid × 7 days ($179) Any of the above with or without prednisone: 60 mg/d po × 7 days, 30 mg/d days 8–14, 15 mg/d days 15–21 (Ann Intern Med 1996;125:376) Pain control: Tricyclics; other options—gabapentin, carbamazepine, lidocaine patch, topical capsaicin, regional nerve block, acupuncture. Narcotics are effective and under-used	Antiviral drugs hasten healing of cutaneous lesions and reduce pain including acyclovir (Am J Med 1988;85:84; NZ Med J 1991; 10 Suppl 102:93); valacyclovir (AAC 1996; 39:1546); and famciclovir (Ann Intern Med 1995;123:89) Patient >50 yr and those with ophthalmic zoster are most likely to benefit Ophthalmic zoster: Consult ophthalmologist (Ophthalmology 1986;793:63) Antiviral treatment should be started within 72 hr of rash onset or while lesions are still forming Meta-analysis of reports of oral acyclovir in 691 patients with zoster showed a 2-fold reduc-tion in duration of pain (CID 1996;22:341) Comparative trial of acyclovir vs. valacyclovir showed slight advantage with valacyclovir (AAC 1995;39:1546) Controlled trial showed prednisone added to acyclovir was associated with more rapid healing, more rapid return to normal sleep, and more rapid return to normal activity (Ann Intern Med 1996;125:376). Others have shown less impressive results (NEJM 1994;330:896) Valacyclovir is superior to acyclovir for re-ducing duration of pain (AAC 1995;39:1546) Post-herpetic neuralgia: Amitriptyline
Acyclovir resistant strains	Foscarnet: 40 mg/kg q8h IV × 10 days ($1050)	Most VZV strains resistant to acyclovir are resistant to ganciclovir and famciclovir
Exposure (zoster or chickenpox); immunosuppressed	Varicella-zoster immune globin, 625 units IM within 96 hr of exposure	Patient susceptible and has substantial exposure (Ann Intern Med 1988;108:221); alternative is to treat chickenpox promptly with acyclovir if it occurs
Susceptible health care workers	None	Must refrain from patient contact during days 8–21 postexposure
Prophylaxis in organ transplant recipients	Acyclovir: 5 mg/kg IV q8h or 200 mg po q6h to 1 yr	Lancet 1983;2:706; NEJM 1989;320:1381 Acyclovir if CMV serology D−R− (Otherwise ganciclovir/valganciclovir × 3–6 mo)

Continued

Virus	Regimen	Comment
CYTOMEGALOVIRUS		
Immunocompetent	None	
Immunosuppressed Pneumonitis, esophagitis, colitis, and CNS infection	<u>Ganciclovir</u>: Induction, 5 mg/kg IV bid × 14–21 days. ($836) Maintenance, 6 mg/kg IV 5 days/wk or oral ($710–836/mo) or valganciclovir (see below) <u>Foscarnet</u>: Induction, 60 mg/kg IV q8h or 90 mg/kg q12h × 14–21 days. ($2250) Maintenance, 90 mg/kg IV qd ($2425/mo) <u>Valganciclovir</u>: 900 mg po bid × 21 days, ($2631) then 900 mg qd (maintenance—$1880/mo) <u>Cidofovir</u> (Vistide) 5 mg/kg IV q wk × 2, then 5 mg/kg IV q 2 wk + probenecid ($1623/mo)	Valganciclovir gives serum levels comparable to those achieved with IV ganciclovir (AAC 2000;44:2811) Efficacy of treatment is established for CMV pneumonitis, esophagitis and radiculopathy; response is less impressive with enteritis and colitis (CID 1993;17:644; JID 1993; 167:278; JID 1993;167:1184; JID 1995; 172;622) Foscarnet is therapeutically comparable with ganciclovir for CMV colitis in AIDS patients (Am J Gastroenterol 1993;88:542). Main problem is poor quality of life because of long hours of infusions
Retinitis	Vitrasert implant ($5000), then valgancyclovir 900 mg po bid × 21 d ($2630) then 900 mg gd ($1880/mo)	
Marrow transplant recipients	<u>Ganciclovir</u>: 7.5–10 mg/kg/d IV × 20 days ± maintenance: 5 mg/kg 3–5×/wk for 8–20 doses or valganciclovir <u>CytoGam</u> (Hyperimmune) in dose of 100–150 mg/kg good for seven doses	<u>Ganciclovir plus hyperimmune globulin</u>: Efficacy best supported for marrow recipients (Ann Intern 1988;109:777; Ann Intern Med 1988;109:783; Transplant 1993;55:1339; JID 1988;158:488; CID 1993;7:S392) <u>Ganciclovir monotherapy</u>: Response rates 22–50% (Pharmacotherapy 1992;12:300) CMV hyperimmune globulin (CytoGam) added by some if severe CMV disease, infection of allograft, recurrent disease, or hypogammaglobulinemia
Solid organ transplants	<u>Ganciclovir, valganciclovir, and CytoGam</u> (as above)	Response rates to ganciclovir in heart, liver, and renal transplant recipients in 14 reports: 67/85 (79%) (Pharmacotherapy 1992;12: 300). Maintenance therapy used in 2 of 14 reports
<u>Prophylaxis</u> Marrow transplant	<u>Allogenic transplant: D−R+</u>: No prophylaxis <u>D+ or R+</u> <u>Ganciclovir</u>, 5–6 mg/kg IV 5–7 days/wk × 3 mo <u>or</u> <u>Acyclovir</u> 10 mg/kg IV q8h × 1 mo, then 800 mg po qid × ≥ 3 mo	<u>Recommendations of ECOG</u> (Ann Intern Med 120:143, 1994); **D, donor; R, recipient; + CMV seropositive** <u>Optimal results</u> are with ganciclovir for 3–4 mo (Ann Intern Med 1993;118:173; Lancet 1994;343:749; Lancet 1995;341:1380) <u>Oral ganciclovir</u> is superior to oral acyclovir for CMV prophylaxis in renal transplants

Continued

Virus	Regimen	Comment
	<u>IVIG</u> 500 mg/kg q2wk × 3 mo + cultures for CMV × 120 days. Positive culture: Ganciclovir + IVIG to day 100 or until 2–3 wk after last culture <u>D−R−:</u> No prophylaxis <u>autologous transplant: R−</u>: CMV negative blood products or leukocyte-filtered products	(Transplantation 1998;66:1682)
Organ transplant recipients		
Renal	<u>Acyclovir</u> 800 mg po qid × 3 mo or <u>Valacyclovir</u> 1 g bid × 3 mo	<u>Supporting data</u> • Oral acyclovir in renal transplants—NEJM 1989;320:1381 • IV ganciclovir in marrow, liver, and heart transplants—NEJM 1996;335:721
Liver	<u>Ganciclovir</u> 1 g po tid × 2–3 mo <u>or</u> <u>Ganciclovir</u> 5–6 mg/kg IV 5–7 days/wk × 3 mo	• Oral ganciclovir in liver transplants—Lancet 1997;350:1729 • Meta-analysis of oral agents—Transplantation 1998;65:641
Heart	<u>Ganciclovir</u> 5 mg/kg IV q12h × 2 wk, then 5–6 mg/kg IV 5 d/wk to complete 3 mo	• Oral valacyclovir—NEJM 1999;340:1462

EPSTEIN-BARR VIRUS

Virus	Regimen	Comment
Oral hairy leukoplakia	<u>Acyclovir</u> 800 mg po 5×/d or valacyclovir	Efficacy established. Relapse rates high; ganciclovir is also effective
EBV-associated lymphomas	No antiviral agent	Acyclovir confers no benefit (NEJM 1984;311:1163)
Infectious mononucleosis	No antiviral agent	Prednisone (80 mg/d × 2–3 days, then taper over 2 wk) in selected cases

HEPATITIS B

Virus	Regimen	Comment
Chronic HBV (see p 193)	Lamivudine: 100 mg/d po × 3 yrs ($2,500/yr) Adofovir: 10 mg/d po × 3 yrs ($6,500/yr) Entecavir: 0.5 gm/d po; 1.0 gm/d for lamivudine resistant strains × 1–3 yrs Interferon alfa-2b 5 mil units/d or 10 mil units 3×/wk SC or IM × 4 mo ($7,300) ($6820) Pegylated interferon 2a (Pegasys) 180 mg SC/wk × 48 wks ($18,700)	Treatment of HBe Ag-neg HBV with any agent gives only temporary benefit for 1 yr; treatment 144 wks gives better results (NEJM 2005;352:2673) High rates of resistance with prolonged treatment with lamivudine: 20% at 1 year and 40% at 3 years Adofovir and entecavir are active vs lamivudine-resistant strains and resistance rates are low Tenofovir is probably as effective as adofovir, or entecavir but not FDA-approved for HBV Peginterferon 2a is superior to interferon (J Viral Hepat 2003;10:298) and to lamivudine for HBeAg-neg HBV infection (NEJM 2004;351:1206) Peginterferon 2b is effective for HBeAg-pos patients; additional lamivudine did not augment response (Lancet 2005;365:123)

Continued

Virus	Regimen	Comment
HEPATITIS C		
Chronic HCV (see p 191)	Pegylated interferon 2b (PegIntron): 1 µg/kg/wk SC × 48 wks ($18,700) or Pegalated interferon 2a (Pegasys) 180 µg/wk SC × 48 wks ($19,000) each plus ribavirin 1000–1200 mg po/d × 48 wks ($10,000)	Peginterferon + ribavirin is the preferred treatment of chronic HCV with sustained viral response rates of 54–63% (Med Letter Guidelines 2005;3:23)
INFLUENZA		
Influenza A & B treatment	<u>Zanamivir</u> 10 mg bid × 5d by inhaler ($58) <u>Oseltamivir</u> 75 mg po bid × 5 days ($73)	Efficacy of all four antivirals required initiation within 48 hrs of onset of symptoms Efficacy in reducing flu-related complications including pneumonia is unknown
Influenza A treatment	<u>Rimantadine</u> 200 mg po qd or 100 mg po bid × 5 days ($20) <u>Amantadine</u> 100 mg po bid or 200 mg po qd × 5 days ($8–16) or 100 mg/day if >65 yrs or renal failure ($4)	There is cross-resistance between amantadine and ramantadine
Influenza A & B prevention (see below)	<u>Oseltamivir</u>: 75 mg/d ($303/6 wks) <u>Ramantadine</u> 100 mg po bid or 200 mg qd ($137) <u>Amantadine</u> 100 mg po bid or 200 mg qd ($66–114)	Efficacy of amantadine or ramantadine prophylaxis is 70–90% (NEJM 2000;343:1778) Oseltamivir is FDA-approved for prophylaxis, is effective vs both influenza A and B, and is less frequently associated with resistance; however, it is more expensive

*Prices are AWP 2002 for lowest dose for designated duration

B. INFLUENZA (MMWR 2000;49(RR-3); Med Letter 2004;46:85)

1. PREVENTION

Vaccination: Preferred method to prevent influenza. Vaccine efficacy in healthy persons shows 70–90% efficacy when there is a good match between vaccine strain and epidemic strain. This has occurred in 13 of the last 14 seasons; the exception was the 1997–98 season when the epidemic was H_3N_2-Sydney. Vaccination "spin off" includes protection of vulnerable elderly residents of nursing homes when the health care workers who serve them have flu vaccine (JID 1997;75:1; Lancet 2000;355:93). The optimal time to vaccinate is Oct—mid November (see p 113 for vaccination guidelines)

2. AVIAN INFLUENZA: Avian influenza strains that have caused human disease since 2003 include H_5N_1, H_7N_2, H_9N_2, H_7N_3, N_7N_7.

- There is no vaccine for humans currently available for any of these strains (Aug 2005)
- Neuraminidase inhibitors are effective against some strains (including H_5N_1) in vitro and in animal models (Antimicrob Ag Chemother 2001;45:1216; Antiviral Res 2000;48:101). There are no adequate and published clinical data (Aug 2005)
  Amantadine and rimantadine are not active vs H_5N_1

Antiviral agents

Agent	Dose (prophylaxis)	Activity	Cost (/6 wks)	Comment
Amantadine	200 mg/d × 6 wk	Flu A	$66	13% had CNS toxicity[a]
Rimantadine	200 mg/d × 6 wk	Flu A	$137	6% had CNS toxicity[a]
Oseltamivir	75 mg/d × 6 wk	Flu A & B	$306	GI side effects in 10–20%[b]

[a]NEJM 1982;307:580.
[b]JAMA 1999;282:1240; NEJM 1999;341:1336.

3. **DIAGNOSIS**
   a. **Clinical:** Physician diagnosed flu is about 70% specific, about the same as the rapid tests. Key clues are fever, epidemic of influenza, and typical respiratory tract symptoms (Arch Intern Med 2000;160; 30
   b. **Rapid tests for office use:** Flu O1A (Biostar), QuickView (Quidel), and Zstatflu (ZymaTx). These cost $15–20/test, results available in 10–20 min, and sensitivity of 57–77%. All three will distinguish influenza A and B. Medical Letter consultants considered QuickVue to be "the easiest and fastest" (Med Lett 1999;41:121)
4. **TREATMENT** MMWR 2000;49(RR-3); JAMA 1999;282:1240; Lancet 2000;355:1845; BMJ 2003;326:1235. Med Letter 2004;46:85
   Meta-analysis of published reports showed neuraminidase inhibitors for treatment had an average 1–2 day reduction in symptoms and a 30% reduction in antibiotic use; for prevention there was 69–92% efficacy for prevention (BMJ 2003;326:1235)
   Medical Letter conclusion: Oseltamivir is superior for the combination of safety and efficacy. Generic amantadine is least expensive, but causes troublesome CNS toxicity, especially in elderly persons.

Comparison of drugs for influenza treament

	Amantadine	Rimantadine	Zanamivir	Oseltamivir
FDA approval	1966	1993	1999	1999
Activity: influenza	A	A	A & B	A & B
FDA approval				
Prophylaxis	+	+	−	+
Therapy	+	+	+	+
In vivo efficacy				
Healthy persons	+	+	+	+
High-risk persons	−	−	−	+
Prophylaxis efficacy	70–90%	70–90%	92%	82%
Treatment duration	3–5 d	3–5 d	5 d	5 d
Need to treat within 48 hr	+	+	+	+
Response–decrease duration by	1–1.5 d	1–1.5 d	1–1.5 d	1–1.5 d
Treatment regimen				
Age 14–64	100 mg bid	100 mg bid	10 mg bid	75 mg bid
>65 yr	100 mg/d	100 mg/d	Same	Same
Renal failure	Dose change	100 mg/d	Same	75 mg/d
Liver failure	Standard	100 mg/d	ND	ND
Prophylaxis regimen	Same	Same	10 mg/d	75 mg/d
Side effects	CNS-moderate	CNS-modest	Bronchospasm	GI
Cost/5 days treatment (AWP)	$2	$20	$48	$63
Cost/6 wks prevention	$13	$171	—	$265

C. HEPATITIS VIRUSES

1. **Hepatitis C:** Current recommendations for management NIH Consensus Conference: Managment of Hepatitis C, 2002 (http://consensus.nih.gov/cons/116/116cdc_statement.htm)
   a. <u>Natural history:</u> 85% develop chronic infection (viral persistence >6 mo usually with elevated ALT). About 10–20% develop cirrhosis within 20 yr, and 1–5% develop hepatocellular carcinoma within 20 yr (NEJM 1992;327:1906; NEJM 1995;332:1463). Extrahepatic manifestations include arthritis, keratoconjunctivitis sicca, lichen planus, glomerulonephritis, and essential mixed cryogobulinemia.
   b. <u>Indications for laboratory test based on risk</u> (MMWR 47 RR-19:1-39)
      (1) Injection drug use (90% prevalence)
      (2) Associated conditions: HIV infection, hemophilia with factor <1987, hemodialysis (ever), unexplained elevated ALT/AST
      (3) Transfusions or organ transplant <1992 (10% prevalence)
      (4) Occupational exposure (2–5% prevalence)
   c. <u>Laboratory tests</u>
      (1) Screening: qualitative HCV RNA—usually with 50 IU/ml limit of detection
      (2) Positive screen: Quantitative HCV RNA such as VERSANT HCV RNA version 3.0 (Bayer Diagnostics; only FDA cleared test) with dynamic range 615–7,700,000 IU
      <u>Note</u>: Many experts routinely screen with the quantitative which is less sensitive since positive qualitative test/negative quantitative test is usually not clinically relevant
      (3) Genotyping for this 6 HCV genotypes
      (4) Liver biopsy: Provides information on stage of fibrosis and degree of hepatic inflammation indicating the stage of disease and urgency of treatment
      <u>Recommendation</u>: Liver biopsy should be done when results will influence if treatment is recommended. "Most experts" do the following:
      • Genotype 1: Routinely biopsy liver to determine indications for treatment
      • Genotype 2 & 3: Do not routinely biopsy liver due to high rate of response.

<u>Grading of liver biopsy</u>

Stage	Metavir	Ishak
0	No fibrosis	No fibrosis
1	Periportal fibrosis expansion	Fibrosis expansion some portal areas ± short fibrosis septae
2	Periportal septae	Fibrosis expansion most portal areas
3	Periportal septae	Fibrous expansion most portal areas + periportal bridging
4	Cirrhosis	Marked bridging
5	—	Marked bridging plus nodules (incomplete cirrhosis)
6	—	Cirrhosis

Indication for treatment: Metavir score ≥2 or Ishak ≥3. With little evidence of fibrosis (Metavir <2 or Ishak <3) biopsies can be used to monitor disease progression.

d. <u>Indications for treatment of HCV</u>

Condition	Recommendation
Acute HCV	Treatment not recommended
Chronic HCV*	More than portal fibrosis on liver biopsy—Metavir ≥2 or Ishak ≥3*
Cryoglobulinemia	Indication for treatment if symptomatic regardless of liver disease

*<u>Widely accepted findings</u>: age >18, abnormal ALT, biopsy features noted, compensated liver disease (bilirubin <1.5 g/dL, INR <1.5, albumin >3.4 g/dL, platelet count >75K/mm^3, no encephalopathy and no ascites), other lab tests acceptable (Hgh 13 g/dL men, 12 g/dL women, ANC >1,500/mm^3, creatinine <1.5 mg/dL, willing to conform to treatment, no depression or depression that is well controlled, and detectable HCV

<u>Contraindications to therapy</u>

Major uncontrolled depression, transplant recipient, autoimmune hepatitis, untreated hyperthyroidism, pregnant or potentially pregnant, severe concurrent disease, age <3 yrs hypersensitivity to drugs

<u>Treatment</u>

Geno-type	Regimen		Duration
	Peginterferon (/wk)	Ribavirin (/d)	
1	Pegasys 180 µg SC	<75 kg 1000 mg	48 wks*
	PegIntron 1.5 µg/kd SC	>75 kg 1200 mg	48 wks*
2–3	Pegasys 180 µg SC	800 mg/d	24 wks
	PegIntron 1.5 µg/kg SC	500 mg/d	24 wks

*May discontinue treatment if early virologic response (EVR) is not achieved. EVR = 2 log decrease in HCV RNA (predicts failure of SVR with specificity of 97%).

e. <u>Goal of therapy</u>: Sustained viral response—No detectable virus at 24 wks after treatment completed. With recommended treatment noted above the following results were achieved (NEJM 2002;347:975; Lancet 2001;258:958):

	Genotype 1	Genotype 2,3
SVR	42–46%	76–82%

2. **Hepatitis B**
   a. <u>Indications to treat</u>: (1) detectable HBsAg±HBeAg; HBV DNA (usually >100,000 c/mL), and (2) liver histology showing necroinflammation (Hepatology 2001;34:1225).
   b. <u>Goal of therapy</u>: Prevent cirrhosis, hepatic failure and hepatocellular carcinoma. (Eradication of HBV is not possible)
   c. <u>Measurable goals</u>: Normal ALT, suppression of HBV DNA, reduction of necroinflammation and eAg seroconversion
   d. <u>FDA - approved drugs for HBV</u>
      Entecavir: Antiviral
      Lamivudine: Antiviral with high rates of resistance
      Adofovir: Antiviral
      Interferon alfa 2b: Immunomodulatory & antiviral
      Pegylated interferon: Immunomodulatory and antiviral
   e. <u>Challenges</u>
      1. Resistance to oral antivirals (especially lamivudine, but also entecavir and adofovir)
      2. Side effects (especially interferon and pegylated interferon)
      3. Cost: $5,000–15,000/year
      4. Treatment for 1–2 years usually results in only temporary improvement (NEJM 2005;352:2673)
   f. <u>Probability estimates</u> (Ann Intern Med 2005;142:821)

	Interferon		Lamivudine		Adofovir	
	eAg+	eAg−	eAg+	eAg−	eAg+	eAg−
Durable response	33%	20%	20%	10%	12%	10%
Drug toxicity	26%	26%	—	—	—	—
Yearly resistance rate	—	—	23%	23%	1%	1%
Cost/month (drug)	$750	—	$160	$160	$530	$530
Duration Rx (wks)	16	48	48**	48–144*	48–144	48–144*

*Treatment of HBeAg neg HBV for 48 weeks with adofovir is associated with high rates of relapse; benefits were maintained with minimal resistance with adofovir for 144 weeks (NEJM 2005;352:2673).

**Treatment of HBeAg pos HBV for 48 weeks with lamivudine is associated with low rates of eAg seroconversion and immediate relapse when treatment is discontinued. Peginterferon was superior (NEJM 2005;352:2682).

3. **Chronic hepatitis D:** Efficacy demonstrated for interferon-alfa in patients with the following criteria: positive HBsAg, anti-HDV IgG and IgM, positive HDV RNA × 3, alanine aminotransferase ≥2 × upper limit of normal × 6 mo, histologic evidence of chronic hepatitis and positive intrahepatic HDV antigen. Patients with advanced cirrhosis were excluded. Optimal regimen was 9 million units IM 3 ×/wk for 48 wk. Response, which was generally transient, was shown by normal alanine transferase and elimination of serum HDV RNA in 7 of 14 patients vs 0 of 13 placebo recipients (NEJM 1994; 330:88; JAMA 1999;282:511).

D. HANTAVIRUS PULMONARY SYNDROME

1. **Definition** (MMWR 2002;51 RR-9; CID 2002;34:1224)
2. **Clinical features:** HPS due to Sin Nombre virus has a median incubation period of 14–17 days, a prodrome of 3–5 days, and clinical features consisting initially of myalgias, GI symptoms (nausea, vomiting, diarrhea), and fever. A clue to the diagnosis in the prodrome stage is thrombocytopenia. The second stage is characterized by cardiopulmonary involvement with tachypnea, tachycardia, cough, and postural hypotension. The complete blood count is highly characteristic with hemoconcentration, leukocytosis with a left shift, thrombocytopenia and circulating immunoblasts that may resemble atypical lymphocytes. By 48 hours postadmission most patients have DIC with typical x-ray changes. The mortality rate is 38% in 344 cases in the U.S.
3. **Diagnosis:** The diagnosis is established with serology (EIA IgM) or RT-PCR for Hantavirus during the first 10 days of illness.
4. **Epidemiology:** Rats and mice are hosts for Sin Nombre virus and transmit it by droppings, saliva, and urine. In the U.S. there were 344 cases reported from 1992 to June 2003 from 31 states, primarily in June and July in the Four Corners area (Arizona, Colorado, New Mexico, and Utah) (www.cdc.gov/ncidod/diseases/hanta.hantavirus.htm). Other areas with HPS are Argentina, Boliva, Brazil, Canada, Chile, Panama, Paraguay, and Uruguay. The average age was 37 years. Person-to-person with nosocomical spread was reported in Argentina (Emerg Infect Dis 1997;3:171).
5. **Treatment:** Supportive care. A trial with ribavirin was unsuccessful (CID 2002;34:304).

E. WEST NILE VIRUS

West Nile Virus (WNV) Infection: Information for Clinicians [CDC www.cdc.gov/ncidod/dvbid/westnile/resources/fact_sheet_clinicians.htm; accessed 7/26/03]: The following is a summary of WNV from the CDC website and other sources:

1. **Clinical Features**
   a. **Mild infection**
      (1) About 80% are asymptomatic and 20% develop mild illness.
      (2) Incubation period is 3–14 days for those with clinical symptoms.
      (3) Symptoms usually last 3–6 days.
      (4) Clinical features are sudden onset of afebrile illness accompanied by malaise, anorexia, nausea, vomiting, eye pain, headache, myalgias, rash and/or lymphadenopathy.
   b. **Severe infection**
      (1) About 1 in 150 cases will cause severe neurologic disease, most commonly encephalitis and less commonly, meningitis
      (2) The major factor for severe neurologic disease is advanced age.
      (3) Features of severe disease are fever, weakness, GI symptoms, and a change in mental status; a minority develop a maculopapular or morbilliform rash involving the neck, trunk, arms, or legs.
      (4) A small number of patients have developed severe muscle weakness and flaccid paralysis or Parkinson's syndrome
      (5) Neurologic presentations include ataxia, cranial nerve abnormalities, myelitis, optic neuritis, polyradiculitis, and seizures.
   c. **Clinical suspicion**
      This diagnosis should be suspected in adults over 50 years who develop unexplained encephalitis or meningitis in summer or early fall, especially if there are local cases or travel to an implicated area.

d. **Neurologic complications**
   (1) Viral encephalitis, characterized by:
      - Fever = 38°C or 100°F, and
      - CNS involvement, including altered mental status (altered level of consciousness, confusion, agitation, or lethargy) or other cortical signs (cranial nerve palsies, paresis or paralysis, or convulsions), and
      - An abnormal CSF profile suggesting a viral etiology (a negative bacterial stain and culture with a mononuclear pleocytosis [WBC 5–1500 cells/mm^3] and/or elevated protein level [>40 mg/dl]).
   (2) Aseptic meningitis (among persons aged 17 years and up), characterized by:
      - Fever = 38°C or 100°F, and
      - Headache, stiff neck and/or other meningeal signs, and
      - An abnormal CSF profile suggesting a viral etiology (a negative bacterial stain and culture with a pleocytosis [WBC between 5 and 1500 cells/mm^3] and/or elevated protein level [=40 mg/dl]).
   (3) Poliomyelitis-like syndromes: acute flaccid paralysis or paresis, (which may resemble Guillain-Barré syndrome), or other unexplained movement disorders such as tremor, myoclonus or Parkinson's-like symptoms, especially if associated with atypical features, such as fever, altered mental status, and/or a pleocytosis. Afebrile patients with asymmetric weakness, with or without areflexia, have also been reported in association with West Nile virus.
2. **Diagnosis**
   (1) The most efficient method is detection of IgM in serum which is usually positive at the time of viral clearance and at the onset of neurologic disease.
   (2) False positive test may be a problem in patients recently vaccinated against or recently infected with related flaviviruses including yellow fever, Japanese encephalitis, or dengue.
   a. **Laboratory findings**
      - Total leukocyte counts are normal or elevated with lymphopenia and anemia.
      - Some have hyponatremia.
      - CSF shows pleocytosis with predominance of lymphocytes, protein is universally elevated and glucose is normal.
      - CT scans of the brain are usually normal, but about one third have MRI demonstrated enhancement of the leptomeninges, the periventricular areas of both.
3. **Treatment:** The usual treatment is supportive. There is an NIH-sponsored trial with hyperimmune globulin, which should be started early.

F. ACTIVITY OF ANTIVIRALS (adapted and updated from NEJM 1999;340:1255)*

Agent	Proven efficacy	Possible efficacy
Acyclovir	HSV, VZV, CMV	EBV, herpes B
Adefovir	HBV	
Amantadine	Influenza A	—
Cidofovir	HSV, VZV, CMV, Molluscum	Small pox virus, monkey pox
Entecavir	HBV	
Famciclovir	HSV, VZV	Hepatitis B
Foscarnet	CMV, HSV, VZV	HHV-8, HIV
Ganciclovir	CMV, HSV	HSV, VZV, EBV, HHV-8, HBV
Interferon-alfa	HBV, HCV, HHV-8, HPV	Hepatitis D
Lamivudine	HBV, HIV	—
Oseltamivir	Influenza A & B	
Penciclovir	HSV	
Ribavirin	Lassa fever, HCV	RSV, paraflu, influenza A & B, measles, Hantavirus, vaccinia
Rimantadine	Influenza A	
Tenofovir	HBV, HIV	
Valacyclovir	HSV, VZV, CMV	EBV
Valganciclovir	CMV, HSV	
Zanamivir	Influenza A & B	

*Antiretroviral agents for HIV are not included

SPECIFIC INFECTIONS

SEPSIS AND SEPSIS SYNDROME

A. CONSENSUS CONFERENCE DEFINITIONS (Crit Care Med 1992;20:864; Chest 1992;161:1644; NEJM 2001;344:707)

<u>**Systemic inflammatory response syndrome (SIRS).**</u> Two or more:
1. Temperature $>38°C$
2. Heart rate >90 beats/min
3. Respiratory rate >20 breaths/min
4. White blood cell count $>12,000/mm^3$, $<4,000/mm^3$, or $>10\%$ immature (bands) forms

<u>**Sepsis.**</u> SIRS plus a documented infection (positive culture for organism).

<u>**Severe sepsis.**</u> Sepsis associated with organ dysfunction, hypoperfusion abnormalities, or hypotension. Hypoperfusion abnormalities include, but are not limited to, lactic acidosis, oliguria, or an acute alteration in mental status.

<u>**Septic shock.**</u> Sepsis-induced hypotension despite fluid resuscitation plus hypoperfusion abnormalities.

<u>**Culture negative populations.**</u>

Culture negative sepsis. SIRS plus empirical antibiotic treatment for a clinically suspected infection but in whom all cultures were negative.

Culture negative severe sepsis. SIRS associated with organ dysfunction, hypoperfusion, or hypotension. However, all cultures were negative. Hypoperfusion abnormalities include, but are not limited to, lactic acidosis, oliguria, or an acute alteration in mental status.

Culture negative septic shock. SIRS associated with hypotension despite fluid resuscitation plus hypoperfusion abnormalities. However, all cultures were negative.

B. EMPIRIC ANTIBIOTIC SELECTION FOR SEPSIS (Med Lett 2001;43:69)
1. **Life-threatening sepsis:** Aminoglycoside (gentamicin, tobramycin, or amikacin) <u>plus</u> one of the following:
   — Third-generation cephalosporin (cefotaxime, cefepime, or ceftriaxone)
   — Ticarcillin-clavulanic acid or piperacillin-tazobactam
   — Imipenem or meropenem

   Suspected methicillin-resistant *S. aureus:* Add vancomycin ± rifampin
2. **Intra-abdominal or pelvic infection:**
   — Any of the following with or without an aminoglycoside: Ticarcillin-clavulanic acid, piperacillin-tazobactam, ampicillin-sulbactam, imipenem, cefoxitin, or cefotetan
3. **Biliary tract source:**
   — Piperacillin + metronidazole ± aminoglycoside
   — Piperacillin-tazobactam or ampicillin-sulbactam ± aminoglycoside
4. **Urinary tract infection** (Nosocomial):
   — Third-generation cephalosporin ± aminoglycoside
   — Fluoroquinolone ± aminoglycoside
   — Ticarcillin/clavulanate or piperacillin/tazobactam ± aminoglycoside
   — Imipenem or meropenem ± aminoglycoside
5. **Meningitis**
   — Community-acquired: Ceftriaxone or cefotaxime + vancomycin 2–4 g/d, ± rifampin
   — Nosocomial: Ceftazidime + vancomycin 2–4 g/d
6. **Nosocomial pneumonia:** Aminoglycoside + cefepime, imipenem, or meropenem ± vancomycin if MRSA suspected

7. **Community-acquired pneumonia:**
   — Ceftriaxone or cefotaxime + macrolide (azithromycin, clarithromycin, or erythromycin)
   — Fluoroquinolone (levofloxacin, gatifloxacin, or moxifloxacin)
   — Aspiration pneumonia suspected: Add clindamycin or metronidazole
8. **Neutropenia + sepsis**
   — Ceftazidime ± aminoglycoside
   — Imipenem, meropenem, or cefepime ± aminoglycoside
   — Piperacillin/tazobactam or ticarcillin/clavulanate, each with amikacin
   — All of above: Add vancomycin if MRSA are suspected
9. **Endocarditis:** Vancomycin + gentamicin

C. DROTRECOGIN (XIGRIS)

Product: Activated protein C exerts antithrombotic effect by inhibition of Factor Va and VIIIa, increases fibrinolysis and inhibits TNF.

Indication: Severe sepsis with: (1) APACHE II score >25, (2) suspected or proven source of infection, and (3) ≥3 signs of systemic inflammation and ≥ one spesis-induced organ dysfunction.

Dose: 24 mcg/kg/hr by continuous infusion × 96 hr (No dose modification for renal or hepatic failure)

Efficacy: In the major clinical trial the 28 day mortality was 25% in drotrecogen recipients compared to 31% in the placebo group (p<0.05) (NEJM 1999;340: 207).

Side effects: Major toxicity causes bleeding; in the large clinical trial the frequency of serious bleeding events was 3.5% in drotrecogen recipients compared to 2% with placebo recipients.

Contraindication: Active, recent, or high risk of bleeding include trauma, epidural catheter, or intracranial lesion. Drug should be stopped 2 hours before invasive procedures and can be started 12 hrs after major surgery if hemostatis is adequate.

D. INTRAVASCULAR CATHETER-RELATED INFECTION: Recommendation of IDSA (CID 2001;32:1249)

Nontunneled central venous catheters

1. Blood culture × 2, remove catheter, culture catheter tip and insert new catheter over guidewire
2. Empiric antibiotics if seriously ill
3. Serious or complicated infection including septic thrombophlebitis, endocarditis or osteomyelitis: Remove CVC and treat 4–6 wks (6–8 wks for osteomyelitis)
4. Uncomplicated infection:
   —Coag-neg staph: Remove CVC and treat 5–7 days or retain catheter and treat 10–14 days ± lock therapy
   —*S. aureus*: Remove CVC and treat 14 days; if TEE is positive: treat for endocaraditis
   —GNB: Remove CVC and treat 10–14 days
   —*Candida*: Remove CVC and treat with antifungal × 14 days

Tunneled central catheters

1. Complicated infections such as port abscesses: Remove CVC and treat with antibiotics 10–14 days
2. Other major complications such as septic thrombophlebitis, endocarditis, or osteomyelitis: Remove CVC and treat with antibiotics 4–6 wks or 6–8 wks for osteomyelitis
3. Uncomplicated infections:
   —Coag-neg staph: Retain CVC and treat with antibiotics for 7 days + antibioitic lock therapy for 10–14 days. If there is persistence or deterioration: Remove CVC.
   —*S. aureus*: Remove CVC and treat 14 days or keep CVC and remove if there is clinical progression

—GNB: Remove CVC and treat 14 days or retain CVC and give systemic
antibiotics + lock therapy. Failure to respond: Remove CVC and treat 10–14
days
—*Candida*: Remove CVC and treat with antifungal therapy 10–14 days

COMPROMISED HOST

PATHOGENS ASSOCIATED WITH IMMUNODEFICIENCY

Condition	Usual conditions	Pathogens
Neutropenia (<500/mL)	Cancer chemotherapy; adverse drug reaction; leukemia	**Bacteria:** Aerobic GNB (coliforms and pseudomonads); *S. aureus, Strep viridans, S. epidermidis* **Fungi:** *Aspergillus, Candida* sp
Cell-mediated immunity	Organ transplantation; HIV infection; lymphoma (especially Hodgkin's disease); corticosteroid therapy	**Bacteria:** *Listeria, Salmonella, Nocardia,* mycobacteria (*M. tuberculosis* and *M. avium*), *Legionella* **Viruses:** CMV, *H. simplex,* varicella-zoster, JC virus **Parasites:** *Pneumocystis carinii; Toxoplasma; Strongyloides stercoralis;* cryptosporidia **Fungi:** *Candida, Cryptococcus, Histoplasma, Coccidioides*
Hypogamma-globulinemia or dysgamma-globulinemia*	Multiple myeloma; congenital or acquired deficiency; chronic lymphocytic leukemia	**Bacteria:** *S. pneumoniae, H. influenzae* (type B) **Parasites:** *Giardia* **Viruses:** Enteroviruses
Complement deficiencies C2, 3 C5 C6–8 Alternative pathway	Congenital	**Bacteria:** *S. pneumoniae, H. influenzae* *S. pneumoniae, S. aureus, Enterobacteriaceae* *Neisseria meningitidis* *S. pneumoniae, H. influenzae, Salmonella*
Hyposplenism	Splenectomy; hemolytic anemia	*S. pneumoniae, H. influenzae,* DF-2
Defective chemotaxis	Diabetes, alcoholism, renal failure, lazy leukocyte syndrome, trauma, SLE	*S. aureus,* streptococci, *Candida*
Defective neutrophilic killing	Chronic granulomatous disease, myeloperoxidase deficiency	Catalase-positive bacteria: *S. aureus, E. coli; Candida* sp

*Patients with primary immune deficiency disorders should receive IV immunoglobulin (200 mg/kg monthly) (Med Lett 1992;34:116).

GUIDELINES FOR USE OF ANTIMICROBIAL AGENTS IN NEUTROPENIC PATIENTS WITH UNEXPLAINED FEVER

(Infectious Disease Society of America, CID 2002;34:730; reprinted with permission)

FIGURE 1: GUIDE TO INITIAL MANAGEMENT

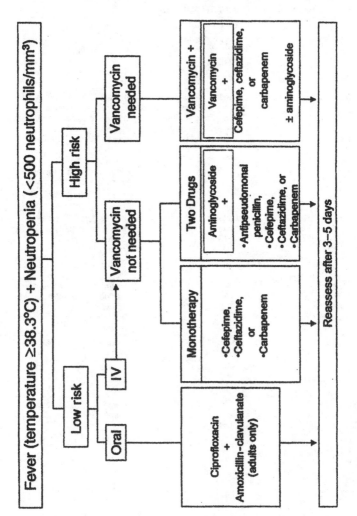

<u>Definition:</u> Fever is defined as a single oral temp of 38.3°C × 1 or 38.0°C for over one hour. Neutropenia is defined as an ANC <500/mm³ or <1000/mm³ with a predicted decrease to <500/mm³.

<u>Evaluation for vancomycin need:</u> (1) suspected catheter-related infection, (2) known colonization with beta-lactam resistant *S. pneumoniae* or MRSA, (3) positive blood cultures for GP bacteria prior to identification, or (4) hypotension.

<u>Assessment for possible oral antibiotic treatment:</u> Patients at low risk for complications may often be treated with oral antibiotics if there is no focus of infection and lack of findings for systemic infection such as rigors or hypotension. If outpatient treatment is to be used, there must be access to medical care 24/7.

<u>Risk assessment:</u> Factors supporting low risk are an ANC exceeding 100/mm³, absolute monocyte count exceeding 100/mm³, normal chest x-ray, nearly normal renal and hepatic tests, neutropenia less than 7 days, malignancy in remission, temperature peak less than 39°C, early evidence of marrow recovery, and none of the following: IV catheter site infection, neurologic or mental status changes, appearance of illness, abdominal pain or cormorbidity/complications.

<u>Antibiotic selection</u> (Figure 1)
1. Low risk, oral treatment: Ciprofloxacin plus amoxicillin-clavulanate.
2. Low risk, IV therapy: Cefepime, ceftazidime, or carbapenem
3. High risk with no need for vancomycin: Monotherapy (see Figure 1) or dual therapy: aminoglycoside plus either an antipseudomonal penicillin, cefepime, ceftazidime, or carbapenem.
4. High risk and vancomycin needed: Vancomycin plus cefepime, ceftazidime, or carbapenem plus/minus aminoglycoside.

Figure 2: Management of patients who become afebrile in first 3–5 days of initial antibiotic therapy.

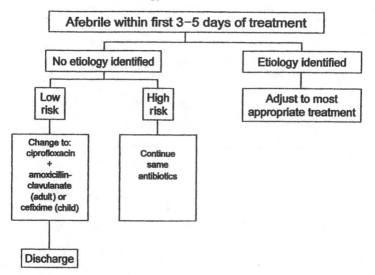

201

Figure 3: Treatment of patients who have persistent fever after 3–5 days of treatment and for whom the etiology of the fever is not found.

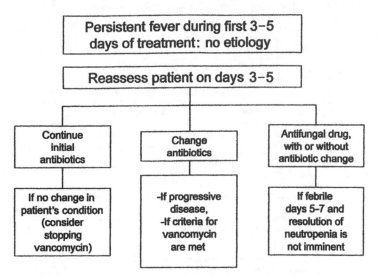

Modifications of therapy based on response at 3–5 days (Figures 2 & 3)
1. Response and pathogen defined: Adjust therapy based on pathogen.
2. Response and no pathogen identified: Oral therapy should be continued. IV therapy may be changed to oral ciprofloxacin plus amoxicillin-clavulanate after 48 hours
3. Persistent fever at 3 days and no change in patient condition: Continue same antibiotics, but consider discontinuing vancomycin if there is no clear need for it.
4. Persistent fever at 3–5 days and progressive disease: Change antibiotic regimen depending on the initial regimen. This includes the addition of vancomycin if it was not initially used and there are criteria for it, or consideration of discontinuing vancomycin if it was included in the initial regimen.
5. Persistent fever at days 5–7: Consider antifungal agent such as amphotericin B, lipid amphotericin B (no more effective, but reduced toxicity), or fluconazole. Fluconazole is acceptable at an institution where *Aspergillus* and azole-resistant *Candida* infections are uncommon, where fluconazole was not used as prophylaxis, and when there is no evidence of pulmonary disease or sinusitis. Recent reviews have not shown clear advantages in efficacy for empiric use of amphotericin B, lipid amphotericin, itraconazole, or fluconazole.

Antibiotic discontinuation (Figure 4): Low risk patients may have antibiotics discontinued when they are afebrile 5–7 days. If the ANC increases above 500/mL, stop antibiotics at 4–5 days. If there is persistent fever at day 3 and persistent ANC <500/mm^3, continue antibiotics for 2 weeks and reasses.

FIGURE 4: DURATION OF ANTIBIOTIC THERAPY

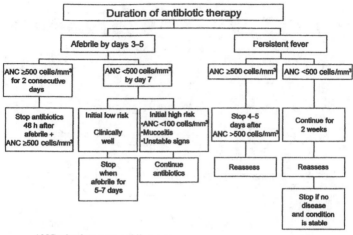

ANC, absolute neutrophil count.

Miscellaneous issues

Antiviral drugs: Not recommended unless there is laboratory or clinical support for use.

Granulocyte transfusions: Not recommended.

G-CSF or GM-CSF: Not recommended for routine use, but may be considered if there is an expected long delay in marrow recovery and those with documented infections who do not respond to antibiotics.

Prophylaxis in neutropenic patients without fever: TMP-SMX is sometimes recommended for PCP regardless of neutropenia. There are good data supporting efficacy of prophylaxis with TMP-SMX, quinolones, fluconazole, and itraconazole for reducing the number of infectious complications of neutropenia, but the Panel recommends against this prophylaxis due to the concerns for antibiotic resistance and the failure of these studies to show reduction in mortality.

FIGURE 5: COMMON INFECTIONS BY TIME AFTER MARROW TRANSPLANTATION*

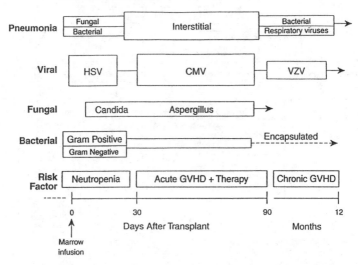

From Infections in Bone Marrow Transplant Recipients. Principles and Practice of Infectious Diseases. Mandell G, Bennett JE, Dolin R (Editors). New York: Churchill Livingstone, 1995: 2718 (reprinted with permission).

TOXIC SHOCK SYNDROME: CASE DEFINITION OF CDC (MMWR 29:229, 1980)

1. Fever: Temperature ≥38.9°C (102°F).
2. Rash: Diffuse macular erythroderma.
3. Desquamation: 1–2 wk after onset, especially palms and soles.
4. Hypotension: Systolic <90 mm Hg for adults or <5th percentile by age for children or orthostatic syncope.
5. Involvement of three or more of the following organs.
   GI: Vomiting or diarrhea at onset
   Muscular: Severe myalgia or creatine phosphokinase >2× normal
   Mucous membrane: Vaginal, oropharyngeal, or conjunctival hyperemia
   Renal: BUN or creatinine ≥2× normal or ≥5 WBC/HPF in absence of UTI
   Hepatic: Bilirubin or transaminase levels ≥ 2× normal
   Hematological: Platelets <100,000/mm³
   CNS: Disoriented or altered consciousness without focal neurologic signs when fever and neurologic signs are absent
6. Negative results for the following (if obtained): Cultures of blood, throat, and cerebrospinal fluid; negative serology for Rocky Mountain spotted fever, leptospirosis, or measles.

GROUP A STREPTOCOCCAL INFECTIONS

Classification and Definition of Group A Streptococcal Toxic Shock Syndrome:
Working Group on Severe Streptococcal Infections (CDC)
(Reprinted with permission from JAMA 269:390, 1993)

Proposed Case Definition for the Streptococcal Toxic Shock Syndrome*

I. Isolation of group A streptococci (*Streptococcus pyogenes*)
    A. From a normally sterile site (e.g., blood, cerebrospinal, pleural, or peritoneal fluid, tissue biopsy, surgical wound)
    B. From a nonsterile site (e.g., throat, sputum, vagina, superficial skin lesion)

II. Clinical signs of severity
    A. Hypotension: Systolic blood pressure ≤ 90 mmHg in adults or <5th percentile for age in children and
    B. ≥2 of the following signs
        1. Renal impairment: creatinine ≥177 μmol/L (≥2 mg/dL) for adults or greater than or equal to twice the upper limit of normal for age. In patients with pre-existing renal disease, a ≥2-fold elevation over the baseline level
        2. Coagulopathy: platelets ≤100 × 10⁹/L (≤100,000/mm³) or disseminated intravascular coagulation defined by prolonged clotting times, low fibrinogen level, and the presence of fibrin degradation products
        3. Liver involvement: alanine amino-transferase (SGOT), asparate amino-transferase (SGPT), or total bilirubin levels greater than or equal to twice the upper limit of normal for age. In patients with preexisting liver disease a ≥2-fold elevation over the baseline level
        4. Adult respiratory distress syndrome defined by acute onset of diffuse pulmonary infiltrates and hypoxemia in the absence of cardiac failure, or evidence of diffuse capillary leak manifested by acute onset of generalized edema, or pleural or peritoneal effusions with hypoalbuminemia
        5. A generalized erythematous macular rash that may desquamate
        6. Soft-tissue necrosis, including necrotizing fasciitis or myositis, or gangrene

* An illness fulfilling criteria IA and IIA and IIB can be defined as a definite case. An illness fulfilling criteria IB and IIA and IIB can be defined as a probable case if no other etiology for the illness is identified.

Therapy of Streptococcal Infections of Skin and Soft Tissue

(NEJM 1996;334:240; AAC 2003;423:104)

1. Antibiotic: *S. pyogenes* is exquisitely sensitive to beta-lactams; penicillin is preferred for pharyngitis, erysipelas, impetigo, and cellulitis. Experimental models of fulminant infections show clindamycin is superior, presumably because it inhibits protein synthesis and activity is independent of inoculum size. Clindamycin or clindamycin plus penicillin is preferred for necrotizing fasciitis, myositis, empyema, and streptococcal toxic shock syndrome. Studies in the mouse myositis model show clindaymcin is superior to penicillin for inhibiting streptococcal toxin production in vivo; penicillin combined with clindamycin showed no antagonism (AAC 1987;31:213; AAC 2003;423:104)
2. IVIG: Anecdotal studies support use for streptococcal toxic shock syndrome at suggested dose of 1g/kg day 1 then 0.5g/kg on days 2 and 3 (CID 2003;37:333)
3. Surgery: Prompt and aggressive exploration and debridement of deep-seated infections are important

ANAEROBIC INFECTIONS

1. Susceptibility in vitro[a]

Susceptibility	B. fragilis group	Bacteroides (other), Prevotella	Fusobacteria	Peptostrep	Clostridia
>95%	Beta-lactam-BL inhibitors Chloramphenicol Imipenem Metronidazole Tigecycline	Same as B. fragilis Cefoxitin Cefoperazone Cefotaxime Clindamycin Trovafloxacin Moxifloxacin Gatifloxacin Tigecycline	Same as B. fragilis Penicillin G Piperacillin Trovafloxacin Moxifloxacin Cefotetan Cefoxitin Tigecycline	Same as B. fragilis Penicillin G Piperacillin Ceftazidime Cefotetan Cefoperazone Ceftriaxone Trovafloxacin Gatifloxacin Moxifloxacin Clindamycin Tigecycline	Ampicillin-sulbactam Chloramphenicol Imipenem Penicillin G Piperacillin Cefotaxime Piperacillin Tigecycline
85–95%	Cefoxitin Gatifloxacin Moxifloxacin	Cefotetan Ceftazidime Ceftriaxone	Cefoperazone Cefotaxime Moxifloxacin Gatifloxacin Clindamycin	Metronidazole Ciprofloxacin Levofloxacin	Cefotetan Cefoxitin Ceftriaxone
70–84%	Piperacillin Ceftizoxime Clindamycin	Penicillin G	Ceftazidime Ciprofloxacin		Cefoxitin Clindamycin
50–69%	Cefotetan Cefoperazone Cefotaxime Ceftazidime Ceftriaxone	Levofloxacin	—	—	Metronidazole Fluoroquinolones
<50%	Levofloxacin Ciprofloxacin Penicillin G	Ciprofloxacin			Ceftazidime

[a]Adapted from: Principles and Practice of Infectious Diseases, AAC 1999;43:2231; AAC 1999;43:2320; CID 2000;30:870; AAC 2001;45:1238; Anaerobe 2001;7:285; CID 2002;35:S126; AAC 2003;47:148.

2. Outcome of *Bacteroides* bacteremia in 128 patients (CID 30:870, 2000)

	Active drug	Inactive drug	P value for difference
Mortality	16%	45%	0.04
Clinical failure	22%	82%	0.002
Microbiological persistence	12%	42%	0.06

3. Susceptibility of anaerobic bacteria.
Modified from National Committee for Clinical Laboratory Standards, Working Group on Anaerobic Susceptibility Testing (J Clin Microbiol 26:1253, 1988; updated Antimicrob Ag Chemother 2001;45:1238)

Metronidazole (except some nonsporulating GPB)
Chloramphenicol
Imipenem/meropenem
Beta-lactam-beta-lactamase inhibitor combinations
 (especially piperacillin-tazobactam)
USUALLY ACTIVE
Clindamycin (increasing in vitro resistance—
 AAC 2001;45:1238; AAC 2003;47:148)
Cefoxitin
Antipseudomonad penicillins
Trovafloxacin/moxifloxacin/gatifloxacin

UNPREDICTABLE ACTIVITY
Cephalosporins (other)
Penicillins (other—especially
 antistaphylococcal agents)
Vancomycin (Gram-positive
 anaerobes only)
Erythromycin (Fusobacteria
 often resistant)
Tetracyclines
VIRTUALLY NEVER ACTIVE
Aztreonam
Aminoglycosides
Trimethoprim-sulfamethoxazole

FEVER OF UNKNOWN ORIGIN

A. Definition

Classic (Medicine 1961;40:1):(1) Illness $\times \geq$ 3 wks, (2) Documented fever $\geq$ 101°F (38.3°C), and (3) Negative diagnostic evaluation with one week in hospital

Contemporary: 2 modifications

1. Emphasis on diagnostic evaluation in outpatient clinic
2. Emphasis on subtypes
   - Nosocomial: Posteroperative complications, drug fever, *C, difficile,* phlebitis pulmonary emboli, ICU sinusitis (Brit J Hosp Med 1996;56:21)
   - Immunodeficient (chemotherapy etc): Infection (JID 1990;161:381)
   - HIV-associated (pre-HAART): MAC, CMV, PCP, TB, lymphoma, Bartonella (J Intern Med 1994;236:529)
   - Elderly: Infections, tumors, and connective tissue diseases (especially temporal arteritis and polymyalgia rheumatica) (J Am Geriatr Soc 1993;41:1187)
   - Young patients: Many undiagnosed (30%) and long-term follow-up shows benign course (Arch Inter Med 2003;163:1033)
   - Prolonged fever (>1 year): Lymphoma, factitious, normal variant, granulomatous hepatitis

B. Etiologic diagnosis in the 5 standard categories: Infection, neoplasm, connective tissue, miscellaneous, and undiagnosed:

Source Period of review Location	Petersdorf[1] 1952–57 U.S.	Larson[2] 1970–80 U.S.	Barbado[3] 1968–81 Spain	Knockaert[4] 1980–89 Belgium	Likuni[5] 1982–92 Japan	DeKleijn[6] 1992–94 Netherlands	Vander[7] 1991–99 Belgium
Number	100	105	133	197	153	167	189
Diagnosis made, %	91	84	78	74	88	69	52
Infection, %*	40	36	39	30	33	37	30
Neoplasm, %*	21	38	25	10	16	18	15
Connective tissue, %*	19	15	19	13	35	33	34
Miscellaneous, %*	21	11	16	29	16	11	20

* % in cases with a final diagnosis
[1]Medicine 1961;40:1
[2]Medicine 1982;61:269
[3]J Med 1984;15:185
[4]Arch Intern Med 1992;152:51
[5]Intern Med 1994;33:67
[6]Medicine 1997;76:392
[7]Arch Intern Med 2003;163:1033

C. Major conditions within categories in most contemporary reviews (Arch Intern Med 2003;16:1033)

1. Infection: Endocarditis, TB, UTI, and intra-abdominal abscess
2. Malignancy ("omas"): Hematologic, solid tumor with hepatic mets
3. Connective tissue: Still disease, polymyalgia rheumatica, and granulomatous disease (sarcoid, Crohn disease, granulomatous hepatitis, and temporal arteritis)
4. Miscellaneous: Pulmonary emboli, drug fever, periodic fever, and "habitual hyperthermia"
5. No diagnosis: Long-term follow-up in 80 cases showed no late sequelae (Arch Intern Med 2003;163:1033)

D. Diagnostic tests (Arch Intern Med 2003;163;545)

Step 1: Confirm fever (daily temps)
　　　　Fever pattern: not helpful (Arch Intern Med 1979;139:1225)
　　　　Stop meds: Fever resolves <72 hrs or there is another cause (Inf Dis Clin N Amer 1996;10:85)

Step 2: Selected tests
- CT abdomen: Cause found in 19% (Radiology 1980;136:407) Repeat scan is not helpful
- Nuclar scans: Variable
- Endocarditis: Duke criteria-sensitivity 82% (CID 1995;21:905)
- Liver biopsy: Yield is 14–17% (Arch Intern Med 1977;137:1001; J Clin Gastro 1993;17:29) (but usually with abnormal LFTs)
- Temporal artery bx: 16% (J Am Gastric Soc 1993;41:1187) (in age >50 yrs)

Continued

- Leg doppler: 2–6% (Intern Med 1994;33:67)

  Tests that are usually not helpful: Ultrasound, bone scan, MRI, D-dimer assay, ESR, and CRP

E. Fever evaluation in critically ill patients Recommendations of the Society of Critical Care Medicine and the ISDA (Clin Infect Dis 1998;26:1042)

Blood culture: Two blood cultures (with 10–15 mL each) from separate sites drawn ≥10 minutes apart. For skin preparation, povidine iodine (10%) should be allowed to dry 2 minutes and tincture of iodine (1–2%) should be allowed to dry 30 seconds. Alcohol with no drying time is an alternative. With an intravenous catheter, one peripheral vein sample and one through the catheter is an alternative to 2 peripheral vein samples, but the results provide less precise information.

Intravascular catheters: The risk of fever with central venous catheters is 5–10 per 1000 catheter days and for peripheral IV catheters the risk is <0.2 per 1000 catheter days. If there is evidence of tunnel infection, emboli events, vascular compromise, or sepsis the catheter should be removed.

Pulmonary infection: The evaluation should include a chest x-ray, Gram stain, and culture of respiratory secretions and pleural fluid evaluation (if present)

C. difficile: If ≥2 loose or watery stools/day there should be one stool sample sent for _C. difficile_ toxin assay. If this is negative a second specimen can be sent. If disease is severe and the toxin test is negative or delayed, it is appropriate to treat empirically with metronidazole.

Sinusitis: If clinical findings support this diagnosis, there should be a CT scan. With evidence of sinusitis on CT scan there should be puncture or aspiration of sinuses under sterile conditions for Gram stain and culture for aerobes, anerobes, and fungi.

Urinary tract infection: Urine should be evaluated by quantitative culture for PMNs. Pyuria should be tested by esterase dipstick and Gram stain of centrifuged urine sediment. Urine should be collected from the urine port of a Foley catheter; UTIs almost always show >10^4 cfu/mL and pyuria with a catheter collection. If the delay in culture of collected urine >1 hr it should be refrigerated or placed in a preservative.

Postop fever: Noninfectious fever is common during the first 48 hrs. post-operative. Unexplained fever >72 hrs post-operative should be evaluated with chest x-ray, urine culture and urinanalysis, and exam for phlebitis, thrombosis, pulmonary emoblism, and wound infection.

Fever due to non-infectious causes: Blood products (especially RBC's & platelets), drugs, pancreatitis, myocardial infarction, pulmonary emboli, and chemical phlebitis.

TREATMENT OF LYME DISEASE AND POTENTIAL EXPOSURES

(Recommendations of Med Letter 2005;47:41; MMWR 1997;46:532; Ann Intern Med 1998;128:37)

Prevention: (NEJM 2003;348:2424): (1) The vaccine (LYMErix has been withdrawn from the market due to poor sales (Nat Med 2002;8:311). (2) Removal of _I. scapularis_ ticks within 36 hrs of attachment using daily tick checks (regarded as most effective preventive strategy) (JID 1997;175:996; NEJM 2001;345:79; Am J Epidemiol 1998;147;391). (3) Prophylactic doxycycline for tick bites (see below). (4) Tick control with acaricide (cardaryl, cyfluthrin, or deltamethrin) in early May reduces _I. scapularis_ nymph population by 68–100% (J Med Entomol 2001;38:344). (5) Note that treatment of early Lyme disease (erythema migrans stage) prevents late sequelae in >95% (Ann

Intern Med 1983;99:22; AAC 1995;39:661; Am J Med 1992;92:396; Ann Intern Med 1996;124:785; NEJM 1997;337:289; Ann Intern Med 2002;136:421)

Tick bite: Prophylactic doxycycline 200 mg po × 1 reduces the risk of Lyme disease if given within 72 hours of a bite from a I. scapularis tick vector especially in a high incidence area, and with bites from nymphal ticks that are partially engorged (NEJM 2001; 344:79). Efficacy is 87%. GI intolerance to doxycycline dose is improved if taken with meal

Epidemiology: In 2002 there were 23,763 cases of Lyme disease reported in the U.S. for a national incidence of 8.2/100,000 (MMWR 2004;53:365). This represents a 40% increase over 2001. The incidence by state in rank order for cases/100,000 was: CT-133, RI-80, PA-32, NY-28, MA-28, DE-24 and WI-20. The peak age was 5–14 yrs for children and 50–59 yrs for adults. Conditions were: EM-68%, arthritis-10%, Bells palsy-8%, radiculopathy-3% and meningitis/encephalitis <1%.

Diagnosis: Recommendations of American College of Physicians (Ann Intern Med 1997;127:110)

Clinical diagnosis: Patients from an endemic Lyme disease area who present with erythema migrans do not require laboratory confirmation. Seroconversion occurs in 27% with symptoms <7 days, 41% with symptoms 7–14 days and 88% with symptoms >14 days (Ann Intern Med 2002;136:421). Confirmation of late Lyme disease requires objective evidence of Lyme disease plus laboratory evidence

Culture: Erythema migrans—saline lavage needle aspiration or 2 mm punch biopsy of the leading edge show *B. burgderfori* by culture or PCR in 60–80% (Ann Intern Med 2002;136:421)

Diagnostic Criteria (2005)

  Endemic areas: Recognition of erythema migrans

  Serology: 1gG detectable at 4–6 wks by EIA or IFA. Confirmation is by Western blot (MMWR 2005;54:125)

Clinical stages

  Erythema migrans

  Early disseminated Lyme disease with carditis and neurologic features including lymphocytic meningitis and radiculoneuropathies

  Late Lyme disease with peripheral neuropathies, chronic encephalopathy, or arthritis with migratory polyarthritis and/or monoarthritis. The term "chronic Lyme disease" (in reference to debilitating fatigue) was first applied in 1985 and has no objective findings, but there is considerable support from Internet site advocacy groups and some physicians (Ann Intern Med 2002;136:413). Multiple studies indicate no evidence of Lyme disease and no benefit from empiric treatment even with long courses of IV antibiotics (NEJM 2001;345:85; Ann Intern Med 1998;128:354; JID 1995;171:356; JID 1995;171:423; CID 2000;31:1107)

TREATMENT OF LYME DISEASE (Med Lett 2005;47:41)

Stage	Preferred	Comment
Erythema migrans	Doxy 100 mg po bid × 10–21 d* (see footnote)	Goal is shorten duration of rash and prevent late sequelae
	Amoxicillin 500 mg po bid × 14–21 d	Doxy is effective vs *Ehrlichia*; beta-lactams are not
	Cefuroxime axetil 500 mg po bid × 14–21 d	Amoxicillin preferred for pregnant/lactating women
		Babesiosis requires clindamycin and quinine

Neurologic

Bells palsy	Doxy 100 mg po bid × 14–21 d	Oral treatment is sufficient for facial nerve palsy alone
	Amoxicillin 500 mg po bid × 14–21 d	Accounted for 11/503 cases (AM J Otolaryn 2002;23:25)
More serious CNS	Ceftriaxone 2 g/d IV × 14–28 d	"More serious" category includes meningitis, encephalitis, cranial nerve palsies, peripheral nerve palsies, etc.
	Cefotaxime 2 g IV q8h × 14–28 d	
Cardiac		
1st degree	Doxy 100 mg po bid × 14–28 d	PR interval <0.3 sec can be treated orally
	Amox 500 mg po tid × 14–28 d	
More serious	Ceftriaxone 2 g/d IV × 14–21 d	PR >0.3 sec gets parenteral drug
Arthritis		
Oral	Doxy 100 mg po bid × 28 d	Oral therapy usually adequate for arthritis
	Amox 500 mg po tid × 28 d	Some require a second course
Parenteral	Ceftriaxone 2 g/d IV × 14–28 d	Alternative to second month of oral therapy
	Cefotaxime 2 gm IV q8h × 14–28 d	Arthroscopic synovectomy may be useful in refractory arthritis of knee

*A subsequent study showed that doxycycline (200 mg/d) given for 10 days was as effective as the same regimen given for 20 days or doxycycline given for 16 days with a single 2 g dose of ceftriaxone (Ann Intern Med 2003;289:1533)

INFECTIONS OF EPIDERMIS, DERMIS, AND SUBCUTANEOUS TISSUE

Condition	Agent	Laboratory diagnosis	Treatment
Superficial erythematous lesions			
Abscess	S. aureus Anaerobes	Culture and Gram stain	Drainage
Acne rosacea	?	Appearance	Doxycycline* Metronidazole (0.75% topical) Isotretinoin (Accutane)
Acne vulgaris	Propionibacterium acnes	Appearance	Tetracycline* Topical clindamycin 1% gel or erythromycin 2% gel Isotretinoin (Accutane) Tretinoin (Retin-A) Benzoyl peroxide Azelaic acid cream (20%) Adapalene 0.1% gel
Cellulitis: Diffuse spreading infection of deep dermis without sharp demarcation	Group A strep; S. aureus (Vibrio sp and Aeromonas sp with freshwater or saltwater exposure; others— S. pneumoniae, H influenzae, anaerobes, legionella, Erysipelothrix rhusiopathiae, Helicobacter cinaedi)	Culture advanced edge of inflammation (rarely positive); 3-mm dermal punch; ulcerated portal of entry, blood; serial DNase titer (Group A strep)	Penicillinase-resistant penicillin*, vancomycin, clindamycin, cephalosporin (first generation), erythromycin, fluoroquinolone MRSA: Vancomycin, daptomycin, linezolid
Erysipelas: Superficial infection with raised and sharply demarcated edge	Group A strep (Groups B, C, and G strep; S. aureus)	Appearance, often at sites of lymphedema	Penicillin*, clindamycin, cephalosporin (first generation)
Lymphangitis	Group A strep	As above	As above
Folliculitis: Infected hair follicle(s)	S. aureus (P. aeruginosa whirlpools, hot tubs, etc)	Culture and Gram stain (usually unnecessary)	Local compresses or topical antibiotics. Fever, cellulitis, or mild face involvement—treat as furunculosis

Continued

Condition	Agent	Laboratory diagnosis	Treatment
Furunculosis/carbuncle: Abscess that starts in hair follicle; carbuncle is deeper and more extensive	S. aureus	Culture and Gram stain	MSSA: Drainage ± penicillinase-resistant penicillin*, clindamycin, vancomycin, cephalosporin (first generation), erythromycin, amoxicillin-clavulanate MRSA (USA 300): TMP-SMX or clindamycin MRSA (nosocomial): Vancomycin, daptomycin, linezolid
Mycobacterial furunculosis	M. fortuitum	Culture negative boils is clue-culture for mycobacteria at 30° & 37° C	Disease of compromised host especially organ transplant recipients and customers of nail salons (NEJM 2002;346:1366)
Recurrent furunculosis	S. aureus		Bathe with hexachlorophene. May be controlled with chronic clindamycin 150 mg qd × 3 mo* Nasal carriers of staph—mupirocin to anterior nares or rifampin 300 mg bid × 5 days
Paronychia: Infection of nail fold	S. aureus	Culture and Gram stain	S. aureus: Incision and drainage ± antistaph antibiotic Candida: Topical nystatin or miconazole
Impetigo: Infection of epidermis with vesicles → pustules on exposed areas ± lymphadenopathy	Group A strep often with S. aureus	Culture and Gram stain Average yield of strep even with biopsy is only 25%	Dicloxacillin, cloxacillin, cephalexin, or amoxicillin + clavulanate, or topical mupirocin (Am J Dis Child 144:1313, 1990; Arch Dermatol 125:1069, 1989)
Whitlow: Infection of distal phalanx finger	S. aureus	Culture and Gram stain	Penicillinase-resistant penicillin*, clindamycin, cephalosporin (first generation)
	H. simplex	Viral culture, Tzanck prep, or FA stain	Acyclovir
Fungal infections: Keratinized tissue—skin, nails, hair (see p 161)	Candida—red, moist, satellite lesions, especially skin folds	Scrapings for KOH prep, culture on Sabouraud medium	Skin: Topical antifungal agent—Miconazole, clotrimazole, econazole, naftifine, or ciclopirox
	Dermatophytes: Epidermophyton, Trichophyton, Microsporum, "ringworm"	Scrapings for KOH prep and culture: Wood's light	Skin: Topical agents (as above) or oral ketoconazole. Nail: Griseofulvin or ketoconazole. Scalp: Selenium sulfide shampoo + griseofulvin
	Tinea versicolor: Malassezia furfur—red or hypo-pigmented macules		Skin: Topical agents (as above), oral ketoconazole, or topical selenium sulfide

Condition	Agent	Laboratory diagnosis	Treatment
Bites			
Dog and cat (NEJM 340:85, 1999)	*P. multocida:* Anaerobes, fusobacteria, bacteroides, porphyromonas, Prevotella streptococci, *Capnocytophaga canimorus*, *S. aureus*	Culture and Gram stain	Risk for tetanus and rabies Lesions should be left open if not potentially disfiguring, if arms or legs involved, or if bite was >6–12 hr before treatment Use of prophylactic antibiotics is controversial (NEJM 340:138, 1999) Amoxicillin + clavulanic acid (Augmentin)*, cefuroxime + metronidazole; TMP-SMX + clindamycin
Human, including clenched-fist injury	Oral flora (strep, anaerobes) *S. aureus, Eikenella corrodens*	Culture and Gram stain	Human bites are usually left open Amoxicillin-clavulanic acid (Augmentin)*, penicillin V ± cephalexin
Rat	*Streptobacillus moniliformis*	*S. moniliformis:* Giemsa stain of blood or pus; culture; serology	Penicillin*, tetracycline
	Spirillum minus	*S. minus:* Giemsa stain of blood or exudate	Penicillin*, tetracycline
Cat-scratch disease	*Bartonella henselae*	Warthin-Starry stain of biopsy	Efficacy of therapy not established. Ciprofloxacin; sulfa-trimethoprim; amoxicillin-clavulanate; macrolides
Burns	*S. aureus*, GNB, *Candida albicans, Aspergillus,* Herpes simplex, group A strep	Quantitative culture and stain of biopsy	Removal of eschar. Topical sulfa (silver sulfadiazine or mafenide) Empiric antibiotics: Aminoglycoside + nafcillin, antipseudomonad penicillin, ticarcillin-clavulanate, vancomycin or cephalosporin *H. simplex*—acyclovir
Sinus tract			
Osteomyelitis	*S. aureus, S. epidermidis,* GNB, anaerobes	Culture of sinus tract drainage does not reliably reflect agent(s) of osteomyelitis	Antibiotics optimally based on bone biopsy
Lymphadenitis	*S. aureus*	Culture and Gram strain	Antistaphylococcal agent
	Mycobacteria (scrofula)	AFB smear and culture	TB—antituberculous drugs MOTT: See pp 185–186

Condition	Agent	Laboratory diagnosis	Treatment
Actinomycosis	*A. israelii, A. naeslundii, A. odontolyticus, Arachnia proprionica*	FA stain, anaerobic culture	Penicillin G*, amoxicillin, clindamycin, tetracycline
Madura foot (tumor masses with draining sinuses)	Actinomycotic: *Nocardia, Actinomadura madurae, A. pelletieri, S. somaliensis*	Culture including AFB stain, culture for *Nocardia*	Antibiotics selected by in vitro sensitivity tests
	Fungi: *Pseudallescheria boydii* (esp U.S.) *Madurella mycetomatis, Phialophora verrucosa*	KOH, culture on Sabouraud's agar	Fungal: Surgical excision; azoles are possibly effective
Nodules/ulcers			
Sporotrichoid (cutaneous inoculation with lymphatic spread)	*Sporothrix schenckii* (thorns)	Histology (PAS, GMS), culture on Sabouraud's agar	Oral SSKI
	M. marinum (tidal water, swimming pool, or tropical fish tank)	Histology, AFB stain and culture (at 30–32°C) TMP-SMX	Rifampin + ethambutol, Minocycline/doxycycline, TMP-SMX
	Nocardia	Histology, AFB stain; culture for *Nocardia*	Sulfonamide, TMP-SMX
Nodules/ulcers (from hematogenous dissemination)	Blastomycosis: Endemic area	Culture biopsy on Sabouraud's agar	Ketoconazole, amphotericin B, itraconazole
	Cryptococcus: Defective cell-mediated immunity	Blood for cryptococcal antigen and culture; histopathology and culture of biopsy	Amphotericin B, fluconazole
	Candida: Defective cell-mediated immunity	Blood culture; histopathology and culture of biopsy	Amphotericin B
Diabetic foot ulcer and decubitus ulcer	Mixed aerobes: Anaerobes *S. aureus* Group A strep	Culture and Gram stain of wound edge or dermal punch biopsy	**Local care:** Debridement, bed rest **Antibiotics:** For moderately severe infection *oral*—cephalexin, clindamycin, moxifloxacin, gatifloxacin, levofloxacin, amoxicillin-clavulanate; *parenteral*—beta-lactam-beta-lactamase inhibitor, ciprofloxacin ± clindamycin, levofloxacin ± clindamycin, gatifloxacin, cefepime. For severe infection—imipenem, vancomycin + metronidazole; severe infections with MRSA— vancomycin, daptomycin, linezolid

* Preferred regimen

DIABETIC FOOT INFECTIONS (IDSA GUIDELINES CID 2004;39:885)

A. **Classification:** PEDIS (International Consensus on the Diabetic Foot CID 2004;39:885)

Infection Category	Description
1	No infection
2	Involves only skin and subcutaneous tissue
3	Extensive cellulitus or deeper infection
4	Systemic inflammatory response syndrome

B. **Microbiology**
   1. Acute infections: S. aureus and Beta-hemolytic strep (especially group B but also A C & G)
   2. Chronic infections: Enterobacteraceae, P. aeruginosa, enterococci (including VRE) anaerobic, S. aureus (including MRSA); sometimes low virulence microbes– coag neg Staph & Corynebacterium sp.

C. **Evaluation**
   1. <u>General status</u> (History, PE): Vital signs, hydration, mental status, Lab: Blood glucose, renal function, acidosis, osmolality.
   2. <u>Foot exam</u>: Biomechanics (deformities)
      Wound evaluation includes exam, debridement and probe (blunt metal probe) to detect tenderness, heat, induration, streaking, bullae, odor, crepitus, cellulitis & pus.
   3. <u>Arterial blood supply</u>: Dorsalis pedis & posterior tibial pulses usually indicate adequate circulation.
      Other tests of arterial supply:
      a) Doppler with waveform analysis
      b) ABI <50—ischemia that will impair healing
      c) Ankle BP <50 mm Hg & toe pressure <30 mm Hg (especially designed cuffs)
      d) $TcpO_2$ <30 mm Hg
   4. <u>Imaging</u>
      a) X ray—osteomyelitis
      b) Ultrasound and CT—good for soft tissue abscesses
      c) MRI—best for osteomyelitis and good for abscesses, involvement of fascia and muscle
      d) Nuclear scans: Sensitive but less specific than MRI
   5. <u>Culture of wound</u>
      a) Obtain culture before antibiotics
      b) Clean and debride prior to culture
      c) Open wound—culture debrided base by curettage or biopsy. Avoid
      d) Avoid swabs
      e) Purulent collections—aspirate
      f) Needle aspiration of cellulitus—rarely positive
      g) Culture should be sent promptly to lab in appropriate container and cultured for aerobes or anaerobes.
      h) Interpretation: Pathogens should have concentrations $>10^5$/gm or ml meaning visualization on gram stain and growth that is moderate or heavy on primary isolation plates

6. Osteomyelitis evaluation
   a) Clues: (1) Nonhealing ulcer despite antibiotics >6 wks; (2) ulcer with bone visible or palpable with blunt metal probe; (3) "sausage toe" (red swollen digit); (4) unexplained elevated WBC ESR or CRP; (5) X ray showing bone destruction below ulcer
   b) Scans: MRi is best
   c) Bone biopsy: For diagnosis or to identify the pathogen(s). Biopsy under fluoroscopic or CT avoidance.

Antibiotics
1. <u>Mild</u> & some moderately severe infections: Empiric selection is oral agent vs aerobic GPC (staph & strep): Dicloxacillin, clindamycin, cephalexin, TMP-SMX, amoxicillin-clavulanate, levofloxacin.
2. <u>Moderately severe</u> where oral or parenteral agents are options:
   a) levofloxacin; b) cefoxitin; c) ceftriaxone; d) ampicillin−sulbactam; e) linezolid + aztreonam; f) ertapenem; g) ticarcillin−clavulanate, h) cefuroxime ± metronidazole
3. <u>Moderately severe or severe</u>: Empiric antibiotics should cover GPC (including MRSA), aerobic GNB and anaerobes: a) Pipercillin + tazobactam; b) levofloxacin/ciprofloxacin + clindamycin; c) imipenem; d) ceftazidime + vancomycin ± metronidazole
4. <u>Duration of antibiotics</u>
   Mild infections: usually 1–2 weeks
   Moderately severe or severe: 2–4 weeks
   Osteomyelitis: 4–6 weeks, shorter if infected bone removed, longer if not
5. <u>Footcare</u>: Debride—sharps preferred to hydrotherapy or topical debriding agents. Pressure off loading is critical
   Dressings that are moist and permit daily inspection
6. <u>Hyperbaric oxygen</u>: Cochrane Library review suggest benefit
7. <u>Surgery</u>:
   Ischemia: Consider angioplasty or vascular by-pass, preferrably early (1–2 days)
   Amputation: Urgent with extensive necrosis or life-threatening infection. Elective if recurrent ulceration despite good care or irreversible loss of foot function

DEEP SERIOUS SOFT TISSUE INFECTIONS
(From Cecil Textbook of Medicine, Philadelphia: Saunders, 1992:1679)

	Gas-forming cellulitis	Synergistic necrotizing cellulitis	Gas gangrene	"Streptococcal" myonecrosis	Necrotizing fasciitis	Infected vascular gangrene	Streptococcal
Predisposing conditions	Traumatic	Diabetes, prior local lesions, perirectal lesions	Traumatic or surgical wound	Trauma, surgery	Diabetes, trauma, surgery, perineal infection	Arterial insufficiency	Traumatic or surgical wound
Incubation period	>3 days	3–14 days	1–4 days	3–4 days	1–4 days	>5 days	6 hr–2 days
Etiologic organism(s)	Clostridia, others	Mixed aerobic-anaerobic flora	Clostridia, esp *C. perfringens*	Anaerobic streptococci	Mixed aerobic-anaerobic flora	Mixed aerobic-anaerobic flora	*S. pyogenes*
Systemic toxicity	Minimal	Moderate to severe	Severe	Minimal until late in course	Moderate to severe	Minimal	Severe
Course	Gradual	Acute	Acute	Subacute	Acute to subacute	Subacute	Acute
Wound findings, local pain	Minimal	Moderate to severe	Severe	Late only	Minimal to moderate	Variable	Severe
Skin appearance	Swollen, minimal discoloration	Erythematous or gangrene	Tense and blanched, yellow-bronze, necrosis with hemorrhagic bullae	Erythema or yellow-bronze	Blanched, erythema, necrosis with hemorrhagic bullae	Erythema or necrosis	Erythema, necrosis
Gas	Abundant	Variable	Usually present	Variable	Variable	Variable	No
Muscle involvement	No	Variable	Myonecrosis	Myonecrosis	No	Myonecrosis limited to area of vascular insufficiency	No
Discharge	Thin, dark, sweetish, or foul odor	Dark pus or "dishwater," putrid	Serosanguineous, sweet or foul odor	Seropurulent	Seropurulent or "dishwater," putrid PMNs	Minimal	None or serosanguineous
Gram stain	PMNs, Gram-positive bacilli	PMNs, mixed flora	Sparse PMNs, Gram-positive bacilli	PMNs, Gram-positive cocci	putrid PMNs, mixed flora	PMNs, mixed flora	PMNs, Gram-positive cocci in chains
Surgical therapy	Debridement	Wide filleting incisions	Extensive excision, amputation	Excision of necrotic muscle	Wide filleting incisions	Amputation	Debridement of necrotic tissue

BONE AND JOINT INFECTIONS

I. OSTEOMYELITIS

A. Classification and Management: Cierney–Mader classification
Comp Orthop 10:17, 1985; see Osteomyelitis. Current Opinion 2:187, 2000

Stage	Example	Microbiology	Therapy
1. Medulary	Hematogenous Infected intramedulary rods	Monomicrobial: *S. aureus* (hematogenous), *S. epid* GNB	Antibiotics × 4–6 wk[a] ± surgery; rod– remove when joint is stable
2. Superficial	Exposed bone at bed of soft tissue wound: Diabetic food ulcer Decubitus ulcer	Polymicrobial: Anaerobes, GNB *P. aeruginosa* Streptococci	Debridement + antibiotics
3. Localized	Entire cortex involved: Infected plates for stabilizing fracture	Polymicrobial: GNB, *S. aureus* streptococci	Debridement[b] + antibiotics × 4–6 wk[a]
4. Diffuse	Through-and-through osteo: Non-union	Polymicrobial: GNB *S. aureus,* strep	Debridement[b] + antibiotics × 4–6 wk[a]

[a]Antibiotics often given parenterally × 2 wk, then orally × 4 wk.

[b]Debridement requires removal of necrotic bone; dead space created may be filled with cancellous bone grafts or tissue flaps or antibiotic impregnated beads. Beads are usually replaced by bone grafts at 2–4 wk.

Empiric treatment:
1. Infected prosthetic material: Vancomycin
2. Hemoglopathy: Nafcillin/oxacillin + ampicillin
3. Vascular insufficiency, diabetic foot ulcer, decubitus ulcer: Ciprofloxacin + clindamycin (po or IV), ciprofloxacin + metronidazole (po or IV), imipenem, piperacillin-tazobactam, cefoxitin, gatifloxacin (po)
4. Human bite: Ampicillin-sulbactam, ceftriaxone

B. Diagnosis:
Surgical sampling or needle biopsy is preferred. Swabs of fistula tracts or ulcers are less reliable (JAMA 239:2772, 1978)

The preferred nuclear imaging method is technetium-99 (sensitivity 70–100%; specificity 20–80%). Favored scans CT and MRI (sensitivity 30–100%; specificity 80–90%; best test with diabetic foot or decubitus ulcer: Probe wound for bone, sensitivity 66%, specificity 85% (see JAMA 273: 721, 1995)

C. Treatment (CID Suppl 1:S155, 1992; NEJM 336:99, 1997)

ANTIBIOTIC TREATMENT OF OSTEOMYELITIS
Adapted from NEJM 336:999 1997

Pathogen	Preferred (parenteral)	Alternative
S. aureus		
Methicillin sensitive	Nafcillin or oxacillin 2 g q6h	Cephalosporin—1st gen; clindamycin, vancomycin
Methicillin resistant	Vancomycin 1 g q12h	
Streptococci	Pen G 4 mil units q6h	Clindamycin, vancomycin
S. epidermidis	Vancomycin 1 g q12h	
Enterobacteriaceae	Quinolone–ciprofloxacin 750 mg q12h	third generation cephalosporin
P. aeruginosa	Ceftazidime 2 g q8h <u>plus</u> aminoglycoside ≥ 2 wk	Imipenem, piperacillin, or cefepime <u>plus</u> aminoglycoside ≥2 wk
Anaerobes	Clindamycin 600 mg IV q6h	Metronidazole, beta-lactam-beta-lactamase inhibitor, imipenem/meropenem
Mixed aerobic anaerobic	Imipenem 500 mg q6h or beta-lactam-beta-lactamase inhibitor	Ciprofloxacin + clindamycin

Empiric treatment:
1. Settings in which S. aureus is anticipated pathogen
   Preferred: Nafcillin or oxacillin, vancomycin, or clindamycin
2. Patient with hemoglobinopathy
   Preferred: Nafcillin or oxacillin plus ampicillin
   Alternatives: Nafcillin or oxacillin plus cefotaxime or ceftriaxone
3. Osteomyelitis with vascular insufficiency, decubitus ulcer, diabetic foot ulcer, etc
   Preferred: Ciprofloxacin plus clindamycin or metronidazole, cefoxitin, imipenem, or beta-lactam-beta-lactamase inhibitor
   Alternatives: Aztreonam plus clindamycin
4. Animal or human bite
   Preferred: Ampicillin or ampicillin-sulbactam
   Alternative: Ceftriaxone or doxycycline

II. BONE AND JOINT INFECTIONS: ASSOCIATIONS

Condition	Bones/joints	Bacteriology
Sickle cell disease	Multiple bones	Salmonella, S. pneumoniae
Injection drug use	Disc space or sternoclavicular joint	S. aureus P. aeruginosa
Penetrating injury of foot	Foot bones	P. aeruginosa
Hemodialysis	Ribs Thoracic vertebrae	S. aureus
Ingestion of unpasteurized dairy products	Knee, hip, sacroiliac joint	Brucella

Condition	Bones/joints	Bacteriology
Rash and arthritis	Multiple	*N. gonorrhoeae* *N. meningitis* *H. influenzae* *Moraxella osloenia* *Streptobacillus moniliformis*
Diabetic foot ulcers	Site of ulcer	Streptococci, anaerobes, GNB
Foreign body	Site of prosthesis	*Staphylococcus epidermidis*
Dog bite or cat bite	Site of trauma	*Pasteurella multocida* Anaerobes
Human bite	Site of trauma	*Eikenella corrodens,* Anaerobes
Tick exposure	Large joints esp knees	*Borrelia burgdorferi*

III. SEPTIC ARTHRITIS (see CID 20:225, 1995)

A. Acute Monarticular Arthritis

1. **Differential diagnosis:** Septic arthritis, rheumatoid arthritis, gout, and chondrocalcinosis (pseudogout). All may cause predominance of PMNs in joint fluid. Need joint fluid aspiration for stain culture and analysis for crystals.
2. **Joint analysis:** WBC $> 50,000/mm^3$ with $> 90\%$ PMNs, protein > 3 g/mL, glucose $<60\%$, poor mucin clot, positive Gram stain and culture
3. **Septic arthritis in adults**

Agent	Treatment (alternatives)[a]	Comment
S. aureus	Methicillin-sensitive: Nafcillin/ oxacillin or cefazolin × 3 wk MRSA or beta-lactam allergy: Vancomycin × 3 wk	Accounts for 50–80% of non- gonococcal septic arthritis cases
N. gonorrhoeae	Ceftriaxone (1 g IV daily); alternatives are cefotaxime (1 g IV q8h), ceftizoxime (1 g IV q8h), or spectinomycin (2 g IM q12h) until 24–48 hr after symptoms have resolved, then cefixime (400 mg po bid) or ciprofloxacin (500 mg po bid) to complete 1 wk Doxycycline 100 mg po bid × 1 wk	Most common cause of monarticular arthritis in young sexually active adults. Skin lesions rarely present and blood cultures usually negative with gonococcal monarticular arthritis; genital or joint fluid culture often positive Doxycycline or azithromycin for presumed *C. trachomatis* infection
Streptococci	Penicillin (cephalosporin-first generation, vancomycin, clindamycin) × 2 wk	Accounts for 10–20% of non- gonococcal septic arthritis cases. Group A is most common; groups B, C, or G, *S. milleri* and *S.* *pneumoniae* are occasional causes

Agent	Treatment (alternatives)[a]	Comment
Gram-negative bacilli	Based on in vitro sensitivity tests. Treat × 3 wk	Accounts for 10–20% of non-gonococcal septic arthritis cases. Most commonly in chronically debilitated host, immunosuppressed, prior joint disease, and elderly. Heroin addicts prone to sacroiliac or sternoclavicular septic arthritis caused by *Pseudomonas aeruginosa*

[a]Duration of antibiotic treatment is 2–4 wk; the exception is gonococcal septic arthritis.

4. **Other therapy:**
   a. ***Drainage:*** Joint aspiration usually advocated (NEJM 312:764, 1985); repeat needle aspiration at 5–7 days often beneficial. Persistence of effusion >7 days is indication for surgical drainage (CID 20:225, 1995)
   b. ***Weight bearing:*** Avoid until inflammation resolves
   c. Passive range of motion first week, active ROM at 1–2 wk
   d. ***Controversies:*** Duration of antibiotics; oral vs parenteral route of antibiotics; splinting vs passive ROM; optimal drainage—aspiration, open drainage, or arthroscopy
5. **Prosthetic joint** (NEJM 2004;351;1645)
   a. **Bacteriology:** Coagulase neg staph (30–43%), S. aureus (12–23%), mixed flora (10–11%), streptococci (9–10%), GNB (3–6%), enterococci (3–7%) and anaerobes (2–4%)
   b. **Classification:**

	Early	Delayed	Late
Time	<3 mo. post op	3–24 mo post op	>24 mo post op
Clinical	Acute hot joint	Subtle implant loosing, joint pain	As with delayed
Source	During surgery	During surgery	Bacteremia

   c. **Diagnosis:**
   - Joint fluid: WBC >1700/mL or >65% PMNs (Am J Med 2004;117:556)
   - Gram stain pos: Specificity 97%, sensitivity 26% (Rev Med Micro 2003;14:1)
   - Culture of joint fluid or tissue with no antibiotic exposure × 14 days: 65–94% sensitive
   - Imaging: X rays (serial), technetium scan (sensitive, not specific), CT (better than X ray), MRI (only in patients with titanium or tantalum implants)
   d. **Treatment**
   <u>Antibiotics</u>: Based on sensitivity tests but favored are bactericidal agents and those with activity vs surface adhering, slow growing, biofilm-producing pathogens such as rifampin (always used with other agents) and fluoroquinolones. Other–IV betalactams and glycopeptides; Oral-TMP-SMX, minocycline and linezolid.
   <u>Surgery + antibiotics</u>
   - Early postop or acute hematogenous: Debridement with retention if symptoms <3 weeks, implant stable and effective antimicrobial agent vs. biofilm pathogen available. Give IV antibiotics × 2–4 wks–then po for a total of 3 months (hip) or 6 months (knee) (JAMA 1998;279:1537)

- Delayed or late Infection with symptoms >3 wks, difficult pathogens, or severely compromised soft tissue: Removal of prosthesis in one or two stages. With 2 stage-reimplant in 2–4 weeks. Antimicrobial treatment should be 3 months (hip replacement) or 6 months (knee replacement). With difficult organisms (enterococci, fungi, multiply-resistant bacteria) delay reimplantation for 6–8 weeks and discontinue antibiotics 2 weeks before reimplantation to obtain a valid intra-operative culture. If no growth: Discontinue antibiotics. If growth: Antibiotics for 3 months (hip) or 6 months (knee). (See J Bone Joint Surg Br 2003;85:637; Clin Infect Dis 2001;32:419; Clin Orthop 1994;298:75)

B. Chronic Monarticular Arthritis
1. **Bacteria:** *Brucella, Nocardia*
2. **Mycobacteria:** *M. tuberculosis, M. kansasii, M. marinum, M. avium-intracellulare, M. fortuitum* (see pp 166–176).
3. **Fungi:** *Sporothrix schenckii* (soil contact), *Coccidioides immitis* (endemic area, non-Caucasian immunocompromised men), *Blastomyces dermatitidis* (endemic area), *Candida* sp (intraarticular steroids or systemic candidiasis), *Pseudallescheria boydii* (penetrating trauma), *Scedosporium* (penetrating trauma) (see pp 151–164).

C. Polyarticular Arthritis
1. **Bacteria:** *Neisseria gonorrhoeae* (usually accompanied by skin lesions, positive cultures of blood and/or genital tract, negative joint cultures); *N. meningitidis*; *Borrelia burgdorferi* (Lyme disease, see pp 213–214); pyogenic (10% of cases of septic arthritis have two or more joints involved).
2. **Viral: Hepatitis B** (positive serum HBsAg, seen in pre-icteric phase, ascribed to immune-complexes often in association with urticaria, symmetric arthritis involving hands most frequently, then knees and ankles); rubella (usually small joints of hand, women more than men, simultaneous rash, and tenosynovitis also seen with rubella vaccine in up to 40% of susceptible postpubertal women); Parvovirus B 19 (symmetric arthritis involving hands/wrists and/or knees; adults more than children; women more than men); mumps (0.5% of mumps cases, large and small joints, accompanies parotitis, men more than women); lymphocytic choriomeningitis virus (adults with aseptic meningitis); arthropod-borne alpha virus: Chikungunya (East Africa, India), O'nyong-nyong (East Africa), Ockelbo agent (Sweden), Ross River agent (Australia), Barmah Forest virus (Australia).
3. **Miscellaneous:** Acute rheumatic fever (Jones' criteria including evidence of preceding streptococcal infection); Reiter's syndrome (conjunctivitis and urethritis, associated infections—*Shigella, Salmonella, Campylobacter, Yersinia*).

OCULAR AND PERIOCULAR INFECTIONS

Condition	Microbiology	Treatment	Comment
Conjunctivitis	S. pneumoniae, S. aureus	Topical bacitracin-polymyxin B, fluoroquinolone, or erythromycin	Guidelines: American Academy of Ophthalmology 1998 Hyperemia ± discharge, photophobia, pain, vision intact
	N. gonorrhoeae	Ceftriaxone, 125 mg IM × 1	Evaluation—4 tests—(1) acuity, (2) external exam, (3) slit lamp biomicroscopy, and (4) diagnostic tests (see below) Most are viral and self-limited
	C. trachomatis	Doxycycline 100 mg bid × 7–14 d Azithromycin 1 g po × 1	Pharyngoconjunctival fever—adenovirus 3 and 7 in children Epidemic keratoconjunctivitis—adenovirus 8
	Adenovirus (types 8, 11 & 19 in adults)	None (highly contagious)	Diagnostic tests—Culture if severe or recurrent purulent conjunctivitis, especially if not responsive. Smears for special stains and cytology—bacteria— PMNs, viral—mononuclear; herpetic—multi- nucleated cells; chlamydia—mixed; allergic— eosinophils
	Allergic or immune-mediated	Topical steroids	C. trachomatis: Inclusion conjunctivitis and trachoma
	Unknown (empiric)	Topical sulfacetamide or neomycin- bacitracin-polymyxin or bacitracin- polymyxin	S. pneumoniae: may cause epidemic conjunctivitis (NEJM 2003;348:1112)
Keratitis	S. aureus, S. pneumoniae, P. aeruginosa, Moraxella, Serratia	P. aeruginosa (contact lens): topical gentamicin, tobramycin or ciproflox- acin eye drops q15–60 min. Staphylococcus, S. pneumoniae, coliforms: topical cefazolin, gentamicin, tobramycin, vancomycin + ceftazidime q15–60 min.	Guidelines: American Academy of Ophthalmology 2000: Management of bacterial keratitis requires the expertise of an ophthalmologist due to the risk of vision loss Pain; no discharge; decreased vision Lab—Culture with corneal infiltrate that extends to deep stroma, is chronic or is unresponsive to broad spectrum antibiotics or has features suggesting *Continued*

Condition	Microbiology	Treatment	Comment
			fungi, amoeba, or mycobacterial infection. Use alginate swab or conjunctival scrapings for stain (Gram, Giemsa, PAS, calcofluor white and methenamine silver) + culture for bacteria and fungi
	Herpes simplex	Trifluridine 1 drop qh (9×/d) for ≤21 d or vidarabine ointment 5×/d ≤21 d; if recurrent—oral acyclovir 400 mg bid	Systemic antibiotics for deep corneal ulcers with bacterial infection Supportive care with cytoplegics, use of corticosteroids controversial For topical antibiotics use solutions Herpes simplex is most common
	Herpes zoster	Valacyclovir 1 g po tid, acyclovir 800 mg 5×/d or famciclovir 500 mg tid ×10 d	
	Fungal: *Fusarium solani, Aspergillus, Candida, Acanthamoeba*	Topical natamycin, (5%) or amphotericin B (0.05–0.15%)	Risks for bacterial keratitis: contact lens, diabetes
	Parasitic: *Acanthamoeba* (contact lens)	Topical propamidine isethionate, 0.1%/ neomycin/gramicidin/polymyxin or polyhexamethylene biguanide 0.02% or chexadine 0.2%: drops qh while awake × 1 wk, then taper	*Acanthamoeba*: Risks or trauma and soft contact lens. Diagnosis by scraping stained with calcofluor white (CID 2002;35:434)
Endophthalmitis	**Bacteria:** Post-ocular surgery: *S. aureus, Pseudomonas, S. epidermidis, P. acnes* Penetrating trauma: *Bacillus* sp. Hematogenous: *S. pneumoniae, N. meningitidis* (others) Injection drug use: *Candida, B. cercus*	Emergent intravitreal antibiotics, and vitrectomy Empiric: Intravitreal vancomycin 1 mg + amikacin 0.4 mg or ceftazidime 2 mg	Lab: Aspiration of aqueous and vitreous cavity for stain (Gram, Giemsa, PAS, methenamine silver) and culture for bacteria and fungi Requires immediate ophthalmology consult: vitrectomy + intravitreal antibiotics Acute: *P. aeruginosa* and *S. aureus* most common Chronic: *P. acnes, S. aureus,* and *S. epidermidis* most common

Condition	Microbiology	Treatment	Comment
Retinitis	**Fungus:** Post-ocular surgery *Neurospora, Candida, Scedosporium, Paecilomyces* Hematogenous: *Candida, Aspergillus*	IV amphotericin + topical natamycin ± corticosteroids; vitrectomy (Ophthalmol 85:357, 1978) IV amphotericin B + flucytosine (Arch Ophthalmol 98:1216, 1980) Aspergillus—removal of infected vitreous (Arch Ophthalmol 98:859, 1980)	
	Histoplasmosis	Systemic corticosteroids	
	Parasites: Toxoplasmosis Toxocara	Systemic + local corticosteroids ± pyrimethamine and sulfadiazine Systemic or intraocular corticosteroids	
Acute reclinal necrosis	**Virus:** *Herpes zoster* (Herpes simplex)	Acyclovir 10–15 mg/kg IV q8h (CID 1997;24:603)	
Periorbital **Lid**			
Blepharitis	Multifactorial: Seborrhea, rosacea *S. aureus*, etc.	Topical corticosteroid ± topical bacitracin or erythromycin Lid hygiene	For rosacea—doxycycline po
Hordeolum	*S. aureus*	¹Oral antibiotic if meibomian gland involvement + warm compresses	Patients with blepharitis should be referred to an ophthalmologist if they experience: vision loss, severe pain, severe or chronic redness, corneal involvement, recurrent episodes or failure to respond (Amer Acad Ophth 1998)
Chalazion	Chronic granuloma	Observation or curettage	
Lacrimal apparatus			
Canaliculitis	Anaerobes, especially *Actinomyces*	Topical penicillin by irrigation	

Condition	Microbiology	Treatment	Comment
Dacryocystitis	**Acute:** S. aureus	Systemic antistaphylococcal agent; then digital massage + antibiotic drops	
	Chronic: S. pneumoniae, S. aureus, Pseudomonas, mixed	Systemic antibiotics; digital massage	
Orbital	S. aureus, (S. pneumoniae, S. pyogenes)	IV antibiotics: Cephalosporin, cefuroxime or third generation (ceftriaxone or cefotaxime)	Over 80% have associated sinusitis Treat sinusitis
	Fungi: Phycomycosis, Aspergillus, Bipolaris, Curvularia, Drechslera	Amphotericin B + surgery	

INFECTIONS OF CENTRAL NERVOUS SYSTEM

I. CEREBROSPINAL FLUID

A. Normal Findings

1. **Opening pressure:** 5–15 mmHg or 65–195 mmH$_2$O
2. **Leukocyte count:** <10 mononuclear cells/mm^3 (5–10/mL suspect); 1 PMN (5%)
   Bloody tap: Usually 1 WBC/700 RBC with normal peripheral RBC and WBC counts; if abnormal: true CSF WBC = WBC (CSF) − WBC (blood) × RBC (CSF)/RBC (blood) **Note:** WBCs begin to disintegrate after 90 min
3. **Protein:** 15–45 mg/dL (higher in elderly)
   Formula: 23.8 × 0.39 × age + 15 mg/100 mL or (more simply) less than patient's age (>35 yr)
   Traumatic tap: 1 mg/1000 RBCs
4. **Glucose:** 40–80 mg% of CSF/blood glucose ratio >0.6 (with high serum glucose, usual ratio is 0.3)

B. Abnormal CSF with Noninfectious Causes

1. **Traumatic tap:** Increased protein; RBCs; WBC count and differential proportionate to RBCs in peripheral blood; clear and colorless supernatant of centrifuged CSF.
2. **Chemical meningitis (injection of anesthetics, chemotherapeutic agents, air, radiographic dyes):** Increased protein, lymphocytes (occasionally PMNs).
3. **Cerebral contusion, subarachnoid hemorrhage, intracerebral bleed:** RBCs, increased protein (1 mg/1000 RBCs), disproportionately increased PMNs (peak at 72–96 hr), decreased glucose (in 15–20%).
4. **Vasculitis (SLE, etc):** Increased protein (50–100 mg/dL), increased WBCs (usually mononuclear cells, occasionally PMNs), normal glucose.
5. **Postictal (repeated generalized seizures):** RBCs (0–500/mm^3), WBCs (10–100/mm^3 with variable percentage PMNs with peak at 1 day), protein normal or slight increase.
6. **Tumors (especially glioblastomas, leukemia, lymphoma, breast cancer, pancreatic cancer):** Low glucose, increased protein, moderate PMNs.
7. **Neurosurgery:** Blood; increased protein; WBCs (disproportionate to RBCs with predominance of mononuclear cells) up to 2 wk post-op.
8. **Sarcoidosis:** Increased protein; WBCs (up to 100/mm^3 predominately mononuclear cells); low glucose in 10%.

C. CSF with Pyogenic Meningitis (NEJM 1993;328:21; Lancet 1995;346:1675)

1. **Findings:** Opening pressure >300 mmH$_2$O 40%; usually 200–500 mmH$_2$O; WBC >100/mm^3 in 96%; most 1000–5000/mm^3; % PMNs >20% in 98%, most >80%; protein >45 mg/dL in 96%; glucose <40 mg/dL in 50–60%; Gram stain pos in 60%, culture positive 73%.
2. **Bacterial studies** in bacterial meningitis
   - <u>Gram stain</u> is positive in 60–90% and shows specificity of 97% (CID 2004;39:1267). Sensitivity depends on bacterial concentrations and is increased 100-fold with cytospin (J Clin Microbiol 1992;30:377). Sensitivity by pathogen: *S. pneumoniae*–90%, *H. influenzae*–86%, *N. meningitis*–75%, GNB–50% and Listeria–33% (Clin Micro Rew 1992;5:130; Medicine 1998;77:313). With prior antibiotics the sensitivity decreases to 20%
   - <u>Latex agglutination:</u> Sensitivity of 75–100% with S. pneumoniae, H. influenzae or *N. meningitidis*. It is rapid (15 min), and simple to do, but not recommended by IDSA because it rarely impacts treatment or outcome, and there are occasional false positives (CID 2004;39:1267)

- **PCR**: Broad based PCR (multiple CNS pathogens) has show sensitivity of 100% and specificity of 98% (CID 2003;36:40). This is likely to be most useful in bacterial meningitis in patients with negative gram stains and for establishing enteroviral infection (Corr Infect Dis Rep 2002;4:309)
- **Lactate concentrations**: Recommended with suspected meningitis in postoperative neurosurgical patients using a threshold of 4.0 mmol/L (CID 1999;29:69)
- **CRP**: Range of sensitivity and specificity in pyogenic meningitis is 18–100% and 75–100%, respectively (Scand J Clin Lab Invest 1998;58:383). May be useful if CSF suggests pyogenic meningitis but gram stain is neg.

3. **Predictors of bacterial meningitis:** Glucose <34 mg/dL, CSF/serum glucose ratio <0.23, protein >220 mg/dL, WBC >2000 mg/dL or 1180 neutrophils/dL each predict bacterial meningitis with 99% certainty (JAMA 1989;262:2700).
4. **Response:** CSF cultures should become sterile within 24–36 hr of appropriate therapy (Pediatr Infect Dis J 1992;11:423).

D. Practical Issues in Management
1. **Need for CT prior to LP:** Review of 301 adult cases of suspected pyogenic meningitis showed evidence that pre-LP scans delayed antibiotic administration by an average of 2 hrs, and showed mass effect in only 2% (NEJM 2001;345:1727). The recommendation was to do the LP with a #22 or #25 needle to minimize risk and restrict pre-LP CT scans to those likely to have an intracranial mass or elevated CSF pressure as indicated by immunosuppression, (AIDS, transplant recipient, cancer chemotherapy), history of CNS disease (mass lesion, stroke or focal infection) dilated or poorly reactive pupils, papilledema, ocular palsy, hemiparesis, arm or leg drift, history of seizures within 1 week, rapid decrease in consciousness with mobility to answer two consecutive questions, bradycardia, irregular respirations, tonic seizures, or decrebrate or decorticate posture (NEJM 2001;345:1768; Arch Dis Child 1992;67:1417)
2. **Dexamethasone in adults with pyogenic meningitis:** Controlled trial showed significant benefit with dexamethasone 10 mg given 15–20 min before first dose of antibiotics and repeated q6h × 4 days. The dexamethasone recipients showed a superior outcome with reduced mortiliaty (11/157 [7%] vs 21/144 [15%]) in placebo recipients (NEJM 2002;347:1549) The results were most striking for the subset with pneumococcal meningitis for mortality (14% vs 34%; p = 0.02) and for unfavorable outcome (26% vs 52%, p = 0.006). It was also particularly useful in those with a moderate-to-severe disease on the Glasgow Coma Scale. The recommendation is 0.15 mg/kg q6h × 2–4 days starting 10–20 minutes before or concurrent with the first dose of an antimicrobial agent for pneumococcal meningitis. It should not be given after antibiotics have been given. Data are inadequate for this recommendation in pyogenic meningitis due to other bacterial pathogens
3. **Rapidity of first antibiotic dose:** There is concensus by experts supported by modest data for rapid antibiotic treatment (Ann Intern Med, 1998;129:862). The British Guidelines recommend the first dose be given parenterally "in the field" while awaiting hospital transfer (J Infect 1995;30:89).
4. **Follow-up LP:** Indication is failure to improve after antibiotics for 48 hours

II. MENINGITIS

A. Pyogenic meningitis: Microbiology
(NEJM 1993;328:21)

Agent	Community acquired (253 cases)	Nosocomial (151 cases)	Mortality (meningitis related)
S. pneumoniae	97 (38%)	8 (5%)	25%
Gram-negative bacilli	9 (4%)	57 (38%)	23%
N. meningitidis	35 (14%)	1 (1%)	10%
Streptococci	17 (7%)	13 (9%)	17%
S. aureus	13 (5%)	13 (9%)	28%
Listeria	29 (11%)	5 (3%)	21%
H. influenzae	9 (4%)	6 (4%)	11%
S. epidermidis	0	13 (9%)	0
Culture negative	34 (13%)	16 (11%)	7%

B. Updated review: 80 cases, Edmonton Canada, 1985–1996 (Medicine 2001;79:360)

1. **Etiology:** S. pneumoniae—42; Listeria—10, H. influenzae—6, S. aureus—5.
2. **CSF** WBC > 100/mm^3—90%; PMN > 50%–91%; glucose < 50 mg/dL—72%; protein > 45 mg/dL—99%; Gram stain positive—48%
3. **Mortality:** 15%
   Mortality in series of pneumococcal meningitis cases was 15/109 (15%) and was unrelated to penicillin susceptibility of the implicated strain.

Continued

C. Initial management (Modified from CID 2004;39:1267)

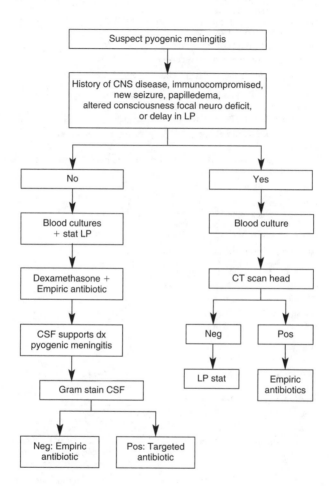

Continued

D. Doses of antimicrobial agents
Cephalosporins:
Cefepime 6 g/d in 8 doses
Cefotaxime: 8–12 g/d in 4–6 doses
Ceftriaxone: 4 g/d in 1–2 doses
Ceftazidime: 6 g/d in 3 doses

Chloramphenicol: 4–6 g/d in 6 doses

Penicillins: Ampicillin: 12 g/d in 6 doses
Nafcillin: 9–12 g/d in 4 doses
Oxacillin: 9–12 g/d in 4 doses
Penicillin G: 24 mil units/d in 4 doses
Aztreonam: 6–8 g/d in 6–8 doses

Trimethoprim-sulfamethoxazole: 10–20 mg/kg/d in 2–4 doses
(trimethoprim) in 4 doses

Vancomycin: 30–45 mg/kg/d in 2–3 doses: maintain trough level of 15–20 mcg/ml

Meropenem: 6 g/d in 3 doses

Fluoroquinolones
Ciprofloxacin 800–1200 mg/d in 3–4 doses
Gatifloxacin 400 mg/d in 1 dose
Moxifloxacin 400 mg/d in 1 dose

Aminoglycosides: Monitor peak and trough levels
Amikacin   15 mg/kg in 3 doses
Gentamicin 5 mg/kg/d in 3 doses
Tobramycin 5 mg/kg/d in 3 doses

Rifampin: 600 mg/d in 2 doses

Intrathecal/intraventricular doses:
Gentamicin 4–8 mg q24h
Tobramycin 4–8 mg q24h
Amikacin 5.0–7.5 mg q24h
Vancomycin 5–20 mg q24h

E. Meningitis: Empiric treatment *(adapted from Med Lett 1999;41:95; NEJM 1996;334:54)*
1. Adults—immunocompetent

Category	Suspected pathogens	Antibiotic
Age Age 2–50 yrs	N. meningitidis S. pneumoniae	Vancomycin + ceftriaxone or cefotaxime ± rifampin if dexamethasone given
Age > 50	S. pneumoniae, N. meningitidis, Listeria monocytogenes, GNB	Vancomycin + ampicillin + ceftriaxone or cefotaxime ± rifampin if dexamethasone given

Continued

Category	Suspected pathogens	Antibiotic
Head trauma		
Basilar fracture	S. pneumoniae, H. influenzae, gr A strep	Vancomycin + cefotaxime or ceftriaxone
Penetrating trauma	S. aureus, S. epider, GNB including P. aeruginosa	Vancomycin + cefepime or ceftazidime or meropenem
Post neuro-surgery	GNB, S. aureus, S. epidermidis	Vancomycin + cefepime or ceftazidime or meropenem
CSF shunt	S epidermidis, S. aureus, GNB P. acnes	Vancomycin + cefepime or ceftazidime or meropenem

2. Adjunctive corticosteroid therapy: Dexamethasone (0.15 mg/kg IV q6h × 2–4 days) starting 10–20 minutes before the first antibiotic for adults with pneumococcal meningitis. This is not recommended for adults with meningitis due to other pathogens or for pneumococcal meningitis already treated with antibiotic (CID 2004;39:1267)

F. Treatment by Organism
IDSA Guidelines (CID 2004;39:1267)

Organism	Antibiotic selection	Comment
S. pneumoniae **Pen-sensitive** (MIC <0.1 μg/mL)	Preferred Penicillin G. Ampicillin Alternative Cefotaxime Ceftriaxone Chloramphenicol	Meningitis is the only clinical condition in which intermediate penicillin reistance is relevant Rates of penicillin resistance in U.S.: Intermediate and high level (MIC ≥ 0.1 μg/mL): 40–50% Chloramphenicol dose should be 6 gm/d Rates of cefotaxime resistance in U.S.
Pen-resistant-intermediate (MIC 0.1 − 1.0 μg/mL)	Preferred Cefotaxime Ceftriaxone Alternative Cefipime Meropenem	(1998–2002), intermediate and high level: 5–10% (CID 1998;27:764; CID 2003; 36:783; CID 2003;36:1013; AAC 2002;46: 2651; AAC 2003;47:1790); great variation by geography
Pen-resistant (MIC >2 μg/ml or Cefotaxime/ Ceftriaxone MIC >1 μg/mL)	Preferred Vancomycin + Ceftriaxone or Cefotaxime Alternative Gatifoxacin Monofloxacin	Rate of vancomycin resistant—0 (Nat Med 2003;9:424) Treat 10−14 days
N. meningitidis **Pen-sensitive** (MIC <0.1 μg/mL)	Preferred Penicillin Ampicillin Alternative Cefotaxime Ceftriaxone Chloramphenicol	Pencillin resistance is rare and found almost exclusively outside U.S. Vaccine reduces infection rate but does not affect outcome (CID 2002;35:1376) Risk in college freshman in dorms (JAMA 2001;286:1894)
Pen-resistant (MIC <0.1 μg/mL)		Intimate and household contacts should receive ciprofloxacin 500 mg × 1 (adults) or rifampin 600 mg po bid × 2 days (adults); 10 mg/kg po bid × 2 days (children) Treat 7 days

Continued

Organism	Antibiotic selection	Comment
H. influenzae **Ampicillin-sensitive**	<u>Preferred</u> Ampicillin <u>Alternative</u> Cefotaxime Ceftriaxone Cefepime Fluoroquinolone Chloramphenicol	Rate of beta-lactamase production 30–40% by type B and nontypable strains (CID 2001; 32:S81) Type B strains: Unvaccinated household contacts <4 yr—rifampin 10 mg/kg po bid × 2 days
Ampicillin-resistant	<u>Preferred</u> Cefotaxime Ceftriaxone <u>Alternative</u> Cefepime Fluoroquinolone Chloramphenicol	Treat 7 days
Listeria monocytogenes	<u>Preferred</u> Ampicillin ± gentamicin Penicillin G ± gentamicin <u>Alternative</u> Meropenem Trimethoprim- sulfamethoxazole	Cephalosporins are active in vitro but are not active in vivo Treat ≥21 days Penicillin or ampicillin are 100 fold more potent when combined with aminoglycoside (J Antimicrob Chemother 1998;41:417) There is no consensus on the need for adding gentamicin to ampicillin. Review of 1808 cases of listerosis showed 47% had CNS infection with 74% immunocompromised, mean age of 50–76 yrs, and mortality of 36% (Emerg Infect Dis 2002;8:305)
Enterobacteriaceae	<u>Preferred</u> Cefotaxime Ceftriaxone <u>Alternative</u> Aztreonam Gatifloxacin Moxifloxacin Ampicillin Trimethoprim- sulfamethoxazole Meropenem	In vitro sensitivity tests required Bactericidal activity desired Chloramphenicol lacks bactericidal activity vs GNB—not recommended Ceftazidime use is usually restricted to GNB resistant to other 3rd gen cephalosporins Treat ≥21 days
P. aeruginosa	<u>Preferred</u> Cefepime ± aminoglycoside Ceftazidime ± aminoglycoside <u>Alternative</u> Aztronam ± aminoglycoside Ciprofloxacin ± aminoglycoside	In vitro sensitivity tests required Monitor peak and trough aminoglycoside levels

Organism	Antibiotic selection	Comment
Staph aureus Methicillin-sensitive	<u>Preferred</u> Nafcillin Oxacillin, <u>Alternative</u> Meropenem Vancomycin	Usually post neurosurgery (Eur J Clin Micro Inf Dis 2002;21:864)
Methicillin- resistant	<u>Preferred</u> Vancomycin ± rifampin <u>Alternative</u> Linezolid TMP-SMX	
S. epidermidis	<u>Preferred</u> Vancomycin ± rifampin <u>Alternative</u> Linezolid	
Enterococcus Ampicillin-sensitive	<u>Preferred</u> Ampicillin + gentamicin	
Ampicillin-resistant	<u>Preferred</u> Vancomycin + gentamicin	
Amp/vanco resistant	<u>Preferred</u> Linezolid	
Strep agalactiae	<u>Preferred</u> Ampicillin ± aminoglycoside Penicillin G ± aminoglycoside <u>Alternatives</u> Cefotaxime Ceftriaxone	

G. Differential diagnosis of chronic meningitis*
(Adapted from Infect Dis Clin Pract 1992;1:158)

Infectious disease		Neoplastic	Miscellaneous
Bacteria	**Fungi**	Leukemia	Systemic lupus**
M. tuberculosis	Cryptococcus	Lymphoma	Wegener's
Atypical mycobacteria	*Coccidioides**	Metastatic	granulomatosis**
*Treponema pallidum**	Histoplasma**	Breast	CNS vasculitis
*Borrelia burgdorferi**	Blastomyces	Lung	Granulomatous vasculitis
Leptospira	*Sporotrichum*	Thyroid	Sarcoidosis
*Brucella**	*Pseudoallescheria*	Renal	Behçet's syndrome
Listeria	*Alternaria*	Melanoma	Vogt-Koyanagi and
Actinomyces/Arachnia	*Fusarium*	Primary CNS	Harada's syndromes
Nocardia	*Aspergillus*	Astrocytoma	Benign lymphocytic

Infectious disease		Neoplastic	Miscellaneous
Parasites	Zygomycetes	Glioblastoma	meningitis
Toxoplasma gondii	Cladosporium	Ependymoma	
Cysticerus	**Viruses**	Pinealoma	
Angiostrongylus	HIV	Medulloblastoma	
Spinigerum	Echovirus		
Schistosoma	HSV (chronic lympho-		
	cytic meningitis and		
	Mollaret's meningitis)		

* Defined as illness present for ≥4 wk with or without therapy; CSF analysis usually shows lympho-cytic pleocytosis. Analysis of 83 previously healthy persons in New Zealand showed 40% had tuberculosis, 7% had cryptococcosis, 8% had malignancy, and 34% were enigmatic (Q J Med 1987;63:283).

** Evaluation: Culture, serum serology, CT scan, or MRI (brain abscess, cysticercosis, toxoplasmosis), cytology CSF (lymphoma, metastatic carcinoma), eosinophilic (parasitic, coccidioidomycosis), CSF serology or antigen (cryptococcosis, coccidioidomycosis, syphilis, histoplasmosis), blind meningeal biopsy (rarely positive), empiric treatment (TB, then penicillin, then amphotericin B, then ? corticosteroids).

H. Aseptic meningitis: infectious and noninfectious causes* (*from American Academy of Pediatrics, Pediatrics 1986;78 Suppl:970 and updated*)

Infectious Agents and Diseases

Bacteria: Partially treated meningitis, *Mycobacterium* tuberculosis, para-meningeal focus (brain abscess, epidural abscess), acute or subacute bacterial endocarditis

Viruses: Enteroviruses, mumps, lymphocytic choriomeningitis, Epstein-Barr, arboviruses (Eastern equine, Western equine, St. Louis), cytomegalovirus, varicella-zoster, herpes simplex, HIV

Rickettsiae: Rocky Mountain spotted fever

Spirochetes: Syphilis, leptospirosis, Lyme disease

Mycoplasma: *M. pneumoniae, M. hominis* (neonates)

Fungi: *Candida albicans, Coccidioides immitis, Cryptococcus neoformans*

Protozoa: *Toxoplasma gondii,* malaria, amebas, visceral larval migrans (*Taenia canis*)

Angiostrongylus cantonensis: Esophinophilic meningitis (NEJM 2002;346: 688) Treat with steroids (CID 2000;31:660)

Nematode: Rat lung worm larvae (eosinophilic meningitis)

Cestodes: Cysticercosis

Noninfectious Diseases

Malignancy: Primary medulloblastoma, metastatic leukemia, Hodgkin's disease

Collagen-vascular disease: Lupus erythematosus

Trauma: Subarachnoid bleed, traumatic lumbar puncture, neurosurgery
Granulomatous disease: Sarcoidosis
Direct toxin: Intrathecal injections of contrast medium, spinal anesthesia
Adverse drug reactions: NSAIDs (Arch Intern Med 1991;151:1309) and rofe-coxib (Arch Intern Med 2002;162:713)
Poison: Lead, mercury
Adverse drug reaction: High dose (2 g/kg) IV immunoglobulin (Ann Intern Med 1994;121:259)
Autoimmune disease: Guillain-Barré syndrome
Unknown: Multiple sclerosis, Mollaret's meningitis, Behçet's syndrome, Vogt-Koyanagi syndrome, Harada's syndrome, Kawasaki disease

* Aseptic meningitis is defined as meningitis in the absence of evidence of a bacterial pathogen detectable in CSF by usual laboratory techniques.

III. BRAIN ABSCESS (CID 1997;25:763)

Associated condition	Likely pathogens	Treatment
Sinusitis	Anaerobic, microaerophilic and aerobic streptococci, *Bacteroides* sp.	Metronidazole + penicillin or cefotaxime + metronidazole
Otitis	*Bacteroides fragilis*, *Bacteroides* sp., streptococci, *Entero-bacteriaceae*, *P. aeruginosa*	Metronidazole + penicillin + ceftazidime
Post-neurosurgery	*Staph. aureus* *S. epidermidis* *Enterobacteriaceae* *P. aeruginosa*	Vancomycin + ceftazidime
Trauma	*Staph. aureus* *Enterobacteraceae*	Nafcillin + cefotaxime or ceftriaxone
Endocarditis	*Staph. aureus*	Penicillinase-resistant penicillin or vancomycin
	Streptococcus sp.	Penicillin or penicillin + aminoglycoside
Cyanotic heart disease	*Streptococcus* sp.	Penicillin or metronidazole + penicillin

RESPIRATORY TRACT INFECTIONS UPPER RTIs: Recommendations of two panels—one representing the CDC and the other representing the American College of Physicians/American Society of Internal Medicine. Both groups published their recommendations in the *Annals of Internal Medicine* and covered the same infections (pharyngitis, bronchitis, sinusitis, and viral URIs). Panel membership overlapped between the two groups, and both said essentially the same thing.

CITATIONS

Topic	Source	Citation
URIs	ACP/ASIM	Ann Intern Med 134:487, 2001
	CDC	Ann Intern Med 134:490, 2001
Pharyngitis	ACP/ASIM	Ann Intern Med 134:506, 2001
	CDC	Ann Intern Med 134:509, 2001
Sinusitis	ACP/ASIM	Ann Intern Med 134:495, 2001
	CDC	Ann Intern Med 134:498, 2001
Bronchitis	ACP/ASIM	Ann Intern Med 134:518, 2001
	CDC	Ann Intern Med 134:521, 2001
Acute exacerbations, chronic bronchitis	ACP/ASIM	Ann Intern Med 134:595, 2001

SUMMARY OF RECOMMENDATIONS (ADULT PATIENTS ONLY)

Diagnosis	Issue	ACP/ASIM	CDC
Sinusitis	Diagnosis	Clinical diagnosis, no imaging	Same
	Cultures	None	None
	Antibiotics Indications	Nasal pus and face pain/ tenderness, + severe symptoms or symptoms >7 d	Same
	Agents	Amoxicillin, doxycycline TMP-SMX	Agents active vs *H. influenzae* and *S. pneumoniae*
Bronchitis	Diagnosis	Rule out pneumonia X-ray if abnormal vital signs or cough >3 wk or rales	Same
	Culture	None	None
	Antibiotic	None	None
		Exception: Pertussis and possibly antiflu agent for ?	Same
Pharyngitis	Strep	10% of cases	5–15%
	Diagnosis	Antigen test No culture	Antigen test No culture
	Antibiotic	Centor score 2–3 (see below) + pos Strep antigen or culture or Centor score 3–4 alone	Same
	Antibiotic	Penicillin	Penicillin
	Alternative	Erythromycin	Erythromycin

Continued

Pharyngitis: Centor criteria and IDSA criteria

Centor criteria for management of streptococcal pharyngitis (Med Decision Making 1981;1:239)

1. *Centor variables*
   - Tonsillar exudate
   - Cervical adenopathy
   - Fever (by history or measurement)
   - Absence of cough

2. Score

Score	Management
1	No strep test and no antibiotic
2–3	Strep test (culture or strep antigen). Treat with penicillin if positive
3–4	Empiric treatment

3. *Pharyngitis Guidelines IDSA* (CID 2002;35:113): Antibiotic treatment of pharyngitis should be restricted in adult patients to patients with pharyngitis and a positive test for group A Streptococcus since: 1) Centor

Centor clinical criteria will overtreat about 50% and the 10% false negative rate of strep tests is inconsequential in adults.

UPPER RESPIRATORY TRACT INFECTIONS

Conditions	Usual pathogens	Preferred treatment	Alternatives	Comment
EAR AND MASTOIDS				
Acute otitis media (Red Book 2000 pg 457)	S. pneumoniae H. influenzae M. catarrhalis (35% sterile)	Amoxicillin	Failure at 3–5 days: Amoxicillin + clavulanate Cefdinir Erythromycin + sulfisoxazole Cefuroxime axetil Parenteral: Ceftriaxone single dose Penicillin–allergy: Erythromycin–sulfisoxazole, clarithromycin, azithromycin	Tympanocentesis rarely indicated Less frequent pathogens: S. aureus, Strep. pyogenes, GNB, and anaerobes Oral or nasal decongestants ± antihistamine
Chronic suppurative otitis media	Pseudomonas Staph. aureus	Neomycin/polymyxin/ hydrocortisone otic drops	Chloramphenicol otic drops	Persistent effusion: Myringotomy
Malignant otitis externa	P. aeruginosa	Ciprofloxacin	Tobramycin + ticarcillin, piperacillin, mezlocillin, cefoperazone, ceftazidime, aztreonam, cefepime, imipenem, or ciprofloxacin	Surgical drainage and/or debridement sometimes required Treat 4–8 wk or longer Oral regimen—see J Arch Otolaryngol Head Neck Surg 1989;115:1063
Acute diffuse otitis externa ("swimmer's ear")	P. aeruginosa Coliforms Staph. aureus	Topical neomycin + polymyxin otic drops	Boric or acetic acid (2%) drops Topical chloramphenicol	Initially cleanse with 3% saline or 70–95% alcohol + acetic acid Systemic antibiotics for significant tissue infection
Otomycosis	Aspergillus niger	Boric or acetic acid drops	Cresylate acetic otic drops	Surgery required for abscess in mastoid bone
Acute mastoiditis	S. pneumoniae H. influenzae S. pyogenes	Same as for acute otitis media	Cefotaxime or ceftriaxone IV	S. aureus is occasional pathogen, especially in subacute cases

Continued

Conditions	Usual pathogens	Preferred treatment	Alternatives	Comment
Chronic mastoiditis	Anaerobes Pseudomonas sp Coliforms S. aureus	None		Surgery often required Pre-op: Tobramycin + ticarcillin or piperacillin
SINUSITIS				
Acute sinusitis (symptoms <4 wk)	H. influenzae S. pneumoniae M. catarrhalis S. aureus	Amoxicillin 500 mg tid (up to 1 g tid)	Telithromycin 800 mg qd × 5 d; Amoxicillin/clav 875 mg po bid Cefditoren 200–400 mg bid Cefuroxime 250 mg bid Levofloxacin 500 mg qd Moxifloxacin 400 mg qd Gatifloxacin 400 mg qd Clarithromycin 500 mg bid or 1 g qd Azithromycin 500 mg, then 250 mg × 5 days ± repeat at day 14–18 Cefpodoxime 200 mg bid Cefprozil 500 mg bid Cefdinir 300 mg bid Doxycycline 100 mg bid	Indications to treat: Symptoms severe or symptoms >7 days Most are viral infections; bacterial superinfection in 0.2–10% Frequency of beta-lactamase-producing bacteria is 20–30%, but amoxicillin appears as effective as alternative agents according to a 1999 meta-analysis of antimicrobial trials (www.ahcpr.gov/clinic/) Bacterial pathogens detected in sinus aspirates in about 50%; dominant are S. pneumoniae (41%), H. influenzae (35%), anaerobes (7%), M. catarrhalis (4%), and S. aureus (3%) (CID 1997;23:1209) No response after 48–72 hours with narrow spectrum agent should lead to an alternative agent such as telithromycin, fluoroquinolones or amoxicillin + clavulanate Frequency of penicillin or macrolide resistant isolates of Streptococcus pneumoniae to penicillin–22%, erythromycin–29%, levofoxacin–0.9%, and telithromycin–0.02%, (PROTEKT US data 2005)
Chronic sinusitis (symptoms >3 mo)	Anaerobes S. aureus S. epidermidis	Amoxicillin	Amoxicillin + clavulanate Clindamycin	Usually reserve antibiotic treatment for acute flares Role of anaerobes is controversial (J Clin Microbiol 1991;29:2396; Am J Otolaryngol 1995;16:303) Endoscopic surgery may be required

Continued

Conditions	Usual pathogens	Preferred treatment	Alternatives	Comment
Nosocomial sinusitis	*Pseudomonas* Coliforms	Aminoglycoside + antipseudo-monad penicillin or aminogly-coside + cephalosporin-3rd generation (ceftazidime)	Imipenem, ceftazidime	Complication of nasal intubation
PHARYNX				
Pharyngitis (see p 238)	*Strep. pyogenes* A. hemolyticum C. diphtheriae, groups C and G strep	Penicillin po (strep only) × 10 days or benzathine penicillin IM × 1	Erythromycin × 10 days Cephalosporin × 5–10 days (cefditoren, ceftibutin, cephalexin, cefaclor, cefadroxil, cefuroxime, cefixime, cefditoren, cefdinir, cefpodoxime) Clarithromycin × 10 days Azithromycin × 5 days	If compliance questionable, use benza-thine penicillin G × 1 IM Penicillin preferred for strep due to established efficacy in preventing rheumatic fever and absence of any penicillin resistance A study of 4782 cases of strep pharyngitis showed a 5-day course of penicillin was as effective as the standard 10-day course (JID 2000;182: 509)
	N. gonorrhoeae	Ceftriaxone 125 mg IM × 1 or ciprofloxacin 500 po × 1		Causes: Viral 50–80%, strep 10%, EBV–1%
	Mycoplasma, C. pneumoniae	Tetracycline or erythromycin (?)		*M. pneumoniae* 2–5%, *C. pneumoniae* 2–5%, *N. gonorrhoeae* 1%
	Viruses (EBV etc)	None except influenza: Amantadine, rimantadine, zanamivir, or oseltamivir		Carrier rate *S. pyogenes* (adults) 2–4% (JAMA 2000;284: 2912) (Scand J Prim HC 1997;15:149) Macrolides: About 5% of group A strep are resistant
	HIV	HAART (indications are unclear)		Acute retroviral syndrome established plasma HIV RNA or p24 Ag

Continued

Conditions	Usual pathogens	Preferred treatment	Alternatives	Comment
Peritonsillar or tonsillar abscess	Strep. pyogenes Peptostreptococci	Penicillin G	Clindamycin	Drainage necessary
Membranous pharyngitis	C. diphtheriae	Penicillin or erythromycin		Diphtheria: Antitoxin
	Epstein-Barr virus	None		Mononucleosis associated with airway closure or severe toxicity should be treated with prednisone
	Vincent's angina (anaerobes)	Metronidazole or clindamycin	Penicillin, amoxicillin, or amoxicillin-clavulanate	
Epiglottitis	H. influenzae S. pyogenes Viruses	Cefotaxime, ceftizoxime, ceftriaxone, cefuroxime Ampicillin-sulbactam		Ensure patent airway (usually with endotracheal tube) Rifampin prophylaxis for household contacts <4 yr (×4 days)
Laryngitis	Viruses (M. catarrhalis)			For M. catarrhalis: Trimethoprim-sulfa, erythromycin, amoxicillin-clavulanate, or cefaclor
PERIMANDIBULAR				
Actinomycosis	A. israelii	Penicillin G or V	Clindamycin Tetracycline Erythromycin	Treat for 3–6 mo
Parotitis	S. aureus (anaerobes)	Penicillinase-resistant penicillin	Cephalosporin-1st gen Clindamycin, vancomycin	Surgical drainage usually required
Space infections	Anaerobes	Clindamycin Amoxicillin-clavulanate	Cefoxitin Penicillin + metronidazole	Surgical drainage usually required
Cervical adenitis				
Acute	Strep. pyogenes	Penicillin	Erythromycin	
	Anaerobes	Clindamycin	Amoxicillin + clavulanate	
	S. aureus	Penicillinase-resistant penicillin	Oral cephalosporin (not cefixime)	

Continued

Conditions	Usual pathogens	Preferred treatment	Alternatives	Comment
Chronic	Mycobacteria	TB: INH, rifampin, PZA + Etham MOTT: see pp 170–171		Noninfectious causes include tumors, lymphoma, saroid cysts
Cat-scratch disease	*Bartonella henselae*	Ciprofloxacin	TMP-SMX Erythromycin	Role of antibiotics is unclear Treat 2 wk Confirm diagnosis with serology
DENTAL				
Periapical abscess Gum boil Gingivitis Pyorrhea	Anaerobes Streptococci	Penicillin Clindamycin	Metronidazole ± penicillin Amoxicillin-clavulanate	Metronidazole often preferred for periodontal disease, i.e., gingivitis, periodontitis
STOMATITIS				
Thrush	*C. albicans*	Oral nystatin (swish and swallow) or clotrimazole troches	Ketoconazole po Fluconazole po	
Vincent's angina	Anaerobes	Penicillin Clindamycin	Metronidazole ± penicillin Amoxicillin-clavulanate	
Aphthous stomatitis	No pathogen identified	Topical corticosteroid (Topicort gel), dyclonine (Dyclone) Miles' solution, viscous lidocaine	Systemic corticosteroids (Prednisone 40 mg/d, then rapid taper) Silver nitrate	Miles' solution: 60 mg hydrocortisone, 20 mL nystatin, 2 g tetracycline, and 120 mL viscous lidocaine
Herpetiform ulcers	*H. simplex*	Acyclovir Valacyclovir or famciclovir		Treatment usually reserved for immunocompromised hosts

Continued

Conditions	Usual pathogens	Preferred treatment	Alternatives	Comment
UPPER RESPIRATORY INFECTION (common cold) (J Clin Microbiol 1999;36:1721; NEJM 2000;343:1715; Ann Intern Med 2001;134:487; Arch Intern Med 2003;163: 278)	Influenza Parainfluenza Rhinovirus Coronovirus	Influenza: Amantadine, rimantadine,oseltamivir, or zanamivir Ipratropium (see comments) Nasal decongestants (see comments)		Antiviral therapy for influenza must be started within 48 hr of onset of symptoms. Amantadine and rimantadine are active against influenza A; oseltamivir and zanamivir are active against influenza A and B Allergic rhinitis—Loratadine 10 mg qd; nasal steroids; avoid allergens Naproxen 500 mg tid × 5 days Ipratropium nasal spray (2 sprays each nostril 3–4 ×/day × 4 days OTC preparations with dexbromphen- iramine 6 mg + pseudoephedrine 120 mg bid × 1 wk Controversial—aspirin and acetamin- ophen, vitamin C, zinc gluconate lozenges Pleconaril is active vs. rhinovirus but failed FDA approval (CID 2003;36: 1523)

COMPARISON OF COMMONLY USED ORAL ANTIMICROBIALS FOR RESPIRATORY TRACT INFECTIONS

Drug	Regimen commonly used			Antimicrobial activity***					Adverse drug reactions (%)****				
	Regimen*	Pill count (10 days)	Cost AWP** (10 days)	Strep. pneumo	H. flu	Gr A strep	Staph. aureus	Anae-robes	Nausea-vomiting	Diar-rhea	Rash	Therapy stopped	Other
Amox-clavulan	875 mg bid	20	$117	++½	+++	+++	+++	+++	1–2	5–10	1	1–3	
Amoxicillin	500 mg tid	30	$13	++½	+	+++	+	++	1–2	5	1	2	
Azithromycin	250 mg qd	6	$48	++	+++	+++	+++	++	1–3	3–4	0.2	1	
Cefaclor	250–500 mg tid	30	$60–130	++	+++	+++	+++	++	1–4	2–6	1–2	2	Serum sickness
Cefdinir	300 mg bid	20	$90	++½	+++	+++	+++	++	3	16	1	3	
Cefditoren	200–400 mg bid	40	$75	+++½	+++	+++	+++	++	1–6	11–15	–	2–3	
Cefixime	200 mg bid	20	$88	++½	+++	+++	++	+	5–7	15–20	1–2	2–3	
Cefpodoxime	200 mg bid	20	$108	++½	+++	+++	+++	++	1–2	4	1–2	2	
Cefprozil	250–500 mg bid	20	$90–180	++	+++	+++	+++	++	2–5	–	–	–	
Cefuroxime	250–500 mg bid	20	$106–196	++	+++	+++	+++	++	2–5	4–8	1	1	
Cephalexin	250–500 mg qid	40	$56	++	+++	+++	+++	++	2–4	1–6	1	1	
Ciprofloxacin	500 mg bid	20	$116	++½	+++	+++	+++	++	2–5	1–2	1–2	1–3	
Clarithromycin	250–500 mg bid	20	$92	++	++	+++	+++	++	3–4	3	–	4	Taste change
Clindamycin	150–300 mg qid	40	$100–200	++½	–	+++	+++	+++	1–2	10–20	–	5–15	C. difficile colitis
Doxycycline	100 mg bid	20	$20	++	+	++	++	++	2–5	1–2	–	1–2	
Erythromycin	250–500 mg qid	40	$11	++	+	+++	++	++	5–30	5	1	5–20	GI intolerance
Gatifloxacin	400 mg qd	10	$94	+++	+++	+++	+++	+++	1–2	1–2	–	1	
Levofloxacin	500 mg qd	10	$106	+++	+++	+++	+++	++	1–2	1–2	–	1–2	
Loracarbef	400 mg bid	20	$128	++	+++	+++	+++	+	2	4	1	1–2	
Moxifloxacin	400 mg qd	10	$98	+++	+++	+++	+++	+++	1–2	1–2	–	1	
Penicillin V	500 mg qid	40	$9	++	+	+++	+	++	3	3	1	2–3	
Telithromycin	800 mg qd	20	$92 est.	+++	+++	+++	+++	++	2–8	10–11	1	4	Headache, dizziness
TMP-SMX	1 DS bid	20	$24	+	++	++	+++	–	10	–	5–10	4–10	Rash

*Typical regimen for respiratory tract infections (otitis, sinusitis, exacerbations of bronchitis, "walking pneumonia").

**AWP, average whole price Sept 2003.

***In vitro activity against community-acquired bacterial pathogens: — indicates minimal activity, + indicates modest activity, ++ indicates moderate activity, +++ indicates activity against nearly all strains or indicates a preferred choice based on clinical trials.

****Adverse reactions according to package inserts (summarized in Infect Dis Clin Pract 4:S103, 1995); "therapy stopped" indicates percentage that discontinued treatment because of adverse drug reaction.

PULMONARY INFECTIONS

A. Specimens and Tests for Detection of Lower Respiratory Pathogens (CID 1998;26:611)

Organism	Specimen	Microscopy (stain)	Culture	Serology	Other/Comment
Bacteria					
Aerobic	Expectorated sputum, blood, TTA, empyema fluid	Gram stain Quellung for *S. pneumo*	X		Pneumococcal urine antigen (JCM 2003;41:2810)
Anaerobic	TTA, empyema fluid	Gram stain	X		
Legionella sp.	Sputum, BAL, pleural fluid	FA (*L. pneumophila*)	X	IFA	Urinary antigen (*L. pneumophila* gr1), PCR (*L. pneumophila* all groups)
Nocardia sp.	Expectorated sputum, bronchial washing, BAL fluid, tissue	Gram and modified carbol fuchsin stain	X		
Chlamydia sp.	Nasopharyngeal swab	—	X[a]	CF for *C. psittaci* MIF for *C. pneumo* ≥ 1:64	PCR for *C. pneumoniae* (experimental)
Mycoplasma sp.	Nasopharyngeal swab	—	X[a]	EIA, CF	
Mycobacteria	Expectorated or induced sputum, bronchial washing, BAL fluid	Fluorochrome stain or carbol fuchsin	X		PPD: PCR for *M. tuberculosis*
Fungi					
Deep-seated					
Blastomyces sp.	Expectorated, sputum, induced sputum, BAL	KOH with phase contrast; Calcofluor white	X	CF, ID	
Coccidioides sp.	As above	As above	X	CF, ID, LA	
Histoplasma sp.	As above	As above	X	CF, ID	Antigen assay: BAL, blood, urine
Opportunistic					
Aspergillus sp.	Lung biopsy	H&E, GMS, Calcofluor white	X	ID	CT scan; EIA expected soon; serum galactomannan
Candida sp.	Lung biopsy	H&E, GMS, Calcofluor white	X		
Cryptococcus sp.	Respiratory secretions, serum, Lung biopsy	H&E, GMS, Calcofluor white	X	LA	Serum or BAL antigen assay
Zygomycetes	Expectorated sputum, tissue	H&E, GMS, Calcofluor white	X		
Pneumocystis carnii	Induced sputum or bronchial brushings, washings, BAL fluid	Toluidine blue, Giemsa, FA, or GMS stain			
Viruses					
Influenza	Nasopharyngeal aspirate	FA: Influenza and RSV	X	CF, EIA, LA, FA	Z-Stat Flu and other rapid tests
Parafu, RSV	Nasopharyngeal aspirate				CMV: Shell viral culture; FA stain of BAL or biopsy
CMV	Bronchial aspirate, BAL, or biopsy (BSL-3 lab)			IFA, EIA	RT-PCR
SARS CoV	Respiratory secretions	EM	X		

CF, complement fixation; PPD, purified protein derivative; ID, immunodiffusion; LA, latex agglutination; H&E, hematoxylin and eosin; CIE, counterimmunoelectrophoresis; EIA, enzyme immunoassay; FA, fluorescent antibody stain; IFA, indirect fluorescent antibody; MIF, microimmunofluorescence test.
[a] Few clinical microbiology labs offer these cultures, and those that do infrequently recover the indicated organisms.

247

B. Criteria for severe CAP based on CURB-65 score (Thorax 2003;58:377)

1. Score: 1 point for each
   C = Confusion − Disoriented in time, place or person
   U = Urea level ≥ 20 mg/mL
   R = Respiratory rate > 30/min
   B = Blood pressure < 90 mm Hg systolic
   65 = Age ≥ 65 years

2. Score   Management

Score	Management
0–1	Outpatient
≥ 2	Admit
≥ 3	ICU often required

C. Preferred antimicrobials by pathogen

S. pneumoniae
     MIC < 2 mcg/ml: Penicillin, amoxicillin
     MIC > 2 mcg/ml: Cefotaxime, ceftriaxone, telithromycin, fluoroquinoline
H. influenzae Beta-lactamase pos: 2nd or 3rd gen cephalosporin, amoxicillin-clavulinate, telithromycin
Mycoplasma pneumoniae: Doxycycline, macrolide, telithromycin
C. pneumoniae: Doxycycline, macrolide, telithromycin
Legionella: Fluoroquinolone, azithromycin, clarithromycin
C. psittaci: Doxycycline
Coxiella burnetii: Doxycycline
Staph aureus:
     MSSA: Nafcillin/oxacillin, telithromycin
     MRSA: Vancomycin, linezolid
     MRSA (USA 300 strain): Vancomycin linezolid ± clindamycin, rifampin
P. aeruginosa: Antipseudomal betalactam, + ciprofloxacin, levofloxacin or aminoglycoside
Enterobacteraceae: 3d generation cephalosporin, carbapenem, fluoroquinolone
Acinetobacter: Carbapenem
B. anthracis (anthrax): Ciprofloxacin or levofloxacin + imipenèm, clindamycin, rifampin, vancomycin or penicillin
Franciella tularensis (tularemia): Doxycycline, gentamicin, streptomycin
Pasteurella pestis (Plague): Gentamicin, streptomycin
Anaerobes: Clindamycin, betalactam-betalactamase inhibitor, carbapenem

D. Empiric Treatment of Lower Respiratory Tract Infections

1. Community-acquired pneumonia: Guidelines of Infectious Diseases Society of America (modified from CID 2003;37:405)
     <u>Outpatient</u>
         Generally preferred: Macrolide*, telithromycin,[†] fluoroquinolone**, or doxycycline
         Modifying factors
             Suspected penicillin-resistant *S. pneumoniae:* Fluoroquinolone**, telithromycin[†]
             Suspected aspiration: Amoxicillin-clavulanate
     <u>Hospitalized Patient</u>
         General medical ward
             Generally preferred: Beta-lactam*** + macrolide* <u>or</u> fluoroquinolone** (alone)

Hospitalized in the intensive care unit for serious pneumonia
　　Generally preferred: Erythromycin, azithromycin, or fluoroquinolone**
　　　plus cefotaxime or ceftriaxone
　Modifying factors
　　Structural disease of lung: Antipseudomonal penicillin, carbapenem, or
　　　cefepime + macrolide or fluoroquinolone** + aminoglycoside
　　Penicillin allergy: fluoroquinolone** + clindamycin
　　Suspected aspiration: fluoroquinolone + clindamycin or beta-lactam-
　　　beta-lactamase inhibitor (alone)

2. **Lung abcess**
   a. **Anaerobic bacteria** (recommendations of IDSA, CID 2000;31:347)
      (1) Clindamycin
      (2) Beta-lactam-beta-lactamase inhibitor
      (3) Imipinem/meropenem/ertapenem
   b. **Other microbial pathogen—see next section**
3. **Acute bronchitis** (Recommendations of ACP and CDC: Ann Intern Med 2001; 134:479 and 521)
   Evaluation of acute cough should focus on ruling out pneumonia
   Chest x-ray if: (1) Abnormal vital signs, (2) "asymetrical lung sounds," or (3) cough ≥3 wks
   Antibiotics are not recommended regardless of duration of cough. Most are viral and self-limited
   Treatment is symptomatic with antipyretics, analgesics, beta-agonist inhalers, antitussives, or vaporizers
   Influenza: Amantadine, rimantadine, zanamivir, or oseltamivir (must start within 48 hr of onset of flu symptoms)
   Pertussis: Erythromycin 500 mg po qid × 14 days or TMP-SMX DS bid × 14 days
   　Antibacterial agents in the absence of pertussis have no documented benefit and should be avoided except with suspected or established pertussis (Am J Med 1999;107:62; Ann Intern Med 2005;142:832)
4. **Exacerbations of chronic bronchitis** (Recommendations of ACP: Ann Intern Med 2001;134:600)
   a. **Chest x-ray:** Useful in hospitalized patients (up to 23% show new findings) and it may be useful in EW visits; there are not data for or against its use in office practice
   b. **Treatment—hospitalized patients**
      Inhaled anticholinergic bronchodilators or short-acting beta$_2$-agonists; anticholinergics are used first and to maximum dose because of fewer side effects
      Systemic steroids for up to 2 weeks
      Noninvasive positive-pressure ventilation supervised by trained physician
      Cautious administration of O_2 to hypoxemic patients
   c. **Antibiotic decision-making**
      Bacteria are responsible for <50% of exacerbations. Most are viral URIs allergic or irritant-associated. When bacteria are implicated the most frequent pathogens are *H. influenzae* (non-typable), *M. catarrhalis* and *S. pneumoniae* in that order (NEJM 2002;347:465; Am J Respir Crit Care Med 2004;170:266; Am J Resp. Crit Care Med 2005;172:195)

---

*Macrolide: Azithromycin, clarithromycin, or erythromycin

**Fluoroquinolone: Levofloxacin, sparfloxacin, gatifloxacin, gemifloxacin, or moxifloxacin or other fluoroquinolone with enhanced activity versus *S. pneumoniae*. Preferably reserve for high-risk patients including those with recent antibiotic exposure, the elderly and those with associated underlying diseases such as CHF, chronic lung disease, renal failure or diabetes.

†Telithromycin is also active against multi-drug resistant *Streptococcus pneumoniae*.

Reserve antibiotics for severe exacerbations

If used, the preference is narrow-spectrum agents. Prior placebo-controlled trials favored amoxicillin, TMP-SMX, and tetracycline (Ann Intern Med 2001;134:595) but they were done prior to emergence of multidrug resistant bacteria and excluded nursing home patients and recent hospital discharges

Interventions without documented benefit: mucolytic therapy, chest physiotherapy, and methylxanthine bronchodilators (the latter two may be harmful)

5. **Nosocomial pneumonia:** ATS/IDSA Guidelines (Am J Respir Crit Care Med 2005;171:388)

   a. **Categories:** Ventilator-associated pneumonia (VAP), Hospital-acquired pneumonia (HAP) and Healthcare-associated pneumonia (HCP)

   b. **Prevention**
      - Semirecumbant position (30–45°) (I)*
      - Infection control (II)*
      - Surveillance
      - Avoid intubation (I)* and reduce duration when necessary (II)*
      - Orotrach/orogastric tubes preferred over nasogastric tubes (to prevent sinusitis) (II)*
      - Continuous aspiration of subglottic secretins is available (III)*
      - Endotracheal cuff at >20 cm H_2O (II)*
      - Oral antibiotics for selective decontamination of GI tract reduces VAP incidence but not recommended for routine use (II)* but may help with outbreaks (I)*
      - Insulin therapy to keep blood glucose at 80–110 mg/dL in ICU patients (I)*
      - For stress bleeding prophylaxis use either H_2 antagonists or sucralfate (I)*
      - Avoid heavy sedation and paralytic agents when possible (II)*

   c. **Diagnosis**
      - Routine: History & physical; O_2 and chest X ray
      - Purulent tracheobronchitis: May need culture and antibiotic therapy but supporting evidence is weak (III); in absence of clinical evidence & infection—don't treat (I)
      - Blood culture if suspected VAP
      - Thoracentesis if effusion is large or patient is toxic (III)
      - Culture based on evidence of infection. No evidence of pneumonia—no culture

        Evidence of HAP—culture respiratory symptoms, endotracheal tube aspirate, BAL or protected brush (II). Sterile culture in absence of antibiotic therapy excludes most pathogens other than Legionella and viruses. Consider these and non-pulmonary sites of infection

   d. **Clinical strategy:** The diagnosis of pneumonia is based on showing a new pulmonary infiltrate plus 2 of the following: 1) Temp $\geq$ 38° C 2) purulent secretions and 3) leukopenia or leukocytosis

      (1) Etiologic diagnosis: Semiquantitative culture or respiratory secretions
      (2) Algorithm

---

*Level 1: Strong supportive evidence
Level 2: Evidence considered moderate
Level 3: Low level evidence

(2) <u>Algorithm</u>

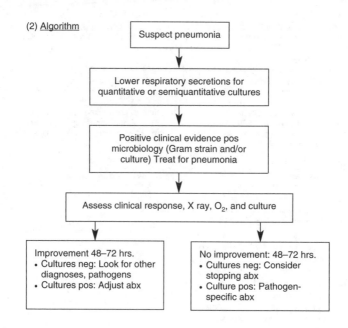

Suspect pneumonia

↓

Lower respiratory secretions for quantitative or semiquantitative cultures

↓

Positive clinical evidence pos microbiology (Gram strain and/or culture) Treat for pneumonia

↓

Assess clinical response, X ray, O_2, and culture

↓

Improvement 48–72 hrs.
• Cultures neg: Look for other diagnoses, pathogens
• Cultures pos: Adjust abx

No improvement: 48–72 hrs.
• Cultures neg: Consider stopping abx
• Culture pos: Pathogen-specific abx

e. **Microbiology strategy:** This approach bases the diagnosis and etiologic agent of HAP or VAP
Review of quantitative culture for HAP and VAT according to metaanalyses of studies using standardized methods including pre-treatment sampling

	Threshold	Sensitivity Specificity
Bronchoscopic	10^4–10^5 c/ml	73 ± 18% 82 ± 19%
Gram stain	Intracellular	69 ± 20% 75 ± 28%
Endotracheal	10^6 c/ml	76 ± 9% 75 ± 28%
Brush catheter	10^3 c/ml	66 ± 19% 90 ± 15%

f. <u>Anticipated Pathogens</u> in HAP, HCAP (Health Care Associated) & VAP
<u>Risk factors for multiply drug resistant pathogens</u>
• Antibiotic therapy in prior 90 days
• Hospital stay >5 days
• High frequency resistance in environment or hospital
• Immunosuppression
• High risk for HCAP: hospitalized ≥ 2 day in past 90 days; residence in chronic care facility, home infusion therapy, chronic dialysis, home wound care family member with multiply drug resistant pathogen

g. Empiric antibiotic based on risk for multiply drug resistant pathogen.
- Pathogens: S. pneumoniae, H. influenzae, MSSA, coliforms (E. coli, K. pneumoniae, Enterobacter, Proteus, S. marcescens
- Antibiotic
  Ceftriaxone or moxifloxacin or Levofloxacin or ertapenem

h. Empiric treatment for patient at risk of resistant pathogens

Pathogens	Antibiotic
• Multiply resistant GNB (P. aeruginosa, ESBL producing K. pneumonia, Acinetobacter	Cefepime or ceftazidine or imipenemin/ microbenem or piperacillin-tazobactium or cipro or levofloxacin or aminoglycoside
• Methicillin resistant S. aureus	Linezolid or vancomycin
• Legionella	Azithromycin or ciprofloxacin or levofloxacin

1. Doses

Antibiotic	Dosage
Cefepime	1–2 gm q 8–12 h
Ceftazidime	2 gm q 8 h
Imipenem	500 mg q 6 h or 1 gm q 8 h
Meropenem	1 gm q 8 h
Pip-tazo	4.5 gm q 6 h
Gentamicin	7 mg/kg/d
Tobramycin	7 mg/kg/d
Amikacin	20 mg/kg/d
Vancomycin	15 mg/kg q 12 h
Linezolid	600 mg q 12 h

ENDOCARDITIS

I. DUKE CRITERIA FOR DIAGNOSIS OF INFECTIVE ENDOCARDITIS
(Am J Med 1994;96:200; CID 2000;30:633)

Note: The Duke criteria have become generally accepted (Am J Med 1994;96:200) and multiple reviews show a specificity of 99% and a negative predictive value of 92% (Am Heart J 1994;128:1200; CID 1998;26:1302).

A. Definite Infective Endocarditis

1. *Pathologic criteria*
   - Microorganisms: Demonstrated by culture or histology in a vegetation, or in a vegetation that has embolized, or in an intracardiac abscess, or
   - Pathologic lesions: Vegetation or intracardiac abscess present, confirmed by histology showing active endocarditis
2. *Clinical criteria* (using specific definitions listed below under "Definitions of Terminology")
   Two major criteria, <u>or</u> one major and three minor criteria, <u>or</u> five minor criteria

B. Possible Infective Endocarditis 1 major 1 1 minor or 3 minor

C. Rejected

1. Firm alternate diagnosis for manifestations of endocarditis, or
2. Resolution of manifestations of endocarditis with antibiotic therapy for 4 days or less, or
3. No pathologic evidence of infective endocarditis at surgery or autopsy, after antibiotic therapy for 4 days or less

Definitions of Terminology

1. <u>Major Criteria</u>
   a. *Positive blood culture for infective endocarditis*
      (1) Typical microorganism for infective endocarditis from two separate blood cultures
         (a) Viridans streptococci, *Streptococcus bovis*, HACEK group, or
         (b) Community-acquired enterococci, in the absence of a primary focus, or
         (c) *S. aureus* bacteremia that is community acquired or nosocomial and with or without a primary focus
      (2) Persistently positive blood culture, defined as recovery of a microorganism consistent with infective endocarditis from
         (a) Blood cultures drawn more than 12 hr apart or
         (b) All of three or a majority of four or more separate blood cultures, with first and last drawn at least 1 hr apart
      (3) Single positive blood culture for *Coxiella burnetii* or antiphase I IgG antibody titer >1:800
   b. *Evidence of endocardial involvement*
      (1) Positive echocardiogram for infective endocarditis
         (a) Oscillating intracardiac mass, on valve or supporting structures, or in the path of regurgitant jets, or on implanted material in the absence of an alternative anatomic explanation, or
         (b) Abscess or
         (c) New partial dehiscence of prosthetic valve, or
      (2) New valvular regurgitation (increase or change in preexisting murmur not sufficient)

2. <u>Minor Criteria</u>
   a. Predisposition: Predisposing heart condition or IV drug use
   b. Fever: ≥38.0°C (100.4°F)

c. Vascular phenomena: Major arterial emboli, septic pulmonary infarcts, mycotic aneurysm, intracranial hemorrhage, conjunctival hemorrhages, Janeway lesions

d. Immunologic phenomena: Glomerulonephritis, Osler's nodes, Roth spots, rheumatoid factor

e. Microbiologic evidence: Positive blood culture but not meeting major criterion as noted previously or serologic evidence of active infection with organism consistent with infective endocarditis

f. Echocardiogram: Consistent with infective endocarditis but not meeting major criterion as noted previously (recommended for deletion)

II. ANTICIPATED AGENTS, ECHO, RISKS

A. Microbiology of endocarditis: Based on literature review (NEJM 2001;345:1318) and international study 2000–2003 (NEJM 2005;293:3012)

	International study 2000–2003 n = 1779	Lit. Review Native valve >16 yrs	Prosthetic valve Time postoperative		
			<60 days	2–12 mo	>12 mo
Streptococcus species	30%	40–65	1	7–10	30–33
Staph. aureus	32%	22–30	20–24	10–15	15–20
Staph. epidermidis	11%	3–8	10–15	2–4	4–7
Enterococcus	11%	5–17	5–10	10–15	8–12
Fungi	2%	1–3	5–10	10–15	1
Gram-negative bacilli	2%	4–10	10–15	2–4	8–12
HACEK and culture negative	10%	3–10	3–7	3–7	3–8

B. Culture negative endocarditis

Microbe	Methods to establish pathogen
Atiotrophia (nutritionally deficient strep)	1) Grow in thioglycolate, and 2) as colonies around *S. aureus* in media supplemented with pyridoxal HCl or L-cysteine
Bartonella	1) Serology, 2) Lysis-centrifugation, and 3) PCR of valve or embolized vegetation (may require > 1 month to culture)
Coxiella burnetti	1) Serology, and 2) PCR, Giemsa stain, or immuno-histologic stains of op specimen
HACEK	Blood cultures to day 7; may require larger incubation and subculture
Chlamydia	Blood culture using specialized technique described
T. whipplei	1) Silver or PAS stain of valve, and 2) PCR or culture of vegetation
Legionella	1) Subculture of blood, 2) Lysis-centrifugation pellet from blood cult, 3) BCYE agar for valve, 4) FA stain of valve, and 5) serology

Brucella	Serology
Fungi	1) Blood culture-*Candida,* 2) Antigen assay urine or blood for *H. capsulatum* or blood for *C. neoformans,* and 3) culture and histology of valve

C. Echocardiography

Transthoracic echo is inadequate in up to 20% of adults due to obesity, chronic lung disease, and chest wall deformities. The sensitivity for vegetations is 60–70% (J Am Coll Cardiol 1991;18:391; Am J Med 1996;100:90). Transesophageal echo increases sensitivity for detecting vegetations to 75–95% and shows specificity of 85–98% (Am J Med 1999;107:198). Guidelines for use (J Am Coll Cardiol 1997;29:862) suggest the preference for transthoracic echo to evaluate native valves in patients who are good candidates for imaging, especially if the probability of endocarditis is less than 4%. For patients with a probability of 4–60%, initial use of transesophageal echo is more cost-effective. TEE is more sensitive for evaluating periovascular extension in myocardial abscesses. <u>*S. aureus* bacteremia</u>: Endocarditis is found in 13–25% (CID 2002;30:633). TEE is useful in determining the duration of therapy in patients with uncomplicated, intravascular-catheter-associated *S. aureus* bacteremia (Am J Med 1999;107:198; Ann Intern Med 1999;130:810; CID 1999;28:106).

D. Endocarditis risk/100,000 person years*

- Native valve: 1.7–6.2
- Prosthetic valve: 60 months: 2,000–3,000
- Injection drug use: 700

E. Health care associated S. aureus endocarditis (NEJM 2005; 293: 3012)

1. Collaborative study in 39 medical centers in 16 countries from 6/00–12/03 S. aureus was the most common pathogen: 558/1779 (31.4%) and healthcare associated was the most common form
2. The 3 categories of S. aureus endocarditis were healthcare associated–218 (39%) community-acquired without IDU–209 (37.5%) and IDU-associated-117 (21%)

	CA-Not IDU n = 209	IDU n = 117	Healthcare assoc n = 218
Age (median)	61 yrs	36 yrs	65 yrs
Invasive procedure	10%	5%	49%
Predominant valve	aortic	tricuspid	mitral
MRSA	13%	10%	49%
Mortality	21%	11%	29%

*NEJM 2005;293:3012

III. TREATMENT OF ENDOCARDITIS

A. Medical Management by Microbial Pathogen (Committee on Rheumatic Fever, Endocarditis and Kawasaki Disease of the American Heart Association's Council on Cardiovascular Disease in the Young: Antimicr254obial Treatment of Infective Endocarditis due to

Viridans Streptococci, Enterococci, and Staphylococci. JAMA 274:1706, 1995)

1. **Streptococci**
   a. **Penicillin-sensitive streptococci** (minimum inhibitory concentration <0.1 μg/mL)
      (1) <u>Penicillin only</u>: Aqueous penicillin G, 12–18 mil units/day either continuously or in 6 equally divided doses × 4 wk.
      (Preferred regimen for patients with a relative contraindication to streptomycin including age >65 yr, renal impairment, or prior 8th cranial nerve damage.)
      (2) <u>Ceftriaxone</u>: 2 g once daily IV × 4 wk
      (3) <u>Two-week course</u>: Aqueous penicillin G 12–18 mil units either continuously or in 6 equally divided doses <u>plus</u> gentamicin 1 mg/kg IM or IV q8h. Peak gentamicin level (1 hr after start of 20- to 30-min infusion) should be 3 μg/mL; trough should be <1 μg/mL. Two-week regimen is not recommended for complicated cases, e.g., extracardiac foci or intracardiac abscesses. Aqueous penicillin G, q12h. (Advocated as most cost-effective regimen by Mayo Clinic group for uncomplicated cases with relapse rates of <1%.)
      (4) <u>Penicillin allergy</u>: Vancomycin, 30 mg/kg/d IV × 4 wk in 2–4 doses not to exceed 2 g/d unless serum levels are monitored. Vancomycin levels 1 hr post dosing should be 30–45 μg/mL with twice daily dosing. Infuse vancomycin over ≥60 min.

Note:
- *Streptococcus bovis* and tolerant streptococci with MIC <0.1 μg/mL may receive any of these regimens
- Nutritionally deficient should be treated as enterococcal endocarditis
- Prosthetic valve endocarditis: IV penicillin for 6 wk and gentamicin for at least 2 wk
- Immediate reaction to penicillin or other beta-lactam is major indication for vancomycin
- Penicillin tolerant strains with MBCs that greatly exceed MICs (>32-fold): Recommend usual therapy, meaning routine MBC determination is not recommended for streptococci
- Gentamicin is now the most frequently used aminoglycoside because of ability to monitor levels and ability to give IV or IM. If streptomycin is preferred, test for high-level resistance (≥1000 μg/mL)
- Two-week treatment regimen is not recommended for complicated cases, e.g., shock, extracardiac foci of infection, or intracardiac abscess
- Desired peak serum levels if obtained: Streptomycin—20 μg/mL, gentamicin—3 μg/mL, vancomycin—20–35 μg/mL (qid), or 30–45 μg/mL (bid)
- Ceftriaxone plus gentamicin once daily × 2 wk may be adequate
- Expected bacteriologic cure rate: >95%; expected survival rate: >90%

   b. **Viridans streptococci and Streptococcus bovis relatively resistant to penicillin G** (minimum inhibitory concentration ≥0.1 μg/mL and ≤0.5 μg/mL)
      (1) Aqueous penicillin G, 18 mil units/d IV either continuously or in 6 divided doses <u>plus</u> gentamicin 1 mg/kg IM or IV q8h × 4 wk
      (2) <u>Penicillin allergy</u>: Vancomycin 30 mg/kg/d × 4 wk in 2 daily doses not to exceed 2 g/d
      (3) <u>Penicillin allergy, cephalosporins</u>: Cefazolin, 1 g IM or IV q8h × 4 wk
   c. **Penicillin-resistant streptococci including enterococci and strains with minimum inhibitory concentrations of >0.5 μg/mL**
      (1) Aqueous penicillin G 18–30 mil units/d IV either continuously or in 6 divided doses <u>plus</u> gentamicin, 1 mg/kg IM or IV q8h × 4–6 wk

(2) Ampicillin 12 g/d IV either continuously or in 6 divided doses <u>plus</u> gentamicin 1 mg/kg IM or IV q8h × 4–6 wk

(3) <u>Penicillin allergy</u>: Vancomycin 30 mg/kg/d IV in 2 doses not to exceed 2 g/24 hr unless serum levels are monitored <u>plus</u> gentamicin 1 mg/kg IM or IV q8h × 4–6 wk. Gentamicin is not required for viridans streptococci

Note:

- Streptococci, groups B, C, and G: Some recommend routine use of penicillin or cephalosporin × 4–6 wk <u>plus</u> gentamicin × 2 wk
- Strep bovis endocarditis is associated with colonic carcinoma
- Patients with symptoms for over 3 mo before treatment and those with prosthetic valve endocarditis should receive combined treatment for 6 wk
- Aminoglycosides: Gentamicin is usually preferred; MIC should be ≤500–2000 μg/mL for gentamicin or ≤2000 μg/mL for streptomycin. Serum levels should be monitored: Desirable peak levels are streptomycin 20 μg/mL and gentamicin 3 μg/mL. Some authorities recommend gentamicin 1.5 mg/kg q8h with goal for peak serum concentration of 5 μg/mL. Usual dose of streptomycin is 7.5 mg/kg IM q12h, not to exceed 500 mg. Streptomycin is more ototoxic, which is often irreversible. Gentamicin is more often nephrotoxic, which is usually reversible.
- For enterococcal endocarditis, shorter courses of aminoglycosides (2–3 wks vs. 4–6 wks) may be adequate (CID 2002;34:159)
- Expected bacteriologic cure rate: >95%; expected survival rate: >90%

2. *Staphylococcus aureus* or *S. epidermidis*

a. *No prosthetic device—methicillin-sensitive*

(1) Nafcillin or oxacillin 2 g IV q4h × 4–6 wk with optional addition of gentamicin 1 mg/kg IV or IM q8h × 3–5 days.

(2) <u>Penicillin allergy, cephalosporin</u>: Cefazolin 2 g IV q8h × 4–6 wk with optional addition of gentamicin 1 mg/kg IV or IM q8h × 3–5 days (should not be used with immediate-type penicillin hypersensitivity).

(3) <u>Penicillin allergy or methicillin-resistant strains</u>: Vancomycin 30 mg/kg/d in two daily doses (not to exceed 2 g/d unless serum levels monitored) × 4–6 wk. With inadequate response, add aminoglycoside × 3–5 days.

(4) <u>Parenteral drug abuse with tricuspid valve endocarditis</u>: Oxacillin or nafcillin + tobramycin parenterally × 2 wk (Ann Intern Med 1988;109:619; Eur J Clin Microbiol Infect Dis 1994;13:559). Vancomycin is not an adequate substitute for nafcillin in this 2-week course (Eur J Clin Microbiol Infect Dis 1994;13:533). Abbreviated course is not recommended for HIV-positive patients or those with persistent fever >7 days or with vegetations >1–2 cm (NEJM 2001;345:1318).

b. *Prosthetic valve or prosthetic material*

(1) <u>Methicillin-sensitive strains</u>: Nafcillin or oxacillin 2 g IV q4h × ≥6 wk plus rifampin 300 mg po q8h × ≥6 wk plus gentamicin 1 mg/kg IV or IM q8h (not to exceed 80 mg) × 2 wk.*

(2) <u>Methicillin-resistant strains</u>: Vancomycin 30 mg/kg/d in 2–4 doses (not to exceed 2 g/d unless serum levels monitored) × ≥6 wk plus rifampin 300 mg po q8h × ≥6 wk plus gentamicin 1 mg/kg IV or IM q8h (not to exceed 80 mg) × 2 wk.*

---

*Surgery often required. If strain is resistant to aminoglycosides, avoid these drugs; use fluoroquinolone if susceptible. If surgery performed, examine in vitro sensitivities because these often change during treatment.

Note:

- Methicillin-resistant staphylococci should be considered resistant to cephalosporins
- Vancomycin is considered inferior to oxacillin or nafcillin for methicillin-sensitive strains of *S. aureus* (Ann Intern Med 1991;115:674)

- Tolerance has no important effect on antibiotic selection
- The occasional strains of staphylococci that are sensitive to penicillin G at <0.1 μg/mL may be treated with regimens advocated for penicillin-sensitive streptococci
- Use of rifampin in prosthetic valve endocarditis will increase required dose of coumadin
- For native valve endocarditis, the addition of gentamicin to nafcillin or oxacillin causes a more rapid clearing of bacteremia in patients with left-sided endocarditis (2.5 vs 4.0 days) but has no impact on cure rates; use of gentamicin (or rifampin) with either methicillin-sensitive or methicillin-resistant strains is sometimes advocated for the first 3–5 days of treatment with a beta-lactam or vancomycin (CID 1993;17:313)
- Duration of treatment: 4–6 wk, 6 wk commonly recommended for left-sided staphylococcal endocarditis
- Coagulase-negative strains infecting prosthetic valves should be considered methicillin-resistant unless sensitivity is conclusively demonstrated
- Aminoglycoside selection for coagulase-negative strains should be selected on the basis of in vitro sensitivity tests; if not active, these agents should be omitted
- Expected outcome: CID 1992;15:589

	Bacteriologic cure	Survival
Left sided	>80%	>50%
Right sided	>90%	>90%

3. **HACEK group:** *Haemophilus parainfluenzae, H. aphrophilus, Actinobacillus actinomycetem comitans, Cardiobacterium hominis, Eikenella corrodens,* and *Kingella kingae*
   a. Ceftriaxone 2 g once daily IM or IV × 4 wk
   b. Ampicillin 12 g/d IV either continuously or in 6 divided doses plus gentamicin 1 mg/kg IM or IV q8h × 4 wk
   c. Recent studies show the most active antibiotics in vitro are third generation cephalosporins, cefepime, meropenem, rifampin, and fluoroquinolones (Diagn Microbiol Infect Dis 1999;34:73)
4. **Fungi** (*Candida* sp and *Aspergillus* sp)* (not included in committee recommendations)
   a. Amphotericin B 0.8–1.0 mg/kg/d IV + flucytosine 100–150 mg/kg/d po
   b. Fluconazole 400 mg/d IV or po (susceptible *Candida* sp. only: Experience limited, but anecdotal experience favorable; experience with fluconazole in combination with flucytosine, rifampin, etc also is limited)
5. **Organisms with special culture requirements:** HACEK (see above), *Coxiella burnetii* (serology), Brucella, *N. gonorrhoeae, Legionella, Bartonella,* corynebacteria, *Listeria,* nutritionally variant streptococci, nocardia, mycoplasma, chlamydia, and mycobacteria
   * **Early surgery virtually always required**

B. Outpatient Treatment

1. Ceftriaxone once daily for penicillin-sensitive viridans streptococci
2. Use of portable computerized pumps for multiple dose or continuous-infusion therapy.
3. Dual-lumen central catheter with two portable pumps permits combination therapy.

C. **Empiric Treatment for Acute Endocarditis** Recommendations of Mayo Clinic (Mayo Clin Proc 1997;72:532)

Setting	Antibiotic regimen	Alternative
Acute onset, native valve	Nafcillin or oxacillin (2 g IV q4h) <u>plus</u> amino-glycoside*	Vancomycin (1 g IV q12h) <u>plus</u> aminoglycoside*
Subacute Native valve	Ampicillin-sulbactam (2 g q4–6h) (ampicillin) <u>plus</u> aminoglycoside*	Vancomycin (1 g IV q12h) <u>plus</u> ceftriaxone (2 g IV q12h) or cefotaxime (4 g IV q6h) + aminoglycoside*
Prosthetic valve	Nafcillin or oxacillin (2 g IV q4h) <u>plus</u> aminoglyco-side* <u>plus</u> rifampin 300 mg IV q12h)	
Intravenous drug use	Nafcillin or oxacillin (2 g IV q4h) plus aminoglycoside*	Vancomycin (1 g IV q12h) + aminoglycoside*

*Aminoglycoside—usually gentamicin 1 mg/kg IV q8h to achieve peak serum levels of about 3 μg/mL.

D. **Monitoring**

1. Serumcidal activity: Not recommended for routine use—may be useful with unusual etiology or unconventional therapy.
2. Blood culture: To verify response and post-treatment to assure cure. Relapses occur within 4 wk.
3. Most relapses occur within 2 months of discontinuing antibiotic treatment

IV. **INDICATIONS FOR CARDIAC SURGERY IN PATIENTS WITH ENDOCARDITIS** (Am J Med 1985;78(suppl 6B):138)

A. <u>Indications for Urgent Cardiac Surgery*</u>

Severe heart failure (especially with aortic insufficiency)
Vascular obstruction
Uncontrolled infection
Fungal endocarditis
Persistent bacteremia (or persistent signs of sepsis)
Lack of effective antimicrobial agents
Unstable prosthetic valve

B. <u>Relative Indications for Cardiac Surgery</u>

1. *Native valve*
   Bacterial agent other than susceptible streptococci (especially *P. aeruginosa, Brucella, Coxiella,* fungi, and resistant enterococci)
   Relapse (especially if nonstreptococcal agent)
   Evidence of intracardiac extension
   Rupture of sinus of Valsalva or ventricular septum
   Ruptured chordae tendineae or papillary muscle
   Heart block (new conduction disturbance)
   Abscess shown by echo or catheterization
   Two or more emboli
   Vegetations demonstrated by echo (especially large vegetation or aortic valve vegetations)

Mitral valve preclosure by echo (correlates with severe acute aortic insufficiency)
2. ***Prosthetic valve:*** Surgical therapy is usually superior to medical treatment (Ann Thorac Surg 1994;58:1073)
   Early postoperative endocarditis (<8 wk)
   Nonstreptococcal late endocarditis
   Periprosthetic leak
   Two or more emboli
   Relapse
   Evidence of intracardiac extension (see above)
   Miscellaneous: Heart failure, aortic valve involvement, new or increased regurgitant murmur or mechanical valve versus bioprosthesis

C. <u>Echocardiographic Findings that Suggest Potential Need for Surgery</u>
   (AHA Committee on Infectious Endocarditis—Circulation 1998; 98:2936):
   1. Persistent vegetations after major embolic event
   2. Large vegetations (>1 cm) mitral valve
   3. Increase vegetation size after 4 wk of therapy
   4. Acute mitral insufficiency
   5. Valve perforation or rupture
   6. Periannular extension of infection

D. <u>Point system:</u> Urgent surgery should be strongly considered with five accumulated points (indications for surgery in infective endocarditis. In Sande MA, Kaye D (Eds). Contemporary Issues in Infectious Disease. New York: Churchill Livingstone, 1984:201–212).

*Note: The validity of these criteria for surgery have never been shown (JAMA 2003;289:1933)

INDICATIONS FOR EMERGENT SURGERY*

	Native valve	Prosthetic valve
Heart failure		
Severe	5	5
Moderate	3	5
Mild	1	2
Fungal etiology	5	5
Persistent bacteremia	5	5
Organism other than susceptible strep	1	2
Relapse	2	3
One major embolus	2	2
Two or more systemic emboli	4	4
Vegetations by echocardiography	1	1
Ruptured chordae tendineae or papillary mm	3	—
Ruptured sinus of Valsalva	4	4
Ruptured ventricular septum	4	4
Heart block	3	3

Early mitral valve closure by echo	2	—
Unstable prosthesis	—	5
Early prosthetic valve endocarditis	—	2
Periprosthetic leak	—	2

*Criterion is ≥ 5 points.

Note: This point system above has never been validated.

Alternative: An alternative point system is based on 6 factors that predict mortality within 6 months: mental status—4; Charlison co-morbidity score—1–6*; CHF-3, pathogen other than *Strep. viridans*—6–8; and medical vs surgical treatment—5.

*1 = myocardial infarct, stroke, dementia, ulcer, mild liver disease, diabetes, chronic lung disease; 2 = severe renal disease, complicated diabetes, hemiparesis, tumor; 3 = severe liver disease; 6 = metastatic cancer, immunodeficiency

Validity testing in 513 patients showed the following mortality data at 6 mo: <6: 6%; 7–11: 17%, 12–15: 31%, >15: 63% (JAMA 2003;289:1933). (This system predicts mortality rather than indications for surgery, but the authors suggest utility in surgical decisions.)

VIRAL HEPATITIS
Types, clinical features, and prognosis

(MMWR 34:313, 1985; MMWR 37:341, 1988; MMWR 39:1, 1990; MMWR 40(RR-12):1, 1991)

Type	Seroprevalence	Incubation period	Diagnosis*	Prognosis/comments
A (HAV)	Person-to-person fecal-oral Contaminated food and water (epidemic) Seroprevalence: Anti-HAV in adults U.S.: 40–50% Acute viral hepatitis: 40–60% Fulminant hepatitis: 8%	15–50 days Avg: 28 days	Acute HAV: IgM anti-HAV Prior HAV: Total (IgM and IgG) anti-HAV *Sequence:* Viral transmission → HAV viremia and fecal shedding at 2 wk, IgM-HAV at 2 wk, IgG-HAV at 8–16 wk	Self-limited: >99% Fulminant and fatal: 0.6% No carrier state or chronic infection Severity increases with age IgM + elevated ALT is presumptive evidence for acute HAV. IgM remains elevated 3–9 mo; IgG persists for life
B (HBV)	Sexual contact or contaminated needles from HBsAg carrier source (transmission via blood transfusions is rare due to HBsAg screening) Efficiency of transmission increased if source is HBeAg positive Seroprevalence (any marker, U.S.) (see p 116) General population: 3–14% blacks: 14%; whites: 3% IV drug abuse: 60–80% Gay men: 35–80% Hemodialysis patients: 20–80% Health care workers (unvaccinated, frequent blood exposure): 15–30% (unvaccinated, no frequent blood exposure): 3–10% Chronic carriers (HBsAg) U.S.: 0.1–0.2%; developing world: 10–30% Acute viral hepatitis: 30–40% Chronic liver disease: 10–15%	45–160 days Avg: 120 days	Acute HBV: HBsAg +, IgM anti-HBc+, anti-HBc+, anti-HBs− Chronic HBV: HBsAg+ × 6 mo, anti-HBc+ IgM anti-HBc−, anti-HBs− HBsAg "window": IgM anti-HBc+, anti-HBc+, HBsAg−, anti-HBsAg− Prior HBV: anti-HBc+, anti-HBs+, HBsAg−, IgM anti-HBc− HBV vaccine response: anti-HBs+, anti-HBc−, HBsAg−, IgM anti-HBc− *Sequence:* Viral transmission → HBsAg at 1–2 mo → IgM-HBc and IgG anti-HBc, anti-HBe at 3 mo → anti-HBs at 4 mo	Fulminant and fatal: 1.4% Carrier state (defined as HBsAg-pos, 2× separated by 6 mo or HBsAg pos and IgM anti-HBc neg): Develops in 6–10% of infected adults, 25–50% of children <5 yr Chronic carriers: 25% develop chronic active hepatitis that progresses to cirrhosis in 15–30%; fatal cirrhosis in 1%/yr, and/or fatal hepatocellular carcinoma in 0.25%/yr Perinatal with HBsAg-pos and HBeAg-pos mother: 70–90% acquire perinatal HBV infection and 85–90% of these carriers will become chronic carriers; >25% of these carriers will develop cirrhosis or hepatocellular carcinoma; perinatal transmission rate is <10% if anti-HBe pos Risk of transmission with needlestick from HBsAg-pos source: 6–30%; highest with HBeAg pos source

Continued

Type	Seroprevalence	Incubation period	Diagnosis*	Prognosis/comments
C (HCV) (parenterally transmitted non-A, non-B) also causes sporadic NANB hepatitis	Contaminated transfused blood: 10%; IVDA—40%; heterosexual contact—10%; unknown—40% Seroprevalence (U.S.): 1.8% Blood donors: 0.2–0.6% General population: 2% Hemophiliacs: 60–90% IV drug abuse: 60–90% Dialysis patients: 15–20% Gay men: 2–6% Health care workers: 0.5–2.0% Sex contacts of HCV patients: 1–10% Chronic hepatitis: 40% Acute sporadic hepatitis in U.S.: 17% Genotype 1: 70–75%	15–150 days (mean 50 days)	Tests: Anti-HCV-EIA-third generation tests show specificity and sensitivity of >99%; can confirm with qualitative HCV RNA (or quantitative HCV RNA) Acute HCV: HCV RNA pos 1–3 wk, anti-HCV at 10–14 wk Active HCV infection: Excluded if ≥2 negative HCV RNA assays over 6 mo *Sequence:* Viral transmission → PCR pos for HCV at 1–3 wk, increased ALT at 4–6 wk and anti-HCV at 10–14 wk	Fulminant and fatal <1% Acute infection: Usually mild with moderate elevation ALT Chronic hepatitis: 85%; cirrhosis: in 10–20% within 20 yr Associated with hepatocellular carcinoma: 1–4%/year with HCV associated cirrhosis Evaluation: 1) Confirmed diagnosis with positive EIA ± positive qualitative HCV RNA; 2) liver function test—ALT; 3) candidates for interferon therapy—quantitative HCV RNA, genotype and liver biopsy Patients with anti-HCV should be considered infectious: should not be blood or organ donors; risk with sex is low—seroconversion rate is 0–0.6%/yr in discordant couples; risk with needlestick injury from HCV infected source is 2%; perinatal transmission rate is 2–7%
Delta	Defective virus that requires presence of active HBV, e.g., co-infection with HBV or superinfection in HBsAg carrier; main source is blood (IV drug abuse, hemophilia) Epidemics: Amazon Basin and Central Africa Endemic areas (Mediterranean Basin, Middle East, Amazon Basin): 20–40%	Superinfection: 30–60 days Co-infection: same as HBV	Acute HBV-HDV co-infection: HDAg+, HBsAg+, IgM anti-HDV+, IgM anti-HBc+, HBV DNA ± HDV RNA Acute HDV superinfection: HDAg+, HBsAg±, IgM antiHDV+, anti-HDV+, IgM antiHBc−, HBV DNA ± HDV RNA	Acute HBV-HDV co-infection with HBV: 1–10% acute fatality, <5% chronic hepatitis Acute superinfection: 5–20% acute fatality, >75% develop chronic hepatitis, with 70–80% developing cirrhosis Epidemics in underdeveloped countries: Fulminant fatal hepatitis in 10–20% of children Chronic delta hepatitis: Worsens prognosis of chronic HBV infection; most likely chronic hepatitis to cause cirrhosis

Continued

Type	Seroprevalence	Incubation period	Diagnosis*	Prognosis/comments
	Nonendemic areas (U.S.): Uncommon		Chronic HDV: HBsAg+, anti-HDV+, and HDV Ag in liver or HDV RNA in serum	Mortality <2% except for pregnant women who have mortality of 10–20%
	Medical care workers and gay men: Low			Usually mild disease predominantly in adults >15 yr; chronic liver disease has not been reported
E (HEV) (enterally transmitted non-A, non-B, or ET-NANB)	Epidemic fecal-oral (Burma, Borneo, Mexico, Somalia, Pakistan, China, India, Russia, Peru, throughout Africa)	20–60 days (mean 40 days)	Anti-HEV (IgM or documented seroconversion). Assays not yet licensed in U.S. but available from CDC (404-639-3048)	No chronic infection
	Sporadic (developing countries) U.S.: no documented cases originating in U.S.		*Sequence:* Viral transmission → HEV Ag in blood → IgM-anti-HEV at 4–8 wk → IgG-anti-HEV at 6–10 wk; duration of IgG-Ab is unknown	Often cholestatic with high alkaline phosphatase
Non A–E	Cause unknown	Unknown	Exclude hepatitis A–E	Candidate virus is SEN virus
	Fulminant hepatitis 30–40%			
	Chronic hepatitis 15–20%			

* Symptoms or signs of viral hepatitis, serum aminotransferase >2.5 × upper limit of normal, and absence of other causes of liver injury.

CDC Hepatitis Hotline: Automated telephone information system concerning modes of transmission, prevention, serologic diagnosis, statistics, and infection control 404-332-4555.

INTRA-ABDOMINAL SEPSIS: ANTIBIOTIC SELECTION

I. PERITONITIS

A. Recommended antibiotics for community-acquired intra-abdominal infections (Guidelines of the Infectious Diseases Society of America, CID— 2003;37:997)

1. Single agent regimens
   a. <u>Beta-lactam-beta-lactamase inhibitors</u>
      - Ampicillin—sulbactam
      - Piperacillin—tazobactam*
      - Ticarcillin—clavulanate
   b. <u>Carbapenems</u>
      - Ertapenem
      - Imipenem*
      - Meropenem*
2. Combination regimens
   a. <u>Cephalosporin-based regimens</u>
      - Cefazolin or cefuroxime + metronidazole
      - Cefotaxime, ceftriaxone, ceftizoxime, ceftazidime or cefepime + metronidazole*
   b. <u>Fluoroquinolone-based regimens</u>
      Ciprofloxacin, levofloxacin, moxifloxacin, or gatifloxacin, each in combination with metronidazole
   c. <u>Monobactam-based regimen</u>
      Aztrenam + metronidazole

---

*Includes severe infections

B. Miscellaneous recommendations

1. <u>Nosocomial intra-abdominal</u> sepsis (healthcare associated): Anticipate resistant pathogens with emperic treatment including *P. aeruginosa* *Enterobacter,* MRSA, enterococci and *Candida.* Treatment should be based on local resistance patterns (emperic) and culture results (pathogen directed)
2. <u>Anaerobes especially *B. fragilis*</u>: Cefoxitin and cefotetan can no longer be recommended
3. <u>Oral therapy of mixed infections:</u>
   - Quinolone + metronidazole
   - Amoxicillin-clavulanate
4. <u>Microbiology</u>
   - Anaerobes: Culture and sensitivity testing is usually unnecessary. Resistance is increasing to clindamycin, cefoxitin, cefotetan, piperacillin, and fluoroquinolones. Consider in vitro sensitivity testing for anaerobes that persist, cause bacteremia, or require prolonged therapy
   - Blood cultures: Not generally recommended
   - Gram stain: Not recommended for community acquired infections. May be recommended for healthcare associated infections to detect MRSA and enterococci
5. <u>Treatment of specific pathogens</u>
   Candida: Antifungal therapy is generally not warranted unless there is immunosuppression, transplantation or with post-op patient
   Enterococcus: Community acquired infection—do not treat; healthcare associated—treat based on in vitro susceptibility tests
6. <u>Biliary tract</u>: Direct therapy at Enterobacteraceae, not enterococci; cover anaerobes only with bile duct—bowel anastomosis

7. <u>Necrotizing pancreatitis</u>: Antibiotics as advocated for intra-abdominal sepsis
8. <u>Duration of antibiotics</u>: Until clinical signs of infection resolve including fever and leukocytosis plus a functioning GI tract

C. Monomicrobial infections

1. Spontaneous peritonitis or "primary peritonitis" (Arch Intern Med 97:169, 1994)*
   a. Aztreonam 1 g IV q8h × 14 days ± agent for Gram-positive bacteria
   b. Cefotaxime 1.5–2.0 g IV q6h or ceftriaxone 1–2 gm IV qd, each ± ampicillin 2 g IV q6h × 14 days
   c. Ticarcillin-clavulanate 3 g IV q6h × 14 days
   d. Gentamicin or tobramycin 2 mg/kg IV, then 1.7 mg/kg q8h <u>plus</u> a beta-lactam: (1) Cefoxitin 2 g IV q6h; (2) cefotaxime 1.5–2.0 mg IV q6h; or (3) piperacillin 4–5 g IV q6h × 14 days

---

*Antibiotics should be adjusted according to sensitivities of implicated strain; rate of positive cultures is 30–40% with blood cultures, 40–65% routine culture of ascites fluid, and 90% with ascites fluid inoculated into blood culture bottles (Gastroenterology 95:1351, 1988).

2. _Candida peritonitis_ (diagnostic criteria and indications to treat in absence of peritoneal dialysis are nebulous): Amphotericin B 200–1000 mg (total dose), 1 mg over 6 hr, then maintenance dose of 20–30 mg/d; utility of fluconazole is not established
3. <u>Tuberculous peritonitis</u>

II. LOCALIZED INFECTIONS

A. Intra-abdominal abscess(es) not further defined: Use regimens recommended for polymicrobial infections with peritonitis (See "I. Peritonitis" above).

B. Liver Abscess

1. <u>Amebic</u>
   a. **_Preferred:_** Metronidazole 750 mg po or IV tid × 10 days plus diloxanide furoate, 500 mg po tid × 10 days or paromomycin 500 mg po bid × 7 days
   b. **_Alternative:_** Emetine 1 mg/kg/d IM × 5 days (or dehydroemetine 1.0–1.5 mg/kg/d × 5 days) <u>followed by</u> chloroquine 500 mg po bid 2 days, then 250 mg po bid × 3 wk <u>plus</u> iodoquinol 650 mg po tid × 20 days
2. <u>Pyogenic</u>: Metronidazole plus ampicillin plus 1) an aminoglycoside, 2) third generation cephalosporin, or 3) aztreonam

C. Biliary Tract Infections

1. <u>Cholecystitis</u>
   a. **_Combination treatment:_** Gentamicin or tobramycin 2.0 mg/kg IV then 1.7 mg/kg IV q8h <u>plus</u> ampicillin 2 g IV q6h, piperacillin 2–5 g IV q6h, or cefoperazone 1–2 g IV q12h*
   b. **_Single agent:_** Cefoperazone 1–2 g IV q12h*. Ampicillin + sulbactam, 1–2 g (ampicillin) IV q6h; ticarcillin-clavulanate 3 g IV q6h; for mild infections the usual recommendation is cefazolin 1–2 g IM or IV q8h, or ampicillin 1–2 g IV q6h
   c. **_Medical Letter consultants_** (Med Lett, 41:95, 1999): (1) Piperacillin or mezlocillin plus metronidazole, (2) piperacillin-tazobactam or ampicillin-sulbactam ± aminoglycoside

---

*Other cephalosporins (second and third generation) are probably equally effective. Some authorities add ampicillin (1–2 g IV q6h) to cephalosporin-containing regimens.

2. <u>Ascending cholangitis, empyema of the gallbladder, or emphysematous cholecystitis:</u> Treat with regimens advocated for peritonitis or intra-abdominal abscess

D. Appendicitis: Recommendations of the Surgical Infection Society (*Arch Surg 127:83, 1992*)

Antibiotic treatment is started pre-op using regimens advocated for peritonitis (p 127)
1. Appendix is normal or inflamed but not perforated: Discontinue antibiotics
2. Gangrene or perforation: Continue antibiotics until clinical improvement with return of bowel function, patient is afebrile, and WBC is <12,000/mm³

E. Diverticulitis: Recommendations of the Surgical Infection Society (*Arch Surg 127:83, 1992*)

1. <u>Hospitalized patients:</u> Use regimens advocated for peritonitis (p 267)
2. <u>Outpatients:</u>
   a. Amoxicillin + clavulanate
   b. Fluoroquinolone plus metronidazole
   c. Trimethoprim-sulfamethoxazole

HELICOBACTER PYLORI: **TREATMENT OF PEPTIC ULCER DISEASE**
(*Adapted from Med Letter Guidelines 2004;2:9; Ann Intern Med 1997;157:87*)

Regimen	Cost	Eradication rate
Diagnosis		

- Breath tests: Specificity 95–100%, sensitivity 88–100%. Documentation of H. pylori eradication with repeat 4 wks after treatment
- Urea breath test: Alternative for patients who cannot do breath test
- Stool antigen: Sensitivity 94%, specificity 90%. Documentation of H. pylori eradication at 6–8 wks post therapy
- Serology: Not reliable
- Biopsy: Permits culture for sensitivity test. Urease test gives rapid diagnosis

Regimen	Cost	Eradication rate
Treatment		
Bismuth subsalicylate 2 tabs tid or qid plus metronidazole 500 mg tid or plus tetracycline 500 mg tid or qid plus ranitidine 150 mg bid or omeprazole 20 mg bid	2 wk	$70	96%
Clarithromycin 500 mg bid plus metronidazole 500 mg bid or amoxicillin 1 g bid plus omeprazole 20 mg bid or lansoprazole 30 mg bid	7–14 days	$260	89–91%
Bismuth subsalicylate 2 tabs qid plus metronidazole 250 mg qid plus tetracycline 500 mg qid	2 wk	$190*	90%
Omeprazole 40–60 mg qd plus amoxicillin 500 mg tid plus metronidazole 500 mg bid	7 days	$111	84%

* Helidac Therapy with 14 blister cards, each with a one day supply

INFECTIOUS DIARRHEA

Source: Guidelines from Infectious Diseases Society of America (CID 2001;32:331)

A. Antimicrobial Treatment

Microbial agent	Preferred	Alternative*	Comment
BACTERIA			
Aeromonas hydrophila	Usually none; if treated: Sulfa-trimethoprim 1 DS po bid × 3 days Ciprofloxacin 500 mg po bid or ofloxacin 300 mg po bid or norfloxacin 400 mg po bid × 3 days	Tetracycline 500 mg po qid × 5 days Gentamicin 1.7 mg/kg IV q8h × 5 days	Efficacy of treatment not established and should be reserved for patients with severe disease, immunosuppression, extraintestinal infection, or prolonged diarrhea
Campylobacter jejuni	Erythromycin 250–500 mg po qid × 5 days	Doxycycline 100 mg po bid × 7 days Furazolidone 100 mg po qid × 7 days Ciprofloxacin 500 mg po bid × 3–5 days	May not alter course unless given early or for severe symptoms Indications include acutely ill, persistent fever, bloody diarrhea, >8 stools/day, dehydration, symptoms <4 days or to prevent transmission. Resistance to erythromycin has been described. Clinical course not altered in trials when treatment started >4 days after onset of symptoms Resistance: Fluoroquinolone resistance is an increasing problem in the U.S. and other parts of the world (NEJM 340:1525, 1999). In Thailand, Spain, and Taiwan the rate of fluoroquinolone resistance is 60–80% (Emerg Infect Dis 7:24, 2001)
Clostridium difficile	Metronidazole 500 mg po tid or 250 mg po qid × 10 days	Vancomycin 125 mg po q6h × 10–14 days Bacitracin 25,000 units po qid × 10–14 days	Diagnosis: Standard is cytotoxin assay for toxin B (most sensitive) or EIA for toxin A and B (less sensitive but more rapid and more generally available) Metronidazole is preferred because of cost, comparable efficacy in clinical trials, and concern for vancomycin-resistant *E. faceum* in nosocomial cases

Continued

Microbial agent	Preferred	Alternative*	Comment
			Discontinuation of implicated antibiotic is often adequate. Some strains are resistant to metronidazole and bacitracin. Expected response is afebrile in 24 hr and resolution of diarrhea in mean of 4–5 days
			When oral treatment is not possible metronidazole 500 mg q8h IV (efficacy not established)
			Antiperistaltic agents: Contraindicated
Multiple relapses	Vancomycin or metronidazole (above doses; ×10 days, then cholestyramine 4 g po tid + lacto-bacillus 1 g qid × 4–6 wk or vancomycin 125 mg po every other day × 4–6 wk)	Vanco 500 mg qid × 10 days, day 7 *Saccharomyces boulardii* 500 mg bid × 4 wk Vanco or metro treatment, then lactobacillus GG ("Culturella") 75 mg bid × 1 mo IVIG 200–300 mg/kg q3wk	Frequency of relapse: 5–50% (average 25%) with any antibiotic treatment *S. boulardii* and lactobacillus GG are not FDA approved and are not readily available Experience with IVIG is limited but supported by studies showing importance of humoral immune response (NEJM 342:390, 2000; Lancet 357:189, 2001)
E. coli Enterotoxigenic *E. coli* (ETEC) and enteroadherent *E. coli* (EAEC)	Ciprofloxacin 500 mg po bid or ofloxacin 300 mg po bid or norfloxacin 400 mg po bid × 3 days TMP-SMX DS po bid × 3 days	Trimethoprim 200 mg po bid × 3 days Bismuth subsalicylate 1048 mg qid × 5 days	Laboratory confirmation *E. coli*-associated diarrhea is usually unavailable Efficacy of antibiotic treatment established for ETEC (traveler's diarrhea). Diagnosis requires demonstration of LT or ST toxins (EIA, DNA probe, rabbit loop, etc). Many ETEC strains are now resistant to doxycycline and TMP-SMX (see traveler's diarrhea, pp 141–142)
Enterohemorrhagic *E. coli* (EHEC)	None	None	Diagnosis: Culture *E. coli* O157:H7 using sorbitol—MacConkey agar; for non-O157 species test stool or supernatant with EIA for Shiga toxin Antibiotic treatment is contraindicated presumably because of increased toxin release with higher rate of HUS in children Life threatening complications: HUS Antiperistaltic agents: Contraindicated and TTP, esp at age extremes

Continued

269

Microbial agent	Preferred	Alternative*	Comment
Enteroinvasive *E. coli* (EIEC)	Usually none, if treated: Sulfa-trimethoprim, 1 DS po bid × 5 days Ciprofloxacin 500 mg po bid or ofloxacin 300 mg po bid or norfloxacin 400 mg po bid × 5 days	Ampicillin 500 mg po or 1 g IV qid × 5 days	Presentation is dysentery as with *Shigella*. Efficacy of treatment not established
Enteropathogenic *E. coli* (EPEC)	Usually none, if treated: Sulfa-trimethoprim, 1 DS po bid × 3–5 days Ciprofloxacin 500 mg po bid or ofloxacin 300 mg po or norfloxacin 400 mg po bid × 3 days	Neomycin 50 mg/kg/d po × 3–5 days Furazolidone 100 mg po qid × 3–5 days	Efficacy of treatment not established. Sensitivity testing necessary
Food poisoning: *Clostridium perfringens, S. aureus, Bacillus cereus, Listeria*	None		Self-limited and toxin-mediated: <u>antimicrobial treatment is not indicated</u> (see p 279)
Plesiomonas shigelloides	Usually none, but if treated: Sulfa-trimethoprim 1 DS po bid × 3 days Ciprofloxacin 500 mg po bid or ofloxacin 300 mg po bid or norfloxacin 400 mg po bid × 3 days	Tetracycline, 500 mg po qid × 5 days	Efficacy of treatment is not established and should be reserved for patients with extraintestinal infection, prolonged diarrhea, or immunosuppression
Salmonella typhi	Chloramphenicol 50 mg/kg/d IV × 10–14 days Ciprofloxacin 500 mg po bid × 10–14 days	Ceftriaxone 1–2 g/d IV × 10–14 days Sulfa-trimethoprim, 1–2 DS po bid × 10–14 days	<u>Steroids:</u> For severe toxicity high-dose antibiotics plus dexamethasone (3 mg/kg × 1, then 1 mg/kg q6h × 48 hr) or prednisone (60 mg/d with taper to 20 mg/d over 3 days) (NEJM 310:82, 1984)

Continued

Microbial agent	Preferred	Alternative*	Comment
Salmonella (other) Enteric fever (non-typhoid *Salmonella*) Metastatic infection Chronic bacteremia Enterocolitis in compromised host See comment	Usually none, if indicated: *Fluoroquinolone:* Ciprofloxacin 500 mg po bid; ofloxacin 300 mg po bid or norfloxacin 400 mg po bid × 5–7 days *Cephalosporin:* Ceftriaxone, 1–2 g/d IV up to 4 g/d × 14 days	Ampicillin 2–6 g/d po or IV × 14 days Amoxicillin 2–4 g/d po × 14 days Chloramphenicol 3–4 g/d IV or po × 14 days Sulfa-trimethoprim 1 DS po bid × 14 days	<u>Antibiotic treatment is contraindicated except with the following:</u> Severe disease, age >50 yr; valvular heart disease, severe atherosclerosis, malignancy, or uremia <u>Duration:</u> 5–7 days unless there is relapsing disease in compromised host—treat ≥14 days
Carrier (*S. typhi*)*	Amoxicillin 6 g/d po + probenecid 2 g/d × 6 wk Ciprofloxacin 500–750 mg po bid × 6 wk	Rifampin 300 mg bid + TMP-SMX 1 DS bid × 6 wk	<u>Definition of carrier:</u> Positive cultures for 1 yr Cholecystectomy for cholelithiasis and carriers who relapse
Shigella	Ciprofloxacin 500 mg po bid or norfloxacin 400 mg po bid or ofloxacilin 300 mg po bid × 3 days Sulfa-trimethoprim 1 DS po bid × 3 days	Ampicillin 500 mg po or 1 g IV qid × 3–5 days Nalidixic acid 1 g po qid × 5–7 days Cefoperazone 1–2 g IV q12h × 5–7 days	Most important of bacterial enteric pathogens to treat because of severe disease and risk of transmission Ampicillin-resistant strains are common; for ampicillin-susceptible strains, amoxicillin should not be used Sulfa-trimethoprim resistance is increasing and is common in strains from some underdeveloped areas. Use only if susceptibility shown Ciprofloxacin in single, 1 g dose is effective for *Shigella*, other than *S. dysenteriae* (Ann Intern Med 117:727, 1992)
Vibrio cholerae	Tetracycline 500 mg po qid × 3 days Doxycycline 300 mg po × 1 Sulfa-trimethoprim 1 DS po bid × 3 days Fluoroquinolone		Rare cause of travelers' diarrhea Oral rehydration often critical

Continued

Microbial agent	Preferred	Alternative*	Comment
Vibrio sp. (*V. parahaemolyticus, V. fluvialis, V. mimicus, V. hollisae, V. furnissii, V. vulnificus*)	Usually none, if indicated: Tetracycline (as above—see comment)	Ciprofloxacin 500 mg po bid × 5 days	Efficacy of treatment is not established and should be reserved for severe disease
Yersinia enterocolitica	Sulfa-trimethoprim 1 DS po bid × 3 days Gentamicin 1.7 mg/kg IV q8h × 3 days Ciprofloxacin 500–750 mg po bid × 3 days Doxycycline 100 mg po bid × 7 days		<u>Efficacy of treatment for enterocolitis or mesenteric adenitis is not established</u>, especially when instituted late; major indications are bacteremia or infection in compromised host <u>Withhold desferoxamine</u>
PARASITES Cryptosporidia	Usually none or symptomatic treatment: Loperamide, lomotil etc plus nutritional support Compromised host: Paromomycin 500 mg po tid × 7 days	Nitrazoxanide 500 mg bid (Unimed Pharmaceuticals, Buffalo Grove, IL)—not approved by FDA Compromised host (AIDS): Paromomycin 1 g bid + azithromycin 600 mg po qd × 4 wk then paromomycin 500 mg po tid	<u>Diagnosis:</u> Stool for acid-fast stain or monoclonal immunoflu-orescent stain; concentration techniques increase yield <u>Treatment:</u> Only for chronic diarrhea in compromised host. Paromomycin is only modestly effective (Am J Med 100:370, 1996) Main treatments in AIDS patient are supportive care and HAART Atovaquone or azithromycin as single agents have not shown good results
*Balantidium coli**	Tetracycline 500 mg po qid × 10 days	Iodoquinol 650 mg tid × 21 days Metronidazole 500 mg po tid × 10 days	No antimicrobial agent has established efficacy

Continued

Microbial agent	Preferred	Alternative*	Comment
*Cyclospora cayetanenis**	Trimethoprim-sulfamethoxazole 1 DS bid × 3 days		Treatment: Efficacy of TMP-SMX is established Diagnosis: Stool for acid-fast stain Reporting: Health departments that identify cases of *Cyclospora* infection should contact CDC 770-488-7760
*Blastocystis hominis** (see comments)	Metronidazole 1.5–2.0 g/ d × 7 days	Iodoquinol 650 mg tid × 20 days	Role as enteric pathogen is unclear
Entamoeba histolytica	Metronidazole 500–750 mg po or IV tid × 5–10 days or tinidazole 2 gm qd × 3–5 days then iodoquinol 650 mg po tid × 21 days or paromomycin 500 mg tid × 7 days	Dehydroemetine 1.0–1.5 mg/kg/d IM × 5 days, then iodoquinol 650 mg po tid × 21 days	Diagnosis: Stool exam × 3 ± endoscopy with biopsy or scraping; serology (IHA) for colitis or hepatic disease. Patients with colitis or extraintestinal disease need drug for tissue phase (metronidazole or dehydroemetine), then a luminal agent (iodoquinol, or paromomycin) Tinidazole is as effective as metronidazole and usually better tolerated (Med Letter 2005;46:70)
Cyst passer			No need to treat because most cases are caused by nonpathogenic organisms now reclassified as *E. dispar*
Giardia lamblia (*G. intestinalis*)	Metronidazole, 250–750 mg po tid × 7–10 days Nitazoxanide 500 mg bid × 3 d or 2 g single dose Tinidazole 2.0 g single dose	Quinacrine 100 mg tid × 7–10 days Furazolidone 8 mg/kg/d po × 10 days	Diagnosis: Stool EIA Metronidazole is less effective than quinacrine, but better GI tolerance and preferred for empiric therapy. Pregnancy: Consider paromomycin 25–30 mg/kg/d × 5–10 days Single dose tinidazole (2 gm) showed 93% cure rate (AAC 1985; 27:227) and higher cure rates than single dose metronidazole (Cochrane Database Syst Rev 2000;2:CD 000217) Med Letter (2005;46:70): Tinidazole is as effective as metronidazole and is usually better tolerated
Isospora belli	Sulfa-trimethoprim, 2 DS po bid × 7–10 days	Pyrimethamine 25 mg + folinic acid, 5–10 mg/d × 1 mo	Diagnosis: Acid-fast stain of stool. Patients with AIDS and other immunosuppressive disorders usually require prolonged maintenance treatment
Microsporidia	Albendazole 400 mg po bid × 3 wk	—	Rare disease in immunocompetent host Response to albendazole is minimal; main treatment in patients with AIDS is support and HAART

APPROACH TO INFECTIOUS DIARRHEA

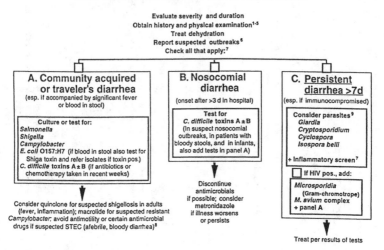

Evaluate severity and duration
Obtain history and physical examination[1-5]
Treat dehydration
Report suspected outbreaks[6]
Check all that apply:[7]

A. Community acquired or traveler's diarrhea
(esp. if accompanied by significant fever or blood in stool)

Culture or test for:
Salmonella
Shigella
Campylobacter
E. coli O157:H7 (if blood in stool also test for Shiga toxin and refer isolates if toxin pos.)
C. difficile toxins A ± B (if antibiotics or chemotherapy taken in recent weeks)

Consider quinclone for suspected shigellosis in adults (fever, inflammation); macrolide for suspected resistant *Campylobacter*; avoid antimotility or certain antimicrobial drugs if suspected STEC (afebrile, bloody diarrhea)[8]

B. Nosocomial diarrhea
(onset after >3 d in hospital)

Test for
C. difficile toxins A ± B
(In suspect nosocomial outbreaks, in patients with bloody stools, and in infants, also add tests in panel A)

Discontinue antimicrobials if possible; consider metronidazole if illness worsens or persists

C. Persistent diarrhea >7d
(esp. if immunocompromised)

Consider parasites[9]
Giardia
Cryptosporidium
Cyclospora
Isospora belli

+ Inflammatory screen[7]

☐ If HIV pos., add:

Microsporidia
(Gram-chromotrope)
M. avium complex
+ panel A

Treat per results of tests

Guidelines from the IDSA (CID 2001; 32:331). (Reprinted with permission)
1. Seafood exposure: culture for vibrio
2. Travelers diarrhea: evaluate if unresponsive to fluoroquinolone or TMP-SMX
3. Abdominal pain: Test for *Yersinia* and enterohemorrhagic *E. coli*
4. Proctitis in gay men: sigmoidoscopy
5. HUS: Test for enterohemorrhagic *E. coli*
6. Outbreaks: Notify health department
7. Fecal lactoferrin test or microscopy
8. Blood diarrhea: Some experts avoid antimicrobials
9. Common tests for parasites: Fluorescence and EIA for *Giardia* and Cryptosporidium, Cyclospora or Mycobacteria; chromotrope of microsporidia

B. Nonantibiotic Management

1. <u>Cholera-like illness:</u> Oral rehydration therapy with Ceralyte, Pedialyte, or generic solutions prepared by mixing in 1L—3.5 g NaCl, 2.5 g NaHCO$_3$, 1.5 g KCl, and 20 g glucose
2. <u>Foods</u> matched to form of stool: <u>Watery</u>—soups, broth, yogurt, soft drinks, vegetables, fresh fruit, Jell-O ± saltine crackers; <u>some form</u>—rice, bread, baked potato, broiled fish or broiled chicken (<u>avoid</u> milk, fried food, spicy food)
3. <u>Drugs:</u> Antiperistaltics are contraindicated with diarrhea because of enterohemorrhagic *E. coli* or *Clostridium difficile*
   a. **Loperamide** 4 mg, then 2 mg/diarrheal stool up to 16 mg/d (avoid with fever and dysentery)
   b. **Diphenoxylate** (no more effective plus potential for opiate toxicity and anticholinergic effects)
   c. **Bismuth subsalicylate:** 30 mL (2 tabs) q 30 min × 8 doses, 1–2 days (good safety profile)
   d. **Attapulgite:** 1.2 g (30 cc) with each diarrheal stool up to 8.4 g (good safety profile and preferred to kaolin/pectin)

C. Fecal Leukocyte Exam (*Lactoferrin test or stool microscopy*)

Often present	Variable	Not present
Campylobacter jejuni	Salmonella	Vibrio cholerae
Shigella	Yersinia	Enteroadherent E. coli
Enteroinvasive E. coli	Vibrio parahaemolyticus	Enterotoxigenic E. coli
Exacerbations of inflammatory bowel disease	C. difficile	Food poisoning: S. aureus, B. cereus, C. perfringens
	Aeromonas	Viral gastroenteritis
	Plesiomonas	Parasitic infection: Giardia,
	Enterohemorrhagic E. coli*	E. histolytica*, Cryptosporidia, Isospora
		Small bowel overgrowth "AIDS enteropathy"

*Frequently associated with blood.

D. Empiric Antibiotic Treatment (IDSA Guidelines—CID 32:331, 2001)

1. <u>Domestically acquired infectious diarrhea</u>
   1. Acute diarrhea: Fever and acute diarrhea (nonbloody)—treat for shigellosis
   2. Chronic diarrhea: Diarrhea >10–14 days—treat for giardiasis
   3. Antibiotic treatment in these settings is arbitrary; antibiotic treatment with diarrhea caused by enterohemorrhagic *E. coli* may be harmful.
2. <u>Travelers' diarrhea</u> (CID 2000; 31:1079; Med Letter 2004;46:75)
   1. <u>Severity</u>
      • Mild (1–2 stools/24 hr) no systemic sx: No therapy or loperamide or bismuth
      • Moderate (>2 stools/24 hr) + no systemic sx: Loperamide or bismuth
      • Moderate (>2 stools/24 hr) + "distressing sx": Loperamide + fluoroquinolone until diarrhea stops (up to 3 days)
      • Severe (>6 stools/24 hr), fever and/or bloody stools: Fluoroquinolone for 3 days
   2. <u>Agents</u>
      • Loperamide 4 mg × 1 then 2 mg with each loose stool (≤16 mg/d) or bismuth subsalicylate (Pepto-Bismol 2 tabs qid, each loose stool)
      • Antibiotic regimens: Norfloxacin 400 mg bid × 3 days or ciprofloxacin ER 1000 mg qd × 3 days or levofloxacin 500 mg qd × 3 days or azithromycin 1000 mg × 1 or 500 mg qd × 3 d or rifamixin 200 mg tid × 3 d (Med Letter 2004;46:75)
      • These antibiotics may be as effective if given for 1 or 2 days

E. Clinical Features of Diarrhea

	Small bowel	Colon
Pathogens	E. coli (ETEC, EPEC, EAEC), cholera, Salmonella, viruses, Cryptosporidium, Cyclospora, Giardia	Shigella, C. difficile, C. jejuni, E. coli 0157:H7 Enteroinvasive E. coli, Aeromonas, Yersinia, E. histolytica, V. parahemolyticus
Pain	Mid abdomen and modest	Lower abdomen with severe cramps Painful defecation
Stools	Watery, large volume	Bloody or mucoid, small volume and frequent
Stool WBC and RBC	Negative	WBC positive; E. histolytica and E. coli 0157:H7—bloody

FOODBORNE OUTBREAKS
(Source: MMWR 2001;50(RR-2))

Agent	Incubation period	Syndrome	Confirmation*
BACTERIAL			
Bacillus anthracis	2 days–wk	Nausea, vomiting, bloody diarrhea, acute abd pain × wks	Blood culture
Bacillus cereus			
Vomiting toxin	1–6 hr	Vomiting ± diarrhea	Test stool or food for toxin
Diarrhea toxin	10–16 hr	Watery diarrhea × 24–48 hr	Test stool or food for toxin
Brucella	7–21 days	Fever, headache, sweats, myalgias, diarrhea, bloody stools × wks	Blood culture and serology
C. jejuni	2–5 days	Diarrhea, abd pain, fever, vomiting × 2–10 days	Stool culture
C. botulinum	12–72 hr	Diploplia, blurred vision, descending paralysis—bilateral vomiting, diarrhea × days–months	Detect toxin in serum, stool, or food Detect C. botulinum in stool or food
C. perfringens	8–16 hr	Diarrhea, cramps × 24–48 hr	Isolate from stool (> 10⁶/g) or food (> 10⁵/g) Detect enterotoxin in stool
E. coli 0157:H7 (EHEC)	1–8 days	Diarrhea—often bloody, cramps no fever × 5–10 days	Stool culture for E. coli 0157:H7 or stool assay for Shiga toxin

Continued

Agent	Incubation period	Syndrome	Confirmation*
Enterotoxigenic (ETEC)	1–3 days	Watery diarrhea, cramps, nausea × 5–10 days	Isolate ST or LT producing *E. coli* from stool
Listeria			
Invasive disease	2–6 wk	Meningitis, fever (elderly, compromised)	Isolate from normally sterile site—blood, CSF
Diarrhea	9–48 hr	Diarrhea, cramps, fever	Listerolysin O antibody
Salmonela			
Non-typhoid	1–3 days	Diarrhea, cramps, fever × 4–7 days	Stool culture
Salmonella typhi	3–60 days, usually 7–14	Fever, malaise, headache, chills	Stool culture
Shigella	24–48 hr	Diarrhea ± blood, cramps, fever × 4–7 days	Stool culture
S. aureus	1–6 hr	Vomiting, cramps ± diarrhea × 24–48 hr	Toxin/organism in stool, food, and vomitus
Streptococcus group A	1–4 days	Fever, pharyngitis	Isolate organism of same M or T type from ≥2 people
Vibrio cholera 01 or 0139	24–72 hr	Severe watery diarrhea ± vomiting × 2–5 days	Stool culture for *V. cholerae*
Vibrio parahemolyticus	2–48 hr	Diarrhea, cramps, vomiting × 2–5 days	Stool culture for *V. parahaemolyticus*
Vibrio vulnificus	1–7 days	Vomiting, diarrhea, cramps, bacteremia (esp liver disease and comp host) × 2–8 days	Stool and blood culture
Yersinia enterocoliticus	24–48 hr	Diarrhea and cramps Appendicitis-like symptoms with fever, abd pain × 1–3 wk	Isolate organism from stool or food
PARASITIC			
Cryptosporidia	2–28 days	Diarrhea, nausea, cramps ± fever × days–weeks	Detect organism in stool or food/water

Continued

Agent	Incubation period	Syndrome	Confirmation*
Cyclospora	1–11 days	Protracted diarrhea, fatigue	Demonstrate organisms in stool
E. histolytica	2 days–4 wk	Bloody diarrhea, abd pain × months	Stool exam
Giardia	1–4 wk	Diarrhea, gas, cramps, nausea × wks	Demonstrate organism or antigen in stool
Toxoplasma gondii	6–10 days	Usually asymptomatic compromised host CNS, myo-carditis, pneumonia × months	Serology IgM
Trichinella	Intestinal phase 1–2 days Systemic phase 2–4 wk	Nausea, vomiting, diarrhea, cramps, then fever × mo	Positive serology or demonstrate larvae in muscle of patient or in meat sources; eosinophilia
VIRAL			
Hepatitis A	15–50 days, median 28 days	Fatigue, anorexia, nausea, jaundice, abnormal LFTs	Detect IgM, ALT
Norovirus**	24–48 hr	Vomiting, cramps, watery diarrhea × 24–60 hr	RT-PCR stool
Astrovirus calicivirus	10–70 hr	Vomiting, cramps, diarrhea, headache fever × 2–9 days	Demonstrate virus by immune electron mi-croscopy, PCR, etc.
CHEMICAL			
Marine toxins			
Ciguatoxin (esp snapper, grouper, or barracuda)	2–6 hr	GI symptoms, then paresthesias lips, tongue, throat, ex-tremities × days–wk	Demonstrate toxin in fish or typical presentation
Scromboid toxin (histamine) (mahi-mahi, scromboidei fish order)	1 min–3 hr usually <1 hr	Flushing, dizziness, burning mouth, headache, GI symptoms, urticaria, pruritis × 3–6 hr	Demonstrate histamine in food or typical presentation
Paralytic or neurotoxic shellfish poison	30 min–3 hr	Parenthesias of lips mouth, face ex-tremities, GI symptoms × days, weakness, dyspnea	Detect toxin in food or water

Continued

Agent	Incubation period	Syndrome	Confirmation*
Puffer fish	<30 min	Parenthesias of lips mouth, face, extremities, ascending paralysis, death in 4–6 hr	Demonstrate toxin in fish or clinical presentation
Heavy metal: Antimony, cadmium, copper, iron, tin, zinc	5 min–8 hr usually <1 hr	Vomiting and metallic taste ± diarrhea	Demonstrate metal in food
Monosodium glutamate (MSG)	3 min–2 hr usually <1 hr	Burning of chest, neck, abdomen, or extremities	Clinical presentation plus ingestion of food with MSG
Mushroom toxins			
Short-acting	<2 hr	Vomiting and diarrhea, confusion, salivation, hallucinations, visual problems, disulfiram reaction	Clinical syndrome in patients who have eaten mushrooms that represent toxic types
Longer-acting *Amanita* sp	6–24 hr	Diarrhea and cramps, × 24 hr, then hepatic and renal failure; often lethal	Clinical syndrome in patients who have ingested the implicated mushroom
Pesticides	Min–few hr	Nausea, vomiting, cramps, diarrhea, blurred vision, twitching convulsions	Analysis of food and blood
Nitrite poisoning	1–2 hr	Nausea, vomiting, dizzy, weak, unconscious, chocolate-colored blood	Food analysis
Mercury	≥1 wk	Numbness, leg paresis, spastic paralysis, blindness	Analysis of blood and hair
Arsenic	Few hrs	Vomiting, diarrhea, cramps	Urine test
Shellfish toxins	Minutes–48 hr	GI symptoms, parethesis, CNS	Detect toxins in shellfish
Sodium floride	Minutes–2 hr	Soapy taste, vomiting, diarrhea, shock	Test vomitus and food

*Confirmation to implicate a cause of an outbreak usually requires documentation in ≥2 persons or demonstration of the organism or toxin in the implicated food.
**Norovirus is the former "Norwalk agent" and is the most common cause of outbreaks of gastroenteritis (JID 2004;190:27)

FOODBORNE ILLNESS BY CLINICAL PRESENTATION
MMWR 2001;50(RR-2)

<u>Watery diarrhea</u>: ETEC, *V. cholera,* enteric virus, *Cryposporidium, Cyclospora*
<u>Dysentery</u>: *Shigella, Salmonella, C. jejuni,* EIEC, EHEC, *Vibrio parahaemolytica, Yersinia enterocolitica*
<u>Persistent diarrhea (≥14 days)</u>: *Cyclospora, Cryptosporidium, E. histolytica, Giardia*
<u>Neurologic syndromes</u> (paresthesias, respiratory suppression): Botulism, poisoning by organophosphate pesticides, thallium, scombroid, ciguatera, tetrodon fish, neurotoxic shellfish, amnesic shellfish, mushroom poisoning, Guillain-Barré syndrome
<u>Systemic illness</u>: *Listeria, Brucella, Trichinella, Toxoplasma, V. vulnificans,* hepatitis A

Continued

URINARY TRACT INFECTIONS

I. CLASSIFICATION BASED ON GUIDELINES ESTABLISHED BY THE INFECTIOUS DISEASES SOCIETY OF AMERICA

(CID 15:S216, 1992; CID 29:745, 1999 and CID 2005;40:643)

Category	Criteria for stated category		Treatment
	Clinical	Laboratory[a]	
Acute, uncomplicated UTI in women	Dysuria, urgency, frequency, suprapubic pain; no urinary symptoms in last 4 wk; no fever or flank pain	>10 WBC/mm³ >10³ cfu/mL uropathogen in MSU	All drugs active vs GNB show cure rates >80% <u>Single dose</u>: No longer favored <u>3-day treatment</u>: Generally preferred. Expected cure rate[b]: >85% at 5–9 days; >65% at 4–6 wk
Acute, uncomplicated pyelonephritis	Fever, chills, dysuria, urgency, frequency, suprapubic pain, CVA tenderness, and/or flank pain Other diagnoses excluded. No history of urologic abnormalities	>10 WBC/mm³ >10⁴ cfu/mL uropathogen in MSU	<u>Mild symptoms</u>: Oral with agent active vs the uropathogen <u>Seriously ill</u>: Parenteral therapy with agent active vs the uropathogen until afebrile 24–48 hr followed by oral agent × 2 wk total therapy. Expected cure rate[b]: >95% at 3–6 days, >80% at 5–9 days post treatment
UTI in male	Any combination of findings in above categories	>10 WBC/mm³ >10⁵ cfu/mL in MSU	UTI in men: Assume tissue invasion—renal or prostate Regimens: TMP-SMX, trimethoprim or fluoroquinolone for 2–6 wk Expected cure rate[b]: >90% at 3–5 days and 50% at 4–6 wk
Complicated UTI	Above + catheter associated, postvoiding residual > 100 mL, calculi, azofemia, or reflux	As above	Regimen: Parenteral—oral or oral using agent active vs uropathogen × 2 wk. Expected cure rate[b]: >90% at 3–5 days, >65% at 5–9 days, and >40% at 4–6 wk
Asymptomatic	No urinary symptoms	>10 WBC/mm³ >10⁵ cfu/mL uropathogen × 2 separated by 24 hr for women and × 1 for men (CID 2005;40:643)	Indications for treatment: Pregnant women, diabetic patients, immunocompromised patients, and children Expected cure rates: >95% at 3–5 days, >75% at 5–9 days, and >50% at 4–6 wk Pyuria combined with asymptomatic bacteruria is not an indication for antibiotic therapy

[a]WBC, white blood cells (unspun urine); MSU, midstream urine culture.
[b]Expected cure refers to eradication of uropathogen and elimination of symptoms. Data provided are expectations based on prior studies with evaluations during treatment at 5–9 days post-treatment and 4–6 wk post-treatment. Positive cultures post-treatment are classified as relapse (same strain), usually indicating renal or prostatic nidus of infection or reinfection indicating new uropathogen.

II. TREATMENT OF CYSTITIS AND PYCLONEPHRITIS Recommendations of SD Fihn (NEJM 2003;349:3) and IDSA guidelines (CID 1999;29:745 CID 2005;40:643))

A. Asymptomatic Bacteruria (CID 2005:40:643)
1. <u>Criteria</u>: See above table
2. <u>Screening</u>: Indications
   - Pregnancy
   - Periodically after therapy
   - Prior to prostate surgery and other urologic procedures with anticipated mucosal bleeding
3. Screening should not be routinely done for diabetic women, premenopausal nonpregnant women, elderly persons, spinal cord injury patients, catheterized patients (until catheter is removed)
4. <u>Treatment:</u>
   - Pregnant women
   - Bacteruria prior to urologic surgery & stopped when surgery is completed unless catheter is left in
   - Catheter acquired UTI that persists ≥ 48 hours after catheter removal in women

B. Uncomplicated Bacterial Cystitis in Non-pregnant Women
Based on recommendations of SD Fihn (NEJM 2003;349:3)
1. **Diagnostic tests:** The urinary dipstick has largely replaced the urine culture and urine microscopy because it is cheaper, faster, and more convenient. The relative merits of these tests are summarized in the following table:
   a. <u>Diagnostic Tests</u>

	Sensitivity	Specificity
Pyuria	95%	71%
Bacteria on Gram stain	40–70%	85–95%
Urinary dipstick	75%	82%
Urine culture	50%	High

Many patients do not need any testing, but can be managed by telephone consultation. Published protocols include women at low risk for complicated infection, who do not have symptoms suggesting vaginitis or cervicitis and in some cases are limited to women <55 years of age (Am J Med 1999;106:636; Br J Gen Prat 2000;50:635; J Fam Pract 2001;50:589).

2. **Treatment:** (see table below) <u>TMP-SMX</u> for three days results in sterile urine within seven days in about 94%; longer courses do not improve efficacy and increase side effects while the single dose is less effective (CID 1999;29:745). The alternative for patients with sulfa allergy is <u>trimethoprim</u>, but this may also cause hypersensitivity, and TMP rashes are commonly misidentified as sulfa reactions in patients who get TMP-SMX (Allergy 1992;47:340). In some areas the pathogens cultured from urine in acute cystitis show rates of TMP-SMX resistance of up to 18% (JAMA 1999;281:736; NEJM 2001;345:1007), especially if this drug has been given within the previous six months (J Gen Intern Med 1999;14:606). The recommendation is a <u>fluoroquinolone</u> if the patient has recently received antibiotics or if the local prevalence of urinary isolates exceeds 15–20%. <u>Nitrofurantoin</u> is another option, preferably using the monohydrate macrocrystal formulation because it is taken just twice daily and causes less GI toxicity compared to the macrocrystalline formulation. This drug may assume more importance if there is increasing resistance to fluoroquinolones. <u>Fosfomycin</u> is less effective than the other agents and should only be used when the others cannot be used (CID 1999;29:745). The expected response rate is symptom relief in 90% within 72 hours and negative cultures (if done) at 7 days in over 90%. Severe dysuria may be treated with phenazopyridine (Pyridium or Uristat) which is now available over-the-counter. Routine follow-up including urine culture is generally not necessary.

3. Regimens:

Agent	Retail Cost	Pregnancy Rating	Major ADRs
Acute uncomplicated cystits			
TMP/SMX 1 DS bid × 3 d*	$2	C	GI intol, rash
Trimethoprim 100 mg bid × 3 d*	$4	C	GI intol

Agent	Retail Cost	Pregnancy Rating	Major ADRs
Norfloxacin 250 mg bid × 3 d	$25	C	Dizzy, GI intol, vaginitis
Levofloxacin 250 mg qd × 3 d	$44	C	As above
Ciprofloxacin 250 mg bid × 3 d	$54	C	As above
Gatifloxacin 400 mg qd × 3 d or 400 mg × 1	$22 $8	C	As above
Nitrofurantoin monohydrate macrocrystals 100 mg bid × 7 d	$30	B	GI intol, pulmonary and liver toxicity
Fosfomycin 3 g po × 1	$34	B	GI intol

C. Pyelonephritis

1. Agent

a. <u>Oral therapy</u>

Oral agent	Comment
Fluoroquinolone	Preferred oral agent for empiric treatment
TMP-SMX	Preferred if pathogen is known to be sensitive

b. <u>Single parenteral dose followed by oral agent</u>
Parenteral agent: Ceftriaxone, gentamicin, or fluoroquinolone

Oral agent	Comment
Gram-positive pathogen	Amoxicillin or amoxicillin-clavulanate
Gram-negative pathogen	Base on in vitro susceptibility tests

c. <u>Hospitalized patients: Parenteral therapy</u>
Parenteral fluoroquinolone (ciprofloxacin was superior to TMP-SMX in terms of clinical response, bacteriologic response, and side effects (JAMA 283:1583, 2000))
Aminoglycoside ± ampicillin
Parenteral extended spectrum cephalosporin ± aminoglycoside
Gram-positive pathogen: Ampicillin-sulbactam ± aminoglycoside
<u>After afebrile 48–72 hr:</u> Oral agent based on susceptibility tests
GNB: Fluoroquinolone or TMP-SMX
GPC: Amoxicillin or amoxicillin-clavulanate

2. Duration: 14 days; 7 days may be adequate in mild or moderately severe cases (JAMA 283:1583, 2000)

D. Management of Bladder Catheter (Infect Dis Clin Pract 1995;4:446)

Incidence of infection: 3–10%/day

Prevention

  Prevention of infection: Maintain closed system

  Prevention of complications of bacteruria: Antibiotics are ineffective

  Prevention of catheterization: Condom catheters; intermittent catheterization
    ± instillations of povidone-iodine and chlorhexidine; suprapubic
    catheterization

Treatment: Treat only symptomatic infections (fever and/or signs of bacteremia)
  (symptoms are rare in this population—Ann Intern Med 160:668, 2000)

Treat 7–10 days: Parenteral or oral antimicrobial

E. Prostatitis (Guidelines of Assoc Genitourinary Med Society of Venereal
Disease London 2002)

1. **Acute prostatitis**
   a. Diagnosis: Midstream urine culture and blood culture; do not do prostatic
      massage (Pathogens are virtually always in urine)
   b. Treatment
      (1) Initial antibiotic treatment: Cefotaxime or ceftriaxone + gentamicin—
          switch to pathogen-specific therapy when sensitivity data available
      (2) Oral antibiotics: Switch to oral agent when clinically improved. Usual agent:
          Ciprofloxacin; alternative: TMP-SMX or trimethoprim × 28 days.
      (3) Adjunctive treatment: Catheterize for urinary retention, hydration,
          analgesics (NSAIDs)
   c. Failure to respond: Possible prostatic abscess—transrectal ultrasound or CT
      scan. Treatment—perineal or transurethral drainage
2. **Chronic prostatitis**
   Diagnosis: Symptoms ≥6 months.
   Urinary localization procedure (Not often done)
   • Patient preparation: No antibiotics × 1 month, no ejaculation × 2 days and
     no distended bladder
   • Specimens: 5–10 mL first voided urine (VB#1), void 100–200 mL then
     midstream (VB#2), vigorous prostatic massage × 1 minute, then post
     prostatic massage (PPM) urine of 5–10 mL (VB#3). All three samples have
     microscopy and quantitative urine cultures.
   • Interpretation
     1. Bacterial infection: Culture of VB#3 ≥10 × that of VB#2 and VB#1 Dx:
        "chronic bacterial prostititis"
     2. Inflammation: >10 PMNs/HPF in prostatic massage specimen or in VB#3.
        Dx: "Chronic bacterial prostatitis" or "chronic abacterial prostatitis/chronic
        pelvic pain syndrome—inflammatory"
     3. Culture and WBC assessment are negative. Dx: "Chronic abacterial
        prostatitis/chronic pelvic pain syndrome—inflammatory".

SEXUALLY TRANSMITTED DISEASES
Recommendations from the CDC (MMWR 2002;51:RR-6)

I. *NEISSERIA GONORRHOEAE* (GONOCOCCAL INFECTIONS)

A. Treatment Recommendations for Uncomplicated Localized Infections (urethral, endocervical, and rectal) (CID 1995;20:S47; Med Lett 1995;37:117)

- Ceftriaxone 125 mg IM × 1 <u>or</u>
- Ciprofloxacin* 500 mg po × 1 <u>or</u>
- Ofloxacin* 400 mg po × 1 <u>or</u>
- Levofloxacin 250 mg × 1 <u>or</u>
- Cefixime 400 mg po × 1

All of the above should be combined with treatment for *C. trachomatis* unless this has been ruled out: Doxycycline 100 mg po bid × 7 days; azithromycin (1 g po × 1) is an alternative.

Alternative: 1) <u>Spectinomycin</u> 2 g IM × 1. (Spectomycin may not be commercially available), 2) Cefotaxime 500 mg IM, 3) Gatifloxacin 400 mg po × 1 or norfloxacin 800 mg po. <u>Azithromycin</u> in a dose of 2 g is effective treatment for both gonorrhea and *C. trachomatis,* but GI side effects are frequent, cost is high, and gonococcal cure rates are relatively low (93%)

---

*Quinolones are contraindicated in persons <17 yr, during pregnancy, and during nursing; they are ineffective vs incubating syphilis; increasing resistance to fluoroquinolones has been reported. (Lancet 2003;262:495)

B. Special Considerations

1. <u>Syphilis:</u> All patients with gonorrhea should be screened for syphilis at initial visit. Regimens with ceftriaxone or a 7-day course of doxycycline or erythromycin may cure incubating syphilis.
2. <u>Follow-up:</u> Patients who respond need no follow-up. Patients with persistent symptoms should have culture for *N. gonorrhoeae* and in vitro susceptibility testing; most are due to re-infection, indicating need for partner referral or nongonococcal urethritis. Expected response rate ≥95%.
3. <u>Infection control:</u> Patients should avoid sexual intercourse until the patient and partner (see below) are cured. This means no sexual contact until therapy is completed *and* both are asymptomatic.
4. <u>Sex partners:</u> Partners should be referred for evaluation and treatment of *N. gonorrhoeae* and *C. trachomatis.* This includes sex partners within 30 days for symptomatic infection and those within 60 days for asymptomatic infection.
5. <u>Reporting:</u> All states require reporting of *N. gonorrhoeae.*
6. <u>Pregnancy:</u> Quinolones and tetracyclines are contraindicated. For *N. gonorrhoeaea* a cephalosporin or spectinomycin is preferred. For *C. trachomatis,* amoxicillin or erythromycin is preferred.
7. <u>HIV infection:</u> Standard recommendations apply.

C. Gonococcal Infections at Selected Sites*

1. <u>Pharyngitis:</u> Ceftriaxone 125 mg IM <u>or</u> ciprofloxacin 500 mg po (both with doxycycline 100 mg po bid × 7 days) or azithromycin 1 g po
2. <u>Conjunctivitis*:</u> Ceftriaxone 1 g IM × 1 plus lavage of infected eye × 1
3. <u>Disseminated gonococcal infections*</u>
   a. Hospitalization is recommended, especially for noncompliant patients, uncertain diagnosis, patients with purulent synovial effusions, or other complications.
   b. Recommended treatment: Ceftriaxone 1 g IV or IM daily
      Alternative regimens: Cefotaxime 1 g IV q8h <u>or</u> ceftizoxime 1 g IV q8h, ciprofloxacin 400 mg IV q12h, ofloxacin 400 mg IV q12h, levofloxacin 250 mg IV/d, or spectinomycin 2 g IM q12h

Duration of parenteral treatment: 24–48 hr after symptoms resolve, then cefixime 400 mg po bid, ciprofloxacin 500 mg po bid, ofloxacin 500 mg po bid, or levofloxacin 500 mg po qd

Duration of oral treatment: To complete a full week of antibiotic treatment

4. <u>Meningitis*:</u> Ceftriaxone 2 gm IV q12h × 10–14 days
5. <u>Endocarditis*:</u> Ceftriaxone 2 gm IV qd × 4 wk
6. <u>Salpingitis:</u> See pelvic inflammatory disease

*Standard recommendations apply for disease control (abstinence from sexual intercourse until treatment completed), partner referral, and concurrent treatment for presumed infection with *C. trachomatis* (doxycycline 100 mg po bid × 7 days).

II. SYPHILIS

A. Classification

1. <u>Primary:</u> Ulcer or chancre at site of infection
2. <u>Secondary:</u> Rash, mucocutaneous lesions, adenopathy
3. <u>Tertiary</u> (late): Cardiac, neurologic, ophthalmic, auditory, or gummatous lesions
4. <u>Latent syphilis:</u> No evidence of disease

    Early latent: Acquired syphilis within 1 yr based on seroconversion ≥4-fold increase in titer, history of primary or secondary syphilis, or sex partner with primary, secondary, or early latent syphilis

    Late latent: Infection >1 yr; syphilis of unknown duration should be managed as late latent syphilis

B. Diagnosis

1. <u>Direct exam</u> (lesion exudate or tissue): Dark-field or direct fluorescent antibody tests
2. <u>Serology:</u> Requires treponemal and nontreponemal tests for diagnosis
    a. ***Treponemal:*** Fluorescent treponemal antibody absorbed FTA-ABS or microhemagglutinin for antibody (MHATP). Reported as reactive or nonreactive, titers do not correlate with assay disease activity; patients who react usually remain reactive for life regardless of treatment or disease activity
    b. ***Nontreponemal:*** Venereal Disease Research Laboratory (VDRL) or rapid plasma reagin (RPR). Results should be reported quantitatively. Titers correlate with disease activity. 4-fold changes in titer are required to demonstrate a significant difference. Sequential tests should be done in the same lab. VDRL and RPR are equally valid, although quantitative results cannot be directly compared. It is expected that this test will become nonreactive with treatment, but some stay reactive for long periods, e.g., serofast reaction
    c. ***Neurosyphilis:***
        (1) Positive CSF VDRL or RPR is considered diagnostic if specimen is not contaminated with blood. This test is negative in about one-third with neurosyphilis. Some advocate CSF FTA-ABS, which is less specific but thought to be highly sensitive
        (2) CSF leukocytosis (>5 WBC/mm^3) is expected in active neurosyphilis and is a sensitive measure of effectiveness of therapy
    d. ***HIV:*** Standard serologic tests are usually accurate but rare false negatives are reported. There is an increased risk of neurosyphilis

C. Treatment: Penicillin G is preferred for all stages

1. **Primary and secondary**
    a. Benzathine penicillin G 2.4 mil units IM × 1
    b. <u>Follow-up:</u> Patients should be re-examined clinically and serologically at 6

and 12 mo. Patients with HIV should have evaluations at 2, 3, 6, 9, 12 and 24 mo ± LP at 6 mo. Treatment failure or reinfection is diagnosed if symptoms persist, symptoms recur, or 4-fold increase in VDRL or RPR titer by 6–12 mo: 1) Evaluate for HIV, 2) perform LP, and 3) retreat with benzathine penicillin 2.4 mil units IM × 3 (weekly)

If titer does not decrease by 4-fold at 6 mo then 1) evaluate for HIV, 2) follow-up clinical and serologic exams at 6 mo (3-mo intervals for HIV-infected patients), and 3) retreat if follow-up cannot be assured— benzathine penicillin 2.4 mil units IM × 3 (weekly)

   c. <u>HIV serology:</u> Indicated in all patients with syphilis; patients in high prevalence areas for HIV should be retested at 3 mo
   d. <u>LP:</u> Indicated in primary and secondary syphilis only if there are clinical signs and symptoms of neurologic involvement (ophthalmic, auditory symptoms, cranial nerve palsies) or with therapeutic failures
      Ophthalmic disease (uveitis): Slit lamp exam
   e. <u>Penicillin allergy:</u>
      Doxycycline 100 mg po bid × 2 wk <u>or</u> tetracycline 500 mg po qid × 2 wk
      <u>Intolerance to tetracyclines</u> (acceptable only in HIV-negative patients): Erythromycin 500 mg po qid × 2 wk <u>or</u> ceftriaxone 1 g/d for 8- to 10-day course
      <u>Pregnancy:</u> Skin test; if positive, desensitize and treat with penicillin*
   f. <u>HIV infection:</u> Benzathine penicillin G: 2.4 mil units ×1
   g. <u>Jarisch-Herxheimer reaction:</u> Acute febrile reaction accompanied by headache and myalgias. There are no proven methods to prevent this. Antipyretics are recommended for treatment. The reaction may induce early labor and cause fetal distress in pregnant women
2. **Latent syphilis** (see "Classification" above)
   a. <u>Early latent</u> (syphilis <1 yr): Diagnosis—documented seroconversion, unequivocal history of primary or secondary syphilis <1 yr previously or sex partner with syphilis <1 yr. <u>Treatment:</u> Benzathine penicillin G 2.4 mil units IM × 1; penicillin allergy, doxycycline 100 mg bid × 4 wk
   b. <u>Late latent</u> (syphilis >1 yr or unknown duration): Benzathine penicillin G 2.4 mil units IM × 3 at weekly intervals; penicillin allergy, doxycycline 100 mg bid × 4 wk
   c. <u>Follow-up:</u> VDRL or RPR at 6, 12, and 24 mo. Patients who develop signs or symptoms of syphilis have a 4-fold increase in titer or an initial titer of ≥1:32 that fails to decrease 4-fold in 12–24 mo should have LP and be retreated
   e. <u>Indications for LP:</u>
      —Neurologic or ophthalmic signs or symptoms (ophthalmic, auditory, cranial nerve symptoms)
      —Other evidence of active disease (aortitis, gumma, iritis, etc)
      —Treatment failure
      —HIV infection
      —Infection >1 yr or unknown duration plus titer ≥1:32
      —Infection >1 yr or unknown duration and nonpenicillin treatment planned
   f. <u>HIV serology:</u> Advocated for all syphilis patients
   g. <u>Penicillin allergy</u> (nonpregnant patients)
      —Infection <1 yr: Doxycycline 100 mg po bid <u>or</u> tetracycline 500 mg po qid × 2 wk
      —Infection >1 yr or unknown duration: Doxycycline 100 mg po bid or tetracycline 500 mg po qid × 4 wk

—Pregnancy: Skin test; if positive, desensitize and treat with penicillin*
(MMWR 1993;42(RR-14):44)

  h. <u>HIV infection:</u> LP, if normal—benzathine penicillin 2.4 mil units IM × 3 (weekly)

  i. <u>Evaluation:</u> Patients with latent syphilis should be evaluated for tertiary disease—aortitis, neurosyphilis, gummas, or iritis

3. **Neurosyphilis and ocular syphilis**
  a. Preferred: Aqueous penicillin G 12–24 mil units/d given as 3–4 mil units q4h × 10–14 days
  b. <u>Alternative</u> if outpatient compliance is assured: Procaine penicillin IM 2.4 mil units/d plus probenecid 500 mg po q6h for 10–14 days
  c. <u>Penicillin allergy:</u>
    —Ceftriaxone 2 g/d IV or IM × 10–14 days
    —Skin test; if positive, desensitize and treat with penicillin*
  d. <u>Follow-up:</u> If CSF initially showed pleocytosis, repeat LP q6mo until normal. Also evaluate CSF VDRL and protein, but these respond less rapidly and are of less certain significance. If cell count has not decreased by 6 mo or CSF is abnormal at 2 yr then retreat.

4. **Late syphilis** (other than neurosyphilis): Gumma, cardiovascular syphilis, etc
  LP: All patients
  Benzathine penicillin 2.4 mil units × 3 at weekly intervals
  <u>Penicillin allergy:</u> Doxycycline 100 mg po bid × 4 wk

---

*Skin test (see desensitization schedule see p 77)

D. Sex partners
1. <u>Patients sexually exposed to primary secondary or early latent syphilis</u> should be evaluated clinically and serologically: Contacts should be treated if seropositive or if seronegative and exposed <90 days. Presumptive treatment should also be given if exposure was >90 days, serologic test results are unavailable, and source had primary, secondary, or early latent syphilis. Patients with syphilis of unknown duration with a nontreponemal test titer of ≥ 1:32 are considered to have early syphilis for purposes of partner notification
2. <u>Long-term partners of patients with late syphilis</u> should be evaluated clinically and serologically
3. <u>Time periods</u> used to identify at-risk sex partners are 3 mo plus duration of symptoms for primary syphilis, 6 mo plus duration of symptoms for secondary syphilis, and 1 yr for early latent syphilis

E. Pregnancy
1. <u>Testing:</u> All women should have screening tests for syphilis in early pregnancy; this should be repeated at 28 wk and at delivery in areas of high prevalence or women with high risk
2. <u>Treatment:</u> Penicillin regimens as summarized above. Penicillin allergy: skin test and desensitize if positive. Note: Some experts recommend a second dose of benzathine penicillin 2.4 mil units at 1 wk for pregnant women with primary, secondary, or early latent syphilis
3. <u>Jarish-Herxheimer reaction:</u> Pregnant women treated for syphilis in the second half of pregnancy who have a Jarish-Herxheimer reaction have increased risk of premature labor and fetal distress

MANAGEMENT OF SYPHILIS: SUMMARY

Form	Initial treatment	LP	Follow-up VDRL/RPR	Expectation VDRL/RPR	Indications to retreat
Primary syphilis	Initial: Benzathine penicillin 2.4 mil units IM × 1 Retreatment: Benzathine penicillin 2.4 mil units IM × 3 (weekly)	Neuro symptoms Treatment failure	3 and 6 mo HIV: 2,3,6,9, 12 and 24 mo	4-fold decrease at 3 mo	Titer increases 4-fold Titer fails to decrease 4-fold at 3 mo + noncompliance or HIV infection Symptoms persist or recur
Secondary syphilis	Initial: Benzathine penicillin 2.4 mil units IM × 1 Retreatment: Benzathine penicillin 2.4 mil units IM × 3 (weekly)	Neuro symptoms Treatment failure	3 and 6 mo HIV: 2,3,6,9, and 12 mo	4-fold decrease at 6 mo	Titer increases 4-fold Titer fails to decrease 4-fold at 6 mo + noncompliance or HIV infection Symptoms persist or recur
Early latent (<1 yr)	Initial: Benzathine penicillin 2.4 mil units IM × 1 Retreatment or HIV infection: Benzathine penicillin 2.4 mil units IM × 3 (weekly)	Neuro symptoms HIV infection Treatment failure	6, 12 mo and q6mo	4-fold decrease if titer ≥1:32 within 6 mo or titer ≥1:4 at 1 yr	Titer increases 4-fold Titer of ≥1:32 fails to decrease 4-fold at 6 mo Develops signs or symptoms of syphilis
Late latent (>1 yr or unknown duration)	Benzathine penicillin 2.4 mil units IM × 3 (weekly)	Neuro sx HIV infection Treatment failure Titer ≥1:32 Non-penicillin treatment	6, 12 mo and q6mo	4-fold decrease if titer ≥1:16 within 12 mo (lower initial titers may remain unchanged)	Titer of ≥1:16 fails to decrease 4-fold at 12 mo with lower initial titer: Increase titer by 4-fold at ≥3 mo
Late syphilis (tertiary, not neurosyphilis)	Benzathine penicillin 2.4 mil units IM × 3 (weekly)	Indicated	6 and 12 mo	As above Granulomatous lesions should heal	As above Documentation of T. pallidum or other histology feature of late syphilis
Neurosyphilis (or ocular syphilis)	Aqueous penicillin G 12–24 mil units/d × 10–14 days	Required	Every 6 mo until negative	CSF WBC decrease at 6 mo and CSF normal at 1 yr	CSF WBC decrease at 6 mo or CSF still abnormal at 2 yr or persisting signs and symptoms of inflammatory response at ≥3 mo or 4-fold increase in CSF VDRL at ≥6 mo or failure of CSF VDRL of ≥1:16 to decrease by 2-fold at 6 mo or 4-fold by 12 mo

III. CHLAMYDIA TRACHOMATIS (MMWR 1993;42(RR-12))

A. Spectrum of disease
- Men: Nongonococcal urethritis, epididymitis, proctitis, and proctocolitis (renal intercourse)
- Women: Mucopurulent cervicitis, salpingitis (PID), postpartum endometritis, cystitis (acute dysuria-pyuria or urethral syndrome), perihepatitis (Fitz-Hugh-Curtis syndrome), proctitis, and proctocolitis
- Infants (postexposure): Conjunctivitis and pneumonitis
- Miscellaneous: Reiter's syndrome (reactive arthritis, conjunctivitis, and urethritis), chronic conjunctivitis, pharyngeal colonization (but not pharyngitis)

B. Screening candidates
- Mucopurulent cervicitis
- Sexually active women <20 yr
- Women 20–24 yr who meet the following criteria and those >24 yr who meet both criteria: Inconsistent use of barrier contraceptives or new or >1 sex partner in past 3 mo
- Pregnant females during third trimester

Screening women is the major element of a chlamydial prevention program. Verification of initial positive test should be performed if the test was not a positive culture and the patient is considered low risk.

C. Detection
1. Polymerase chain reaction (PCR) (Roche Molecular Systems, Branchburg, NJ) and ligase chain reaction (LCR) (Abbott Laboratories, Abbott Park, IL). These assays require about 8 hr and show sensitivity of 86–98%; specificity is 99–100%, and they can be performed on urine. The cost is $14–28/specimen (although commercial labs charge more)
2. Conditions that warrant presumptive diagnosis of chlamydial infection*

Condition	Chlamydia patients	Prevalence in partners
Nongonococcal urethritis	30–40%	10–43%
Pelvic inflammatory disease	8–54%	36%
Epididymitis (<35 yr)	50%	10–43%
Gonococcal infection: Men	5–30%	40%
Gonococcal infection: Women	25–50%	Unknown

*Patients with these conditions should be immediately treated, including an antibiotic for chlamydia. Sex partners should be treated without waiting for results of tests. Chlamydia tests are encouraged even if a presumed diagnosis is made to 1) ensure proper care, especially if symptoms persist; 2) facilitate counseling; 3) provide better grounds for partner notification; and 4) improve compliance.

3. Conditions that may not warrant presumptive diagnosis of chlamydial infection

Condition	Chlamydia patients	Prevalence in partners
Mucopurulent cervicitis	9–51%	2–27%
Proctitis (homosexual men)	8–16%	Unknown
Acute urethral syndrome	13–63%	Unknown

D. Treatment (CID 1995;20:S66)
  1. Preferred*
     - Azithromycin 1 g po × 1 day
     - Doxycycline 100 mg po bid × 7 days (contraindicated in pregnancy and growing children)
  2. Alternatives
     - Levofloxacin 500 mg po qd × 7 days or ofloxacin 300 mg po bid × 7 days (Both are contraindicated in pregnancy and children ≤17 yr)
     - Erythromycin ethylsuccinate 800 mg po qid × 7 days
     - Erythromycin base 500 mg po qid × 7 days
  3. Pregnancy
     Preferred: Erythromycin base 500 mg po qid × 7 days or amoxicillin 500 mg po tid × 7 days
     - Erythromycin ethylsuccinate 800 mg po qid × 7 days or
     - Erythromycin ethylsuccinate 400 mg po qid × 14 days or
     - If amoxicillin or erythromycin not tolerated: Azithromycin 1 g po
  4. HIV infection: As above

---

* Azithromycin has the advantage of single dose observed therapy. A comparative trial with doxycycline for PID showed azithromycin was significantly better, presumably because of reduced compliance with tetracycline. Ofloxacin is equally effective compared with azithromycin and doxycycline but is relatively expensive and offers no dosing advantage. Erythromycin is less efficacious than azithromycin or doxycycline and causes substantial gastrointestinal toxicity.

E. Follow-up: Not indicated unless symptoms persist or recur or erythromycin is used. Failure rates with doxycycline regimen are 0–3% for men and 0–8% for women.

F. Disease prevention: Patient should avoid sex for 7 days from initiation of treatment, and until all partners are treated and cured

G. Partner referral: Evaluation and treatment of partners within 60 days. Last sex partner should be evaluated, tested, and treated regardless of the time interval

H. Reporting: *C. trachomatis* has required reporting in most states

I. Prevention of ophthalmic neonatorum (*N. gonorrhoeae* and *C. trachomatis*): Instill into the eye <1 hr after birth: Silver nitrate (1%) aqueous solution × 1 or erythromycin (0.5%) ophthalmic ointment × 1

IV. LYMPHOGRANULOMA VENEREUM

A. Agent: Biovar (strain) of *C. trachomatis,* invasive serotypes L1, L2, L3

B. Symptoms: Tender inguinal and/or femoral lymphadenopathy; protocolitis in women and gay men

C. Diagnosis: Serology: CF titer ≥ 1:64

D. Treatment:
  1. Drainage: Bubos may require incision or aspiration
  2. Preferred antibiotic: Doxycycline 100 mg po bid × 21 days
  3. Alternatives: Erythromycin 500 mg po qid × 21 days
     Expected responses: 50% have healed ulcers at 7 days, 80% at 14 days, and 100% at 28 days. Relapse rate is 3–5%
  4. Pregnancy: Use erythromycin regimen

5. <u>Sex partners</u>: Examine and treat partners of 30 days prior to onset of symptoms
6. <u>HIV infection</u>: As above

E. Sex Partners: Examine, test, and treat partners within 30 days

F. Reporting: Required in most states

V. GENITAL HERPES SIMPLEX

A. Treatment

	Duration	Acyclovir	Valacyclovir	Famciclovir
First episode	7–10 days	400 mg tid	1 g bid	250 mg tid
Recurrent	5 days	400 mg tid or 800 mg bid	500 mg bid	125 mg bid
Suppressive	>5 yr	400 mg bid	500 mg qd or 1 g/d	250 mg bid
Severe disease	2–7 days*	5–10 mg/kg IV q8h		

* Then oral therapy to complete 10 days

1. <u>First episode:</u> Acyclovir treatment shortens duration of pain, viral shedding, and systemic symptoms. Treatment has no effect on rate or frequency of relapses
2. <u>Recurrent episodes:</u> Should be started with the prodrome or within 1 day of onset of lesions
3. <u>Prophylaxis:</u> Consider with ≥6 recurrences/yr: Safety and efficacy are documented for continuous prophylaxis up to 10 yr without cumulative toxicity or risk of resistance (JID 1994;169:1338). There is also a significant reduction in viral shedding. Suppressive treatment is contraindicated in pregnancy
4. <u>HIV infection</u>

	Duration	Acyclovir	Valacyclovir	Famciclovir
Recurrent	5–10 days	400 mg tid	1 g bid	500 mg bid
Suppression	—	400–800 mg 2–3 ×/d	500 mg bid	500 mg bid

4. <u>Pregnancy:</u> Registry to report exposure experiences with acyclovir or valacyclovir: 800-722-9292, ext 58465. To date the experience shows no risk to the infant with 601 exposures to acyclovir; this sample size is adequate to detect a 2-fold teratogenic risk over the 3% baseline rate of birth defects (MMWR 1993;42:806). There are sparse data about famciclovir or valacyclovir in pregnant women, so acyclovir is preferred. Indications for acyclovir in pregnancy:
   • First episode of genital herpes
   • Severe genital HSV or extragenital HSV disease (encephalitis, disseminated disease, etc.)
5. <u>Perinatal infections:</u> Most perinatal HSV infections occur with mothers who have no history of HSV. Risk of transmission is highest with delivery at the time the mother has <u>primary HSV</u> (30–50%); risk with recurrent HSV at the time of delivery is about 3%. Women at risk (HSV negative pregnant woman and HSV infected partner) should be warned of risk of unprotected sexual contact in late pregnancy

B. Management of pregnancies complicated by genital herpes simplex
1. No signs of genital HSV at onset of delivery—vaginal delivery
2. HSV lesions at onset of labor—most recommend C-section
3. Severe genital HSV during pregnancy—oral or IV acyclovir

C. Neonatal herpes: Treat infant with acyclovir 30–60 mg/kg/d × 10–21 days

VI. CHANCROID

A. Agent: *Haemophilus ducreyi*

B. Clinical features: Painful genital ulcers ± tender inguinal adenopathy with or without suppuration; uncommon in U.S. (MMWR 1995;44:567)

C. Diagnosis: Culture requires specialized media that are not commercially available. Even with these media, the yield is <80%. PCR may soon be available. Presumptive diagnosis: Typical clinical findings <u>plus</u> no evidence of syphilis (dark-field of lesion exudate or negative serology at least 7 days after onset of ulcer) <u>and</u> atypical for herpes simplex or negative tests for herpes simplex. Presence of suppurative inguinal adenopathy is nearly diagnostic

D. Treatment (CID 1995;20:539)
1. <u>Preferred:</u>
   - Azithromycin 1 g po × 1 or
   - Ceftriaxone 250 mg IM × 1 or
   - Erythromycin base 500 mg po qid × 7 days
   - Ciprofloxacin 500 mg po bid × 3 days (contraindicated in pregnant or lactating women and with age <18 yr)
2. <u>Alternatives:</u> None
3. <u>HIV infection:</u> All regimens are less effective—azithromycin and multiple dose regimens are preferred (STD 1994;21:231)

E. Follow-up: Symptoms improve within 3 days, and objective improvement is seen within 7 days. Examine 3–7 days after treatment. If not improved, consider wrong diagnosis, co-infection (10% coinfected with HSV or *T. pallidum*), HIV infection, noncompliance, *H. ducreyi*, resistance to (rare with recommended treatments), need for needle aspiration of fluctuant adenopathy.

F. Partner referral: Examine and treat partners <10 days

G. HIV infection: Longer treatment or close follow-up

VII. GRANULOMA INGUINALE (DONOVANOSIS)

A. Agent: *Calymmatobacterium granulomatis*

B. Geography: Rare in U.S.; endemic in India, Australia, South Africa, New Guinea

C. Clinical presentation: Painless, progressive genital ulcer that is highly vascularized (beefy red) and bleeds easily

D. Treatment
- Trimethoprim-sulfamethoxazole 1 DS bid until healed (≥21 days)
- Doxycycline 100 mg bid until healed (≥21 days)
- Alternative: Ciprofloxacin 750 mg bid × 21 days, erythromycin 500 mg po qid × 21 days, or azithromycin 1 g/wk × 3

E. **Sex partners:** Examine partners within 60 days and treat those with symptoms

F. **Pregnancy:** Erythromycin ± aminoglycoside (gentamicin)

G. **HIV infection:** Consider adding gentamicin to treatment regimen

VIII. PEDICULOSIS PUBIS (PUBIC LICE)

A. **Treatment**
- Permethrin (1%) cream rinse (Nix) applied to affected area and washed after 10 min or
- Lindane (1%) shampoo applied 4 min and then thoroughly washed off (not recommended for pregnant or lactating women) or
- Pyrethrins and piperonyl butoxide (nonprescription) applied to affected areas and washed off after 10 min

Note: Permethrin has less potential toxicity with inappropriate use; lindane is least expensive and non-toxic if used correctly

B. **Adjunctive:** Retreat after 7 days if lice or eggs are detected at hair–skin junction. Clothes and bed linen of past 2 days should be decontaminated (machine washed or machine dried using hot cycle or dry cleaned) or removed from body contact at least 12 hr

C. **Follow-up:** Evaluate at 1 wk if symptoms persist. Retreat if lice or eggs are seen at hair–skin junctions

D. **Pregnancy:** Permethrin or pyrethrins

E. **Sex partners:** Treat sex partners within preceding month as above

IX. SCABIES (*SARCOPTES SCABIEI*)

A. **Symptoms:** Pruritus

B. **Recommended:** Permethrin (5% cream, 30 g) massaged and left 8–14 hr (preferred—Semin Dermatol 12:22, 1993). Lindane considered preferable drug for scabies by *Medical Letter* consultants (Med Lett 1995;37:117)

C. **Alternatives:** Lindane (1%) 1 oz lotion or 30 g cream applied thinly to all areas of the body below neck and washed thoroughly at 8 hr (not recommended for pregnant or lactating women) or sulfur (6%) ointment applied thinly to all areas nightly × 3; wash off previous application before new applications and wash thoroughly 24 hr after last application. Ivermectin (200 μg/kg po × 1 or 0.8% topical solution) appears to be effective (NEJM 1995;333:26)

D. **Sex partners and close household contacts:** Treat as above

E. **Pregnancy:** Avoid lindane

F. **Adjunctive:** Clothing and bed linen contaminated by patient should be decontaminated (machine washed or machine dried using hot cycle or dry cleaned or removed from body contact × 72 hr)

G. **Outbreaks:** Control can usually be achieved only by treating the entire population at risk

X. HEPATITIS B

Rates and risk of HBV are high in patients with STDs. Serologic tests of STD clinic patients show evidence of past infection in 28% of persons ≥25 yr and

7% in those <25 yr. HBV vaccination is recommended for 1) sexually active homosexual and bisexual men; 2) men and women diagnosed with another STD, and 3) persons with more than one sex partner in the prior 6 mo (MMWR 1999;48:33) Usual regimen is three doses at 0, 1, and 6 mo at a cost of about $50/dose (see p 114).

XI. HUMAN PAPILLOMAVIRUS: WARTS

A. Types: Exophytic warts are usually benign and caused by HPB types 6 and 11. Types 16, 18, 31, 33, and 35 are associated with genital dysplasia and carcinoma; these types are usually subclinical

B. Treatment goals: No treatment is known to eradicate HPV, reduce risk of cervical dysplasia or cervical carcinoma, or prevent recurrence (CID 1995;20:S91). The goal of therapy is to eliminate the symptoms and emotional distress associated with exophytic warts

C. Treatments: Determined by wart area, wart count, anatomic site, morphology, cost, patient preference, and provider experience. Most treatments are 60–70% effective in clearing exophytic warts and show recurrence rates > 25% (Int J Dermatol 1995;34:29)

1. Patient applied
   - Podofilox 0.5% soln or gel (Condylox) apply bid × 3 days, then no therapy × 4 days; repeat cycle up to 4 times. This treatment is relatively brief, inexpensive, safe, and simple. Local pain is common. The wart area should be <10 cm^2 and the total volume of podofilox should be <0.5 mL
   - Imiquimod 5% (Aldara) cream (see Med Lett 1997;39:118)
     Apply hs 3×/wk—daily for up to 16 wk. Wash with mild soap and water 6–10 hr after application. Local inflammation is common. More expensive than podofilox (AWP $432/16 wk vs $56/4 wk for podofilox)
2. Provider applied
   - Cryotherapy: liquid nitrogen or cryoprobe, repeat q1–2wk. Requires technical expertise
   - Podophyllin resin 10–25% applied to wart and air-dried. Repeat weekly
   - Trichloroacetic acid or bichloroacetic acid 80–90% applied to wart and air-dried
3. Alternative treatments
   - Laser surgery
   - Intralesional interferon: Rarely recommended because of systemic reactions and requirement for multiple visits
   <u>Management by anatomical site</u>
   - Cervical warts: Must consult expert to exclude high-grade SIL
   - Vaginal warts: Cryotherapy or podophyllin
   - Meatal warts: Cryotherapy or podophyllin 10–25%
   - Anal warts: Cryotherapy, surgical removal, or TCA/BCA 80–90%
   - Oral warts: Cryotherapy or surgical removal

D. Follow-up: Not mandatory after warts have cleared

E. Sex partners: Not necessary because there is no curative therapy and treatment does not reduce transmission.

F. Pregnancy: Use of podofilox, podophyllin, and imiquimod is contra-indicated in pregnancy. HPV types 6 and 11 can cause laryngeal papillomatosis in offspring, but mechanism of transmission is unclear. Cesarean section should not be performed to prevent this complication.

G. **Subclinical warts:** Indirect tests are Pap smear, colposcopy, biopsy, or acetic acid application; definitive diagnosis requires detection of HPV DNA or RNA or capsid proteins. Pap smear diagnosis does not correlate well with detection by HPV DNA in cervical cells; cell changes caused by HPV are similar to mild dysplasia and often regress spontaneously. Therefore, screening for subclinical HPV with nucleic acid or capsid antigen tests for detection of HPV is not recommended. Management is based on results of dysplasia on Pap smear.

H. **Education:** Genital HPV infection is common, usually sexually transmitted, and has a variable incubation period. Most warts are benign; exophytic genital warts are not associated with carcinoma. Recurrence in 3 months post-treatment is common; likelihood of transmission post-therapy is unknown. The value of disclosure to prior partners is also unknown.

XII. GENITAL ULCER DISEASE

Agents	Diagnosis	Treatment*	Comment
Herpes simplex	Culture or antigen test for HSV	See p 293	Most common cause in U.S.
Syphilis	Dark-field exam or direct immuno-fluorescence test	See p 288	Second most common identifiable cause in U.S.
Chancroid	Culture for H. ducreyi	See p 294	Most labs do not have the appropriate media; rare in U.S.

*Based on results of above tests. About 25% will have no laboratory confirmed diagnosis; in this case treat for the most likely agent.

XIII. URETHRITIS

A. **Diagnosis:** Any of the following
   — Mucoid or purulent urethral discharge
   — Positive leukocyte esterase test on first voided urine or microscopic exam of first voided urine showing ≥10 WBC/HPF
   — Urethral Gram stain showing >5 WBC/HPF

B. **Microbiology:** Evaluate for gonococcal and chlamydial infection.
   Gonococcal: Presumptive evidence is urethral discharge with >5 WBC/HPF plus typical Gram-negative diplococci.
   Nongonococcal: *C. trachomatis* (20–55%), *Ureaplasma urealyticium* (20%), *Trichomonas vaginalis* (2–5%), HSV (rare)

C. **Management**
   1. Gram stain of discharge
      a. Gram-negative intracellular displococci + >5 WBC/HPF: Treat for *N. gonorrhoeae* and *C. trachomatis;* refer partners
      b. Negative Gram stain + > 5 WBC/HPF: Test for *N. gonorrhoeae* and *C. trachomatis;* treat for *C. trachomatis;* refer partners if tests are positive
      c. Negative tests: Test for *N. gonorrhoeae,* and *C. trachomatis;* defer treatment pending test results unless patient is at high risk and unlikely to return: treat patient and partner for *N. gonorrhoeae* and *C. trachomatis*

2. Gram stain unavailable: Test for *N. gonorrhoeae* and *C. trachomatis;* treat for *N. gonorrhoeae* and *C. trachomatis;* refer partners if tests are positive
3. Nongonococcal urethritis: Treat for *C. trachomatis*

D. Sex partners: Evaluate and treat sex partners within ≤ 60 days of symptomatic patients or last sex partner if last sex preceded intervals.

E. Follow-up and disease prevention: Avoid sex until patient and partner have completed 7 days of therapy.

F. Persistent or recurrent urethritis
1. Reexposure or noncompliance with original regimen: Retreat
2. Compliant and no reexposure: Intraurethral swab for wet mount and culture for *T. vaginalis.* Treatment is metronidazole 2 g po × 1 plus either Erythromycin base 500 mg po qid × 7 days <u>or</u> Erythromycin ethylsuccinate 800 mg po qid × 7 days

XIV. EPIDIDYMITIS

A. Microbiology
Men <35 yr: *N. gonorrhoeae, C. trachomatis;* gay men are likely to have enteric pathogens as well
Men >35 yr: *E. coli* and other urinary tract pathogens

B. Diagnosis: (1) Urethral smear for Gram stain for *N. gonorrhoeae* and nongonococcal urethritis (≥5 WBC/OIF) suggests gonococcal infection, (2) urine LCR for *N. gonorrhoeae,* and *C. trachomatis,* (3) uncentrifuged urine for WBCs and Gram stain for GNB.

C. Treatment
- *N. gonorrhoeae:* Ceftriaxone 250 mg IM × 1 plus doxycycline, 100 mg po bid × 10 days
- *C. trachomatis:* Ofloxacin 300 mg po bid × 10 days or levofloxacin 500 mg qd

D. Follow-up: Expect improvement within 3 days; swelling >1 wk—evaluate for testicular cancer, TB, fungal infections, abscess, or infarction.

E. Sex partners: Evaluate and treat sex partners with sexually transmitted epididymitis if contact was within 60 days and gonococci or *C. trachomatis* is suspected or confirmed. Patient should avoid sexual intercourse until patient and partner are cured.

XV. PROCTITIS, PROCTOCOLITIS, AND ENTERITIS

A. Classification

Condition	Symptoms	Microbiology
Proctitis*	Anorectal pain, tenesmus, constipation, rectal discharge	*N. gonorrhoeae, C. trachomatis,* syphilis, HSV
Proctocolitis*	Symptoms of proctitis plus diarrhea ± cramps and inflammation of colonic mucosa to 12 cm	*Shigella, E. histolytica, Campylobacter* sp, LGV; *C. trachomatis* (rare)
Enteritis	Diarrhea without signs of proctitis or colitis	*Giardia;* HIV infection—CMV, *M. avium,* microsporidia, *Cryptosporidium, Isospora, Salmonella*

*Proctitis indicates inflammation limited to the distal 10–12 cm of the colon. Proctocolitis shows inflammation extending beyond 12 cm.

B. **Diagnosis** (proctitis): Anoscopy with evaluation of anorectal pus for PMNs, Gram stain, and evaluation for gonococci, *C. trachomatis,* syphilis, and HSV

C. **Treatment** (proctitis with history of recent receptive anal intercourse plus anorectal pus): Ceftriaxone 125 mg IM *plus* doxycycline 100 mg po bid × 7 days

XVI. MUCOPURULENT CERVICITIS (MPC)

A. **Agents:** Can be caused by *N. gonorrhoeae* or *C. trachomatis,* but most cases involve neither. Most women with gonococcal and chlamydial infections do not have MPC. MPC is not a sensitive predictor of infection.

B. **Diagnosis:** Yellow endocervical exudate in endocervical canal or in an endocervical swab specimen. Some women have no symptoms, some have vaginal discharge, and some have abnormal vaginal bleeding, especially postcoital bleeding.

C. **Test:** Chlamydia trachomatis and *N. gonorrhoeae*

D. **Treatment:** Recommendations based on results of tests of *N. gonorrhoeae* and *C. trachomatis* unless likelihood of infection with either organism is high or patient is unlikely to return for treatment.
   1. Gonococcal endocervicitis: see p 285
   2. Chlamydia endocervicitis: see p 290
   3. Treat for both if high prevalence of both infections, e.g., many STD clinics
   4. Treatment may be delayed for laboratory test results if prevalence of both infections is low and compliance with return visit is likely

E. **Sex partners:** Partners of women treated for gonorrhea or *C. trachomatis* should be examined and treated; patients should avoid sex until treated, i.e., 7 days.

XVII. PELVIC INFLAMMATORY DISEASE

A. **Conditions:** PID includes endometritis, salpingitis, tubo-ovarian abscess, and pelvic peritonitis.

B. **Microbiology:** Most common—*N. gonorrhoeae* and *C. trachomatis*; less common—endogenous bacteria including anaerobes, Gram-negative bacilli, and streptococci. Role of mycoplasma is unclear.

C. **Diagnosis:** Sexually active women with uterine/adnexal tenderness or cervical motion tenderness. Additional supporting findings are: (1) oral temperature $\geq 101°F$, (2) cervical/vaginal mucopurulent discharge, (3) WBC's in vaginal secretions, (4) increased ESR, (5) elevated CRP, or (6) lab documentation of *N. gonorrhoeae* or *C. trachmatis*

D. **Indications for hospitalization and/or parenteral antibiotics:**
   1. Surgical emergency such as possible acute appendicitis
   2. Pregnancy
   3. Patient failed oral therapy
   4. Patient is unable to follow or tolerate oral therapy
   5. Severe illness as indicated by high fever, nausea, and vomiting
   6. Tubo-ovarian abscess

E. **Treatment**
   1. <u>Parenteral regimen</u>
      • Cefoxitin 2 g IV q6h or cefotetan 2 g IV q12h until at least 24 hr after clinical improvement *plus* doxycycline 100 mg bid po or IV × 14 days*

- Clindamycin 900 mg IV q8h *plus* gentamicin 2 mg/kg IV or IM followed by 1.5 mg/kg q8h at least 24 hr after clinical improvement then doxycycline 100 mg po bid × 14 days or clindamycin 450 mg po qid × 14 days (clindamycin preferred for tubo-ovarian abscess)
  Alternatives/parenteral regimen
  - Ofloxacin 400 mg IV q12h or levofloxacin 500 mg IV qd *plus* metronidazole 500 mg IV q12h
  - Ampicillin/sulbactam 3 g IV q6h *plus* doxycycline 100 mg IV or po q12h
  - Ciprofloxacin 200 mg IV q12h *plus* doxycycline 100 mg IV or po q12h *plus* metronidazole 500 mg IV q12h
  2. Oral therapy
    - Single dose parenteral plus oral:
      Ceftriaxone 250 mg IM × 1 or cefotaxime or
      Cefoxitin 2 g IM plus probenecid 1 g po
      Plus metronidazole 500 mg po bid × 7 days or
    - Oral regimen: Ofloxacin 400 mg po bid or levofloxacin 500 mg qd × 14 days plus metronidazole 500 mg po bid × 14 days

F. Follow-up: Patients should show substantial clinical improvement within 3 days. Outpatient evaluation: Follow-up in 72 hr with expectation of substantial clinical improvement or hospitalization. Patients should be examined 7–10 days after therapy.

G. Sex partners: Examine all sex partners and treat for *N. gonorrhoeae* and *C. trachomatis*.

H. Expected clinical cure rates with suggested antibiotic regimens: 85–95% for PID with most failures ascribed to tubo-ovarian abscesses (CID 1994;19:720). Response expected within 3 days. Major concern is late sequelae with infertility (16%) and ectopic pregnancy (9%) (STD 1992;19:185)

XVII. VAGINITIS/VAGINOSIS

A. Diagnostic tests:
Requirement: pH paper and 2 slides for microscopy—one with 2 drops of normal saline and the second with 10% KOH
Interpretation
  - pH >4.5: Bacterial vaginosis or trichomoniasis
  - Saline mount—*T. vaginalis* or clue cells of bacterial vaginosis
  - KOH—*Candida* pseudohyphae or release of amine odor with bacterial vaginosis

B. Trichomoniasis (almost always an STD)
  1. Clinical features: Women—malodorous yellow-green discharge with vulvar irritation
  2. Diagnosis: Wet mount or culture. PMNs, pH > 4.7, and a positive amine odor test. Sensitivity of wet mount is 60–70%; culture is more sensitive.
  3. Usual treatment: Metronidazole 2 g po as single dose
     Alternative: Metronidazole 375 mg or 500 mg po bid × 7 days
     Allergy to metronidazole: Desensitization (Am J Obstet Gynecol 174:934, 1996).
     Topical metronidazole is not recommended.
  4. Treatment failure: Repeat metronidazole 2 g/d × 3–5 days; if treatment fails again consult CDC 770-488-4115 or http://www.cdc.gov/std
  5. Asymptomatic women: Treat as above
  6. Pregnant women: Metronidazole 2 g × 1. Note: Treatment of

asymptomatic trichomoniasis in pregnant women does not reduce preterm delivery and may do harm. Routine screening and treatment should not be done (NEJM 2001; 345:487)

7. Lactating women: Treat with 2 g metronidazole and suspend breastfeeding × 24 hr
8. Sex partners: Treat with 2 g metronidazole or 500 mg po bid × 7 days
9. Disease prevention: Patient and partner should avoid sex until both are cured
10. Treatment failures: Retreat with metronidazole 500 mg po bid × 7 days
    Persistent failures: 2 g dose daily × 3–5 days

C. Bacterial vaginosis

1. Etiology: Dysbiosis of the vaginal flora with reduction in H_2O_2 producing lactobacilli by anaerobic bacteria, *G. vaginalis,* and *Mycoplasma hominis*. Cause is unknown. Frequency is increased with multiple sex partners, but rare cases are seen in virgins. Treatment of male sex partners is not helpful.
2. Frequency: Frequency in sexually active women in STD and gynecology clinics is 5–20% (J Obstet Gynecol 1993;169:446).
3. Clinical symptoms: Malodorous vaginal discharge; over half of cases are asymptomatic.
4. Diagnosis: Three of the following:
   1. Homogeneous, white non-inflammatory discharge that adheres to vaginal walls
   2. Presence of clue cells
   3. pH of vaginal fluid > 4.5
   4. Fishy odor of vaginal discharge with or without addition of 10% KOH ("whiff test")
5. Microscopic exam shows no polymorphonuclear cells, sparse lactobacclli, and numerous coccobacillary forms on epithelial cells (clue cells). Cultures are not indicated.
6. Complications: There is an association between BV and adverse outcome of pregnancy (postpartum endometritis, amnionitis, preterm delivery, preterm labor, premature rupture of membranes) and infectious complications of gynecologic surgery. A large trial designed to examine this issue failed to demonstrate any benefit with metronidazole therapy (NEJM 2000;342:534).
7. Goals of treatment:
   Non-pregnant women: Relieve symptoms.
   Pregnant women: Relieve symptoms and prevent adverse outcome of pregnancy (especially those with prior preterm birth or maternal age > 50).
8. Treatment
   a. Non-pregnant:
      • Metronidazole 500 mg po bid × 7 days
      • Clindamycin 2% (5 g) intravaginal hs × 7 days
      • Metronidazole gel 0.75% (5 g) intravaginal bid × 5 days
      • Alternative: Metronidazole 2 g po × 1 or clindamycin 300 mg po bid × 7 days or clindamycin ovules 100 mg intravaginally qd hs × 3 days
        Cure rates for preferred regimens: 75–84%
   b. Pregnant: Bacterial vaginosis is associated with increased risk of preterm delivery. Some studies show treatment is associated with reduced rates of preterm delivery (NEJM 1995;333:1732; Am J Obstet Gynecol 1994;171:345) and some do not (NEJM 2000;342:5334). Therefore, some recommend screening and

treatment at the first visit. Recommendations for treatment are:
Preferred: Metronidazole 250 mg po tid × 7 days
Alternatives
- Metronidazole 2 g po × 1
- Clindamycin 300 mg po bid × 7 days
- Metronidazole gel 0.75% (5 g) intravaginal bid × 5 days
- Metronidazole 250 mg po tid × 7 days
9. <u>Sex partners:</u> No evaluation

D. Vulvovaginal candidiasis (not considered an STD)

Includes CDC 2002 guidelines and IDSA Guidelines (CID 2000;30:672)

1. <u>Clinical features:</u> Vaginal discharge and vulvar pruritis
2. <u>Diagnosis:</u> Vulvovaginal erythema and white discharge. KOH wet prep or Gram stain showing yeast or pseudohyphae, or positive culture. (Culture is non-specific) Vaginal pH is usually <4.7 and PMNs increased. About 10–20% of healthy women harbor *Candida* sp in the genital tract.
3. <u>Classification:</u> (CID 2000;30:672) Uncomplicated–mild to moderate severity, sporadic, *C. albicans,* normal host. Complicated: Severe disease, recurrent, non-albicans species, abnormal host (uncontrolled diabetes, immunosuppression, corticosteroids, HIV, etc)
4. <u>Treatment:</u> Douching is contraindicated (Obstet Gynecol 1993;81:601) Intravaginal preparation (3- to 7-day regimens are usually more effective than single dose). Topical agents are oil based and may weaken latex condoms and diaphragms. Longer regimens and azoles are advocated for complicated cases.
<u>Topical agents:</u>
- Butoconazole 2% cream (5 g)* at hs × 3 days or 2% sustained release (5%) × 1
- Clotrimazole 1% cream* (5 g)* daily × 7–14 days.
- Clotrimazole 100 mg vaginal tab* daily × 7 days or 2 tabs daily × 3 days or 500 mg tab × 1.
- Miconazole 2% cream* (5 g) daily × 7 days.
- Miconazole 200 mg supp* daily × 3 days or 100 mg supp* daily × 7 days.
- Nystatin 100,000 unit vaginal tablet, one/day × 7–14 days.
- Tioconazole 6.5% ointment (5 g)* × 1.
- Terconazole 0.4% cream (5 g) daily × 7 days or 0.8% cream (5 g) daily × 3 days.
- Terconazole 80 mg supp daily × 3 days.

---

* Available over-the-counter.

<u>Systemic agents:</u>
- Preferred: Fluconazole 150 mg po × 1
- Alternatives: Itraconazole 200 mg bid × 1 day or ketoconazole 500 mg po × 5 days (CID 2000;30:672)
<u>Severe disease:</u>
- Topical azole × 7–14 days
- Fluconazole 150 mg po and repeat at 3 days
5. <u>Expected response rate:</u> 70–90% within 48–72 hr. Patients may be classified as uncomplicated vulvovaginitis (mild to moderate, sporadic, normal host, and sensitive *C. albicans*) vs complicated vulvovaginitis (severe disease, abnormal host, reduced susceptibility of *Candida*). Uncomplicated disease responds well to azoles including single dose and short course (7 days). Patients with complicated vulvovaginitis often require longer therapy (10–14 days).

6. <u>Sex partners:</u> No evaluation
7. <u>Pregnancy:</u> Topical azoles (clotrimazole, miconazole, butoconazole, and terconazole) × 7 days
8. <u>HIV serology:</u> Not indicated for vaginal candidiasis per se.
9. <u>Recurrent or complicated and refractory vulvovaginal candidiasis:</u>
   Topical agent × 7–14 days or fluconazole 150 mg po and repeat 3 days later ± maintenance: Clotrimazole 500 mg topically q wk × 6 mo <u>or</u> itraconazole 400 mg q month <u>or</u> itraconazole 100 mg po qd × 6 mo. IDSA guideline is for azole therapy po in standard dose ×2 wk, then fluconazole 150 mg q wk, ketoconazole 100 mg qd, itraconazole 100 mg qod, or daily topical azole. Treatment of sex partners is not effective and should not be conducted unless there is symptomatic balanitis or penile dermatitis
10. <u>HIV infection:</u> Incidence of vaginal candidiasis is increased, but response to therapy is usually good. Standard treatment should be given

XVIII. PAP SMEARS

A. **Frequency** (American College of Obstetrics/Gynecology and American Cancer Society): Annually for sexually active women
B. **HIV infection:** Pap smear on initial evaluation; at least one additional Pap smear should be obtained in the next 6 mo to rule out a false-negative test. If negative, repeat testing at least annually. Results of Pap smears should be managed similarly to those from patients without HIV infection
C. **Classification of results** (Bethesda System, JAMA 1989;262:931; JAMA 1994;271:1866):
   Low-grade squamous intraepithelial lesion (SIL): Includes cellular changes associated with HPV and mild dysplasia/cervical intraepithelial neoplasia 1 (CIN 1)
   High-grade SIL: Includes moderate dysplasia/CIN 2, severe dysplasia/CIN 3, and carcinoma in situ (CIS/CIN 3)
D. **Results:**
   — Severe inflammation with reactive cellular changes: Repeat within 3 mo, then repeat every 4–6 mo until there are three consecutive negative smears
   — Low-grade SIL or atypical squamous cells of undetermined significance (ASCUS): Referral for colposcopy; an acceptable alternative is repeat Pap smear every 4–6 mo for 2 yr until there are three consecutive negative smears. If smears are persistently abnormal, refer for colposcopy and biopsy
   — High-grade SIL or persistent low-grade SIL or ASCUS: Refer to physician who can perform colposcopy

XIX. PREGNANCY

<u>Hepatitis B</u>: Screen for HBsAg (surfase antigen) at first visit
N. gonorrhoeae: Screen in first trimester; repeat in third trimester for high-risk patients
C. trachomatis: Screen in first trimester; repeat in third trimester for high-risk patients
<u>HIV</u>: Test with informed consent at first visit
<u>Bacterial vaginosis</u>: Screen with Gram stain at first visit if history of preterm delivery
<u>Pap smear</u>: First visit if none in prior year
<u>Herpes simplex</u>: Routine cultures are not indicated; see p 295

Continued

XX. SEXUAL ASSAULT

A. Evaluation

1. <u>Initial evaluation</u>
   a. Cultures of any sites of penetration or attempted penetration for *N. gonorrhoeae* and *C. trachomatis* (a non-culture test that is positive for *C. trachomiatis* must be confirmed with another test using different technology)
   b. Wet mount for *T. vaginalis*. If vaginal discharge: Examine wet mount for bacterial vaginosis and *Candida* sp
   c. Serum sample for HIV, hepatitis B, and syphilis
   <u>Follow-up evaluation at 2 wk</u>: Repeat evaluation
   <u>Subsequent evaluation</u>: Serology for syphillis and HIV at 6, 12, and 24 wk

B. Treatment

- Ceftriaxone 125 mg IM × 1
- Metronidazole 2 g po × 1
- Azithromycin 1 g po × 1 or doxycycline 100 mg po bid × 7
- Hepatitis B vaccination

DURATION OF ANTIBIOTIC TREATMENT

Location	Diagnosis	Duration (days)
Actinomycosis	Cervicofacial	4–6 wk IV, then po × 6–12 mo
Arthritis septic	*S. aureus,* GNB	14–28 days
	Streptococci, *H. influenzae*	14 days
	N. gonorrhoeae	7 days
Bacteremia	Gram-negative bacteremia	10–14 days
	S. aureus, portal of entry known	2 wk
	S. aureus, no portal of entry	4 wk
	Line sepsis: Bacteria	3–5 days (post-removal)
	Candida	≥10 days (post-removal)
	Vascular graft	4 wk (post-removal)
Bone	Osteomyelitis, acute	4–6 wk IV
	chronic	≥3 mo or until ESR is normal
Bronchi	Exacerbation of chronic bronchitis	7–10 days
Brucella	Brucellosis	6 wk
Bursitis	*S. aureus*	10–14 days
Central nervous system	Cerebral abscess	4–6 wk IV, then oral 10 days
	Meningitis: *Listeria*	14–21 days
	N. meningitidis	7 days
	S. pneumoniae	10–14 days
Ear	Otitis media, acute	5–10 days (JAMA 1998; 279:1736)
Gastrointestinal	Diarrhea: *C. difficile*	10 days
	C. jejuni	7 days
	E. histolytica	5–10 days
	Giardia	5–7 days
	Salmonella	14 days
	Shigella	3–5 days or single dose
	Traveler's	3 days
	Gastritis, *H. pylori*	10–14 days
	Typhoid fever	5–14 days
	Sprue	6 mo
	Whipple's disease	1 yr
Heart	Endocarditis: Pen-sensitive strep	14–28 days
	Pen-resistant strep	4 wk
	S. aureus	4 wk
	Microbes, other	4 wk
	Prosthetic valve	≥6 wk
	Pericarditis (pyogenic)	28 days

Location	Diagnosis	Duration (days)
Intra-abdominal	Cholecystitis	3–7 days post-cholecystectomy
	Primary peritonitis	10–14 days
	Peritonitis/intra-abdominal abscess	≤7 days after surgery
Joint	Septic arthritis, gonococcal	7 days
	Pyogenic, non-gonococcal	3 wk
	Prosthetic joint	6 wk
Liver	Pyogenic liver abscess	4–16 wk
	Amebic	10 days
Lung	Pneumonia: *C. pneumoniae*	10–14 days
	Legionella	14–21 days
	Mycoplasma	10–14 wk
	Nocardia	6–12 mo
	Pneumococcal	Until febrile 3–5 days
	Pneumocystis	21 days
	Staphylococcal	≥21 days
	Tuberculosis	6–9 mo
	Lung abscess	Until x-ray clear or until small stable residual lesion; usually >3 mo
Nocardia	Nocardiosis	6–12 mo
Pharynx	Pharyngitis—group A strep	10 days
	Pharyngitis, gonococcal	1 dose
	Diphtheria	7–14 days
Prostate	Prostatitis, acute	2 wk
	chronic	3–4 mo
Sexually transmitted diseases	Cervicitis, gonococcal	1 dose
	Chancroid	7 days
	Chlamydia	7 days (azithromycin—1 dose)
	Disseminated gonococcal infection	7 days
	H. simplex	7–10 days
	Lymphogranuloma venereum	21 days
	Pelvic inflammatory disease	10–14 days
	Syphilis	10–21 days
	Urethritis, gonococcal	1 dose
Sinus	Sinusitis, acute	10–14 days
Systemic	Brucellosis	6 wk
	Listeria: Immunosuppressed host	3–6 wk
	Lyme disease	14–21 days
	Meningococcemia	7–10 days
	Rocky Mountain spotted fever	Until afebrile, 2 days

Continued

Location	Diagnosis	Duration (days)
	Salmonellosis	10–14 days
	Bacteremia	≥3–4 wk
	AIDS patients	4–6 wk
	Localized infection	6 wk
	Carrier state	6–9 mo
	Tuberculosis, pulmonary	
	extrapulmonary	9 mo
	Tularemia	7–14 days
Urinary tract	Cystitis	3 days
	Pyelonephritis	14 days
Vaginitis	Bacterial vaginosis	7 days or 1 dose
	Candida albicans	Single dose fluconazole
	Trichomoniasis	7 days or 1 dose

TRADE NAMES OF ANTIMICROBIAL AGENTS
For: For trade names see Antimicrobial Agents pp 1–17

Trade name	Generic name	Trade name	Generic name	Trade name	Generic name
Abelcet	amphotericin lipid complex ABLC	Cefadyl	cephapirin	Flagyl	metronidazole
		Cefanex	cephalexin	Floxin	ofloxacin
Abreva	docosanol	Cefizox	ceftizoxime	Flumadine	rimantadine
Achromycin	tetracycline	Cefobid	cefoperazone	Fortaz	ceftazidime
A-cillin	amoxicillin	Cefotan	cefotetan	Fortovase	saquinavir
Aerosporin	polymyxin B	Ceftin	cefuroxime axetil	Forvade	cidofovir gel
Aftate	tolnaftate			Foscavir	foscarnet
Agenerase	amprenavir	Cefzil	cefprozil	Fulvicin	griseofulvin
A-K-chlor	chloramphenicol	Ceptaz	ceftazidime	Fungizone	amphotericin B
Ala-Tet	tetracycline	Chero-Trisulfa-V	trisulfa-pyrimidines	Furacin	nitrofurazone
Albamycin	novobiocin			Furadantin	nitrofurantoin
Albenza	albendazole	Chloro-mycetin	chloramphenicol	Furamide	diloxanide furoate
Aldara	imiquimod				
Alferon N	interferon alfa-n3	Cinobac	cinoxacin	Furatoin	nitrofurantoin
Alinia	nitazoxanide	Cipro	ciprofloxacin	Furoxone	furazolidone
AmBisome	amphotericin liposomal	Claforan	cefotaxime	G-Mycin	gentamicin
		Cleocin	clindamycin	Gantanol	sulfamethoxazole
Amcap	ampicillin	Cloxapen	cloxacillin	Gantrisin	sulfisoxazole
Amficot	ampicillin	Cofatrim	TMP-SMX	Garamycin	gentamicin
Amikin	amikacin	Coly-Mycin M	colistimethate	Geocillin	carbenicillin indanyl sodium
Amoxil	amoxicillin	Concidas	caspofungin		
Amphotec	amphotericin lipid complex ABCD	Copegus	ribavirin	Germanin	suramin
		Cotrim	TMP-SMX	Grifulvin	griseofulvin
Amplin	ampicillin	Crixivan	indinavir	Grisactin	griseofulvin
Ancef	cefazolin	Cubicin	daptomycin	Gulfasin	sulfisoxazole
Ancobon	flucytosine	Cytovene	ganciclovir	Halfan	halofantrine
Anspor	cephradine	D-Amp	ampicillin	Hepsera	adofovir
Antepar	piperazine	Daraprim	pyrimethamine	Herplex	idoxuridine
Antiminth	pyrantel pamoate	Declomycin	demeclocycline	Hetrazan	diethyl-carbamazine
Aoracillin B	penicillin G	Denavir	penciclovir		
Aralen	chloroquine	Diflucan	fluconazole	Hiprex	methenamine hippurate
Arsobal	melarsoprol	Doryx	doxycycline		
Atabrine	quinacrine	Doxy-caps	doxycycline	HIVID	zalcitabine
Augmentin	amoxicillin + clavulanic acid	Doxy-D	doxycycline	Humatin	paromomycin
		Duricef	cefadroxil	Ilosone	erythromycin estolate
Avelox	moxifloxacin	Dycill	dicloxacillin		
Azactam	aztreonam	Dynabac	dirithromycin	Ilotycin	erythromycin
Azulfidine	sulfasalazine	Dynapen	dicloxacillin	Intron A	interferon alfa-2b
Bactrim	trimethoprim/sulfamethoxa-zole	E-mycin	erythromycin	Invanz	ertapenem
		EES	erythromycin ethylsuccinate	Invirase	saquinavir
				Jenamicin	gentamicin
Bactroban	mupirocin	Elimite	permethrin	Kaletra	lopinavir/rectonavir
Baraclude	entecavir	Emtet-500	tetracycline		
Beepen-VK	penicillin V	Epivir	lamivudine	Kantrex	kanamycin
Biaxin	clarithromycin	Erothricin	erythromycin	Keflex	cephalexin
Bicillin	benzathine peni-cillin G	ERYC	erythromycin	Keflin	cephalothin
		Ery-Tab	erythromycin	Keftab	cephalexin
Biltricide	praziquantel	Erythrocot	erythromycin	Kefurox	cefuroxime
Bio-cef	cephalexin	Eryzole	erythromycin-sulfisoxazole	Kefzol	cefazolin
Bitin	bithionol			Ketek	telithromycin
Brodspec	tetracycline	Factive	gemifloxacin	Kwell	lindane
Cancidas	caspofugin	Famvir	famciclovir	Lamisil	terbinafine
Capastat	capreomycin	Fansidar	pyrimethamine + sulfadoxine	Lampit	nifurtimox
Caropen-VK	penicillin V			Lamprene	clofazimine
Ceclor	cefaclor	Fasigyn	tinidazole	Lanacillin	penicillin V
Cedax	ceftibutin	Femstat	butoconazole	Lariam	mefloquine

Continued

307

Trade name	Generic name	Trade name	Generic name	Trade name	Generic name
Ledercillin VK	penicillin V	Ornidyl	eflornithine	Roferon-A	interferon alfa-2a
Levoquin	levofloxacin	Ovide	malathion		
Lice-Enz	pyrethins	Paludrine	proguanil	Rovamycine	spiramycin
Lincocin	lincomycin	Panmycin	tetracycline	Seromycin	cycloserine
Lincorex	lincomycin	PAS	aminosalicylic acid	Silvadene	silver sulfadiazine
Lorabid	loracarbef	Pathocil	dicloxacillin	Soxa	sulfisoxazole
Lotrimin	clotrimazole	Pediamycin	erythromycin ethylsuccinate	Spectrobid	bacampicillin
Lyphocin	vancomycin			Spectracef	cefditoren
Macrobid	nitrofurantoin	Peflacine	pefloxacin	Sporanox	itraconazole
Macrodantin	nitrofurantoin	Pegasys	peginterferon alfa 2a	Staphcillin	methicillin
Malarone	atovaquone and proguanil			Sterostim	somatropin
Mandelamine	methenamine mandelate	PEG-Intron	peginterferon alfa 2b	Storz-G	gentamicin
				Stoxil	idoxuridine
Mandol	cefamandole	Pen G	penicillin G	Stromectol	ivermectin
Marcillin	ampicillin	Pen-V	penicillin V	Sulfamar	TMP-SMX
Maxaquin	lomefloxacin	Pen-VK	penicillin V	Sulfamylon	mafenide
Maxipime	cefixime	Penamp	ampicillin	Sulfametho-prim	TMP-SMX
Mectizan	ivermectin	Penetrex	enoxacin		
Mefoxin	cefoxitin	Pentam 300	pentamidine isethionate	Sulfimycin	erythromycin-sulfisoxazole
Mepron	atovaquone				
Merrem	meropenem	Pentids	penicillin G	Sumycin	tetracycline
Metric	metronidazole	Pentostam	sodium stibo-gluconate	Suprax	cefixime
Metro-IV	metronidazole			Suspen	penicillin V
Mezlin	mezlocillin	Permapen	penicillin G benzathine	Sustiva	efavirenz
Minocin	minocycline			Symadine	amantadine
Mintezol	thiabendazole	Pipracil	piperacillin	Symmetrel	amantadine
Monocid	cefonicid	Plaquenil	hydroxychloro-quine	Synercid	quinupristin-dalfopristin
Monodox	doxycycline				
Monistat	miconazole	Polycillin	ampicillin	Tamiflu	oseltamivir
Monurol	fosfomycin	Polymox	amoxicillin	TAO	troleandomycin
Myambutol	ethambutol	Povan	pyrvinium pamoate	Tazicef	ceftazidime
Mycamine	micafungin			Tazidime	ceftazidime
Mycelex	clotrimazole	Priftin	rifapentine	Teebactin	aminosalicylic acid
Mycobutin	rifabutin	Primaxin	imipenem + cilastatin		
Mycostatin	nystatin			Tegopen	cloxacillin
MyE	erythromycin	Principen	ampicillin	Teline	tetracycline
Nafcil	nafcillin	Proloprim	trimethoprim	Tequin	gatifloxacin
Nallpen	nafcillin	Pronto	pyrethrins	Terramycin	oxytetracycline
Natacyn	natamycin	Prostaphlin	oxacillin	Tetracap	tetracycline
Nebcin	tobramycin	Protostate	metronidazole	Tetracon	tetracycline
NebuPent	pentamidine aerosol	Pyopen	carbenicillin	Tetralan	tetracycline
		Rebetrol	ribavirin	Tetram	tetracycline
NegGram	nalidixic acid	Rebatol	ribavirin	Tiberal	ornidazole
Netromycin	netilmicin	Relenza	zanamivir	Ticar	ticarcillin
Neutrexin	trimetrexate	Retrovir	zidovudine	Timentin	clavulanic acid + ticarcillin
Niclocide	niclosamide	RID	pyrethrins		
Nilstat	nystatin	Rifadin	rifampin	Tinactin	tolnaftate
Nix	permethrin	Rifamate	rifampin-INH	Tindamax	tinidazole
Nizoral	ketoconazole	Rifater	rifampin, INH, pyrazinamide	Tobrex	tobramycin
Noroxin	norfloxacin			Trecator SC	ethionamide
Nor-Tet	tetracycline	Rimactane	rifampin	Triazole	TMP-SMX
Norvir	ritonavir	Robicillin VK	penicillin V	Trimox	amoxicillin
Nydrazid	INH	Robimycin	erythromycin	Trimpex	trimethoprim
Nystex	nystatin	Robitet	tetracycline	Trisulfam	TMP-SMX
Omnipen	ampicillin	Rocephin	ceftriaxone	Trizivir	AZT and 3TC and ABC
		Rochagan	benznidazole	Trobicin	spectinomycin

Continued

308

Trade name	Generic name	Trade name	Generic name	Trade name	Generic name
Trovan	trovafloxacin	Veetids	penicillin V	Wycillin	penicillin G
Truxcillin	penicillin G	Velosef	cephradine	Wymox	amoxicillin
Tygacil	tigecycline	Vermox	mebendazole	Xifaxan	rifaximin
Virazole	ribavirin	Vfend	voriconazole	Xigris	drotrecogin
Ultracef	cefadroxil	Vibramycin	doxycycline	Yodoxin	iodoquinol
Unasyn	ampicillin/ sulbactam	Vibratabs	doxycycline	Zagam	sparfloxacin
		Videx	didanosine	Zartan	cephalexin
Unipen	nafcillin	Vira-A	vidarabine	Zefazone	cefmetazole
Urex	methenamine hippurate	Viracept	nelfinavir	Zentel	albendazole
		Viramune	nevirapine	Zerit	stavudine (d4T)
Uri-tet	oxytetracycline	Virazole	ribavirin	Ziagen	abacavir
Uroplus	TMP-SMX	Viroptic	trifluridine	Zinacef	cefuroxime
V-Cillin	penicillin V	Vistide	cidofovir	Zolicef	cefazolin
Valcyte	valganciclovir	Vitravene	fomivirsen	Zosyn	piperacillin/ tazobactam
Valtrex	valacyclovir	Wesmycin	tetracycline		
Vancocin	vancomycin	Win-cillin	penicillin V	Zovirax	acyclovir
Vancoled	vancomycin	Wintrocin	erythromycin	Zithromax	azithromycin
Vansil	oxamniquine	Wyamycin S	erythromycin	Zyvox	linezolid
Vantin	cefpodoxime proxetil				

Index

313

315

Levofloxacin—*Continued*
  for pneumonia, 248, 252
  for pulmonary infections, 30
  in renal failure, 50
  for respiratory tract infections, 246
  for sinusitis, 241
  for traveler's diarrhea, 143
  for tuberculosis, 156
  for ulcers, 215
  for urinary tract infections, 283
Levoquin. *See* Levofloxacin
Lice, 171
  pubic, 294
Lice-ENZ. *See* Permethrin
Ligases chain reaction (LCR), for *Chlamydia*
    trachomatis, 290
Lincocin. *See* Lincomycin
Lincomycin, 10
Lindane
  cost of, 10
  dosing regimens for, 10
  for pubic lice, 294
  for scabies, 294
Linezolid
  adverse reactions, 70
  cost of, 10
  during dialysis, 57
  dosing regimens for, 10
  drug interactions, 91
  in hepatic disease, 60
  for infected prosthetic devices, 36
  for meningitis, 235
  for pneumonia, 248, 252
  in renal failure, 50
  for septicemia, 36
  for ulcers, 215
  for wound infections, 36
Liquifilm. *See* Idoxuridine
Listeria,
  in endocarditis, 258
  in food poisoning, 270, 277
  in meningitis, 228, 230, 232, 234, 235
Lisseria monocytogenes, 29, 234
Liver abscess
  antibiotics for, 305
  description of, 266
  treatment of, 27, 266
Loa loa, 169
Lobectomy, antibiotic prophylaxis for,
    133
Lomefloxacin
  adverse reactions, 75
  cost of, 10
  dosing regimens for, 10
  in renal failure, 56

Loperamide
  for infectious diarrhea, 272, 275
  for traveler's diarrhea, 144, 275
Lorabid. *See* Loracarbef
Loracarbef
  cost of, 10
  during dialysis, 57
  dosing regimens for, 10
  in renal failure, 50
  for respiratory tract infections, 246
Lotrimin. *See* Clotrimazole
Lower respiratory infections, 247–252
Lung abscess
  antibiotic treatment for, 305
  description of, 249
Lung fluke, 170
Lyme disease. *See also* Borrelia burgodorferi
  aseptic meningitis and, 236
  treatment of, 21, 209–211
Lymphadenitis, 214
Lymphangitis, 212
Lymphogranuloma venereum, 23, 291–292,
    305
Lyphocin. *See* Vancomycin

Macrobid. *See* Nitrofurantoin
Macrodantin. *See* Nitrofurantoin
Macrolides. *See also specific agent*
  for actinomycosis, 18
  for cat scratch disease, 214
  for dental infections, 32
  for gynecologic infections, 32
  for infected prosthetic devices, 36
  for oral infections, 32
  for pneumonia, 22, 37, 248, 249
  for pulmonary infections, 32
  for sepsis, 32
  for septicemia, 24, 32, 36
Madura foot, 215
Mafenide, 10
Malaria
  aseptic meningitis and, 236
  countries with risk of, 146
  prevention of, 144–145, 172
  treatment of, 171–172
Malarone. *See* Atovaquone-proguanil
Malassezia furfur, 153, 213
Malignant otitis externa, 240
Mandelamine. *See* Methenamine mandelate
Mandol. *See* Cefamandole
Mansonella ozzardi, 169
Mansonella perstans, 169
Mansonella streptocerca, 169
Mastectomy, antibiotic prophylaxis for, 139

332

Rocephin. *See* Ceftriaxone
Rochalimaea henselae. See Bartonella
henselae
Rochalimaea quintana. See Bartonella
quintana
Rocky Mountain spotted fever, 34, 236, 305
Roferon-A. *See* Interferon alfa; Interferon
alfa-2a
Roundworm. *See* Ascariasis
Rubella vaccine. *See also* MMR vaccine
for health care workers, 107
for homeless, 107
for immigrants, 108
during pregnancy, 106
recommendation by age, 99, 104–105
route of administration, 103

Salmonella
in infectious diarrhea, 270, 271, 275
in sickle cell disease, 220
treatment for, 35
Salmonella typhi
in infectious diarrhea, 270, 271, 274, 275
treatment for, 34–35
Salpingitis, 23, 286, 298–299, 305
Sandoglobin. *See* IVIG
Sarcopes scabiei, 174, 294
Scabies, 174, 294
Schistosomiasis, 174
Scrub typhys, 34
Selenium sulfide, for fungal infections, 153,
215
Sepsis, 197–199
intra-abdominal, 265–267
treatment of, 18, 20, 23, 25, 26, 27, 28, 32,
33, 197–198, 265–267, 305
Septic arthritis
antibiotics for, 304
description of, 221–223
treatment of, 27, 28, 32, 221– 223, 305
Septic shock, 197
Septicemia, 18, 20, 21, 22, 23, 24, 26, 28, 29,
32,
33, 35, 36, 39, 40
Septra. *See* Trimethoprim-sulfamethoxazole
Seromycin. *See* Cycloserine
Serratia marcescens, 35
Sex partners, syphilis and, 288
Sexual assault, 303
Sexually transmitted diseases, 285–303
antibiotic treatment for, 305
pregnancy and, 302
Sheep liver fluke, 169
Shellfish toxins, 278, 279
Shigella sp., 35, 271, 274, 275, 276, 277

Silvadene. *See* Silver sulfadiazine
Silver sulfadiazine, 15
Sinusitis, 238, 241–242
acute, 241
in brain abscess, 237
chronic, 241
nosocomial, 242
treatment of, 27, 29, 305
SIRS. *See* Sepsis
Skin abscess, 32
Skin infections
streptococcal, 205
treatment of, 30
Skin test
for penicillin allergy, 80–82
for syphilis, 288
Sleeping sickness. *See* Trypanosomiasis
Smallpox vaccination, 126–128
Sodium fluoride, 279
Sodium stibogluconate
adverse reactions, 76
for parasitic infections, 170
Soft tissue infections
deep serious, 218
streptococcal, 205
treatment of, 30, 31
Southeast Asian liver fluke, 170
Soxa Gulfasin. *See* Sulfisoxazole
Spectinomycin
adverse reactions, 76
for arthritis, septic, 221
cost of, 14
dosing regimens for, 14
for gonococcal infections, 285
in renal failure, 53
for septic arthritis, 221
Spectracef. *See* Cefditoren
Spectrobid. *See* Bacampicillin
Spinal surgery, antibiotic prophylaxis for,
138
Spirillum minus, 35
Sporanox. *See* Itraconazole
Sporothrix schenckii, 223
Sporotrichosis, 149, 215
Staphcillin. *See* Methicillin
Staphylococcus aureus
in blepharitis, 226
in bone/ joint infections, 220–221
in cervical adenitis, 243
in dacryocystitis, 227
in endocarditis, 254–255, 257–258
in endophthalmitis, 225
in infectious diarrhea, 270, 275, 277
in keratitis, 224
in mastoiditis, 240–241